# THE RUNNER'S HANDBOOK

Bob Glover, a sub-three-hour marathoner and competitive runner for fifteen years, has had a multifarious athletic career. In Vietnam in 1969 he organized and directed the "Hue Olympics," attracting thousands of visitors to a burned-out stadium that had once been headquarters for the North Vietnamese Army. As fitness director of New York City's West Side Y.M.C.A., he developed and led the country's largest fitness program, with over three thousand participants. He has run in twenty-six marathons, one fifty-kilometer race, and one fifty-miler on a track, as well as in the Mount Washington Race (eight miles up the Northeast's highest peak). He is also founder and coach of the Greater New York Athletic Association, whose women's team is now of national caliber. Recently, he founded Robert H. Glover and Associates, Inc., a physical-fitness consulting firm serving a variety of corporate and community clients.

Jack Shepherd was graduated from Haverford College and Columbia University but says, "I really got my education as a senior editor at *Look* magazine during the 1960s, when I covered the civil-rights movement, drugs, Berkeley, etc." As an author-journalist he has traveled in forty-six of the fifty United States and the Far East, Europe, the Caribbean, and Africa. Articles by him have appeared in *Newsweek, Harper's,* the *Saturday Review, Reader's Digest, The New York Times Sunday Magazine,* and other periodicals; he is the author or coauthor of seven previous books—among them *The Forest Killers,* nominated for a National Book Award, and his second bestseller *The Adams Chronicles.* After a recent trip to East Africa he began Bob Glover's running program, which, he soon decided, deserved to be the subject of a book.

# THE RUNNER'S HANDBOOK

## A COMPLETE FITNESS GUIDE
## FOR MEN AND WOMEN ON THE RUN

**BOB GLOVER** *and* **JACK SHEPHERD**

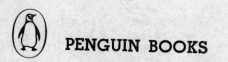

**PENGUIN BOOKS**

Penguin Books Ltd, Harmondsworth,
Middlesex, England
Penguin Books, 625 Madison Avenue,
New York, New York 10022, U.S.A.
Penguin Books Australia Ltd, Ringwood,
Victoria, Australia
Penguin Books Canada Limited, 2801 John Street,
Markham, Ontario, Canada L3R 1B4
Penguin Books (N.Z.) Ltd, 182–190 Wairau Road,
Auckland 10, New Zealand

First published in the United States of America
in simultaneous hardbound and paperbound editions by
The Viking Press and Penguin Books 1978
This edition reprinted 1978 (twice)

Copyright © Jack Shepherd and Robert Glover, 1977, 1978
All rights reserved

LIBRARY OF CONGRESS CATALOGING IN PUBLICATION DATA
Glover, Bob.
    The runner's handbook.
    Bibliography: p. 404
    Includes index.
    1. Running—Training.    2. Running—Psychological    aspects.
I. Shepherd, Jack, joint author.    II. Title.
GV1061.5.G55    1978b    796.4'26    78-1888
ISBN 0 14 046.325 9

Printed in the United States of America by
Offset Paperback Mfrs., Inc., Dallas, Pennsylvania
Set in Linotype Electra

The authors acknowledge with thanks *The New England
Journal of Medicine* for permission to reprint the article that
appeared in the January 20, 1977, issue.

Except in the United States of America,
this book is sold subject to the condition
that it shall not, by way of trade or otherwise,
be lent, re-sold, hired out, or otherwise circulated
without the publisher's prior consent in any form of
binding or cover other than that in which it is
published and without a similar condition
including this condition being imposed
on the subsequent purchaser

## DEDICATION

To Alexander Melleby, who taught me by his example that a man's most important possession is his pride in his work, and that if a man stands tall and fights for what he believes in, he will always be a winner.

And to Hans Kraus, M.D., who has spent more than half a century promoting the concept that our nation needs exercise, not drugs, to be healthy and high; a man who taught me that tension is the root of all evil.

# CONTENTS

ACKNOWLEDGMENTS  ix

INTRODUCTION: DOWN THE ROAD TO FITNESS  1

1. THE RUN-EASY METHOD: A BASIC
   PROGRAM FOR ALL RUNNERS  17

2. BEGINNER AND INTERMEDIATE RUNNERS  51

3. THE BEGINNER COMPETITOR AND BEYOND  67

4. THE ULTIMATE FITNESS CHALLENGE: THE MARATHON  94

5. RUNNING STYLE  110

6. SUPPLEMENTAL EXERCISES  121

7. NEVER TOO YOUNG, NEVER TOO OLD  137

8. WOMEN ON THE RUN  152

9. RUNNING WITH MOTHER NATURE AND HER CHILDREN  171

10. ANALYZING RUNNING SHOES: IF THE SHOE FITS . . .  201

11. Injuries: Diseases of Inactivity, Diseases of Excellence   218

12. The Heart-Lung Machine   273

13. Eat, Drink and Be Merry   291

14. Food and Drink for Racing   317

15. Stress and Tension   331

16. Running Inside Your Head   347

17. Where to Run When You're on the Run: Twenty-One Cities   358

18. Runners Make Better Lovers   389

Appendices   396
    Running Publications   396
    Runner's Aids   396
    Road Runner's Clubs and Officers   396
    Reading List   403
    Pacing Charts   406–407

Index   408

## ACKNOWLEDGMENTS

I grew up in the running revolution. People like Lydiard, Bowerman, Ross, Corbitt and Kleinerman encouraged me and others like me to make Earth a runner's world. Later, Sheehan, Schuster, Ullyot, Henderson, Lebow, Kuscsik, Switzer and others spread the revolution.

I once saw Tom Fleming of the New York Athletic Club, a world class long-distance runner, give a trophy he had just won to the man most responsible for encouraging his running: Road Runner's Club official, Joe Kleinerman. I have few trophies to give away. But during my two decades of running, I have made many friends. Many of them have helped with this book, and I can only reward them with the trophy of praise.

After he started attending my beginner's classes, Jack Shepherd suggested that we do this book. I'm glad he did, although I had no idea how much work it would be. It's worse than an uphill marathon. But along the way, as with any race, we had a lot of help from other runners.

We would like to thank several members of the medical profession for the time they spent gathering material for this book, and for reading the chapters as we completed them.

Dr. Hans Kraus, M.D., developed "The Y's Ways to a Healthy Back" program and wrote the book *Backache, Stress and Ten-*

*sion,* which served as a guideline for the stretching and relaxation exercises in this book. Dr. Kraus serves as an important member of the President's Council on Physical Fitness and Sports. He also spent a great deal of time reviewing the chapters on injuries and exercises. I deeply appreciate that, and also his concern for me as my personal physician and self-adopted "grandfather."

Dr. Richard Schuster, D.P.M. has been a pioneer in the field of sports podiatry. He developed inserts for my feet that saved me from a crippling knee injury; without his professional services and personal encouragement I wouldn't be running today. His extensive reviews of the chapters on injuries and shoes aided the accuracy of this book.

Dr. Norbert Sander, M.D. was my supervisor at the City Island Fitness and Medical Center in New York City, New York. As medical director of the center, he believes his patients need fitness more than medicine, and it is that philosophy that forms the backbone of his unique sports medicine practice. Dr. Sander's knowledge of sports medicine both as a runner-doctor and as a national class long-distance runner has been an invaluable assistance to us.

Dr. Murray Weisenfeld, D.P.M. and Dr. Dennis Richard, D.P.M. also helped with the chapters on injury, which we very much appreciate.

Dr. George Sheehan, M.D. is a cardiologist-runner-writer. His lectures and writings have opened new paths for sports medicine in our running world, and his personal advice to me has been of major value to this book.

Dr. Edward Dwyer, M.D. is a cardiologist who has served as medical director of my YMCA cardiac rehabilitation program. His guidance over the years and with sections of this book has been invaluable.

Dr. Milton Brothers, M.D. is the author of *Diabetes*, and contributed his knowledge to this area of the book. I am greatly indebted to him for his help to me personally and for his valued medical advice in my work.

Dr. Edward Colt, M.D. a runner-doctor and chairman of the medical committee of the 1977 New York Marathon, reviewed sections of this book. His contribution to both is very much welcomed and needed.

Many of these doctors also worked with me as speakers at Road Runner's Club clinics, and their lectures added ideas to this book. I'm especially indebted to the internationally-known physician-coach-promoter, Dr. Ernst van Aaken, M.D., and the highly respected coach of Olympic champions, Arthur Lydiard of New Zealand, for their thoughts at our clinics.

Several members of the National YMCA also helped develop this book and my program.

Alexander Melleby is director of Physical Education for the Pacific Region YMCA. He developed, with Dr. Kraus, "The Y's Way to a Healthy Back" program, is co-author of *Jogging Away from Heart Disease*, and is one of the nation's top fitness experts. In 1971, he introduced me to physical fitness and began guiding my career. As my supervisor for two years at the West Side YMCA in New York City, Al Melleby guided me down the road to fitness programming. We gratefully appreciate his review of much of this book.

Dr. Clayton Myers, Ph.D. is the National YMCA Fitness Director and author of the book *The Official YMCA Physical Fitness Handbook*. His work in developing the "Y's Way to Physical Fitness" program guided us in this book, and his friendship and direction were invaluable.

George Goyer gave me direction and inspiration in my career

with the Rome, New York, Family Y. Dee Howell, Fitness
Director of the Rome Family Y, was a great help in the women's
chapter, and her friendship and support are always welcome.
Robert Elia, executive director of the Enterprise, Alabama,
YMCA, was my first employer when I returned, without direction or prospects, from Vietnam. He guided me into "people
work," and showed me the satisfaction of helping others.

Other fitness experts also pitched in.

Dr. Richard Warner, Ed.D., supervisor of the Physical Fitness Laboratory at New York City's Exxon Corporation, served
as advisor and class leader of my fitness programs at the YMCA.
His review of the physiology in this book was very beneficial
and is appreciated. Also reviewing physiology material in this
book was my graduate school advisor, Dr. Bernard Gutin, Ed.D.
Director of Applied Physiology at Teacher's College, Columbia
University, who gave his time freely.

Others whose work contributed include: Dr. Lawrence Gold-
ing, Ph.D., Director of Applied Physiology at the University of
Nevada, Las Vegas, whose classroom lectures on fitness and
personal discussions with me served as important background
for this work; James Rumsey, R.P.T., whose work with Dr.
Kraus and position as athletic trainer at Florida State University
gave him a special viewpoint in reviewing the exercise and
injury sections; Pete Schuder, a doctoral student in exercise
physiology at Columbia University, and a former all-America
quarter-miler and coach of Columbia's distance runners, helped
greatly with the beginner's-fitness and the competitive-runner
sections.

Hundreds of members of the Road Runner's Club of New
York have also pitched in. Special mention must cover:

Fred Lebow, president of the Road Runner's Club of New

York and race director for the New York City Marathon, whose leadership in the development of the entire road running program in that city spearheaded the growth in running all across the nation. His review of the beginner runner chapter is greatly appreciated.

Barry Geisler, the National Road Runner's Club Age-Group Chairman, gets a special thanks for working on our chapter about kids.

Nina Kuscsik, R.N., is a good running friend, a national class marathoner for the Greater New York AA., and a pioneer in the development of women's running. She assisted with several parts of this book, especially the women's chapter, and we are very much in her debt.

Other women runners have also helped us, including Kathryn Lance, author of *Running for Health and Beauty*.

Gary Muhrcke a long-distance runner–shoe salesman, helped with the shoe chapter.

Ted Corbitt, R.P.T., a former Olympic marathoner and record holder for ultra-marathon events, worked as the first president of the Road Runner's Club of New York, and got the running revolution off on the right foot. He was of great help in the injury, shoe and Mother Nature chapters.

I must thank all of the "guinea pigs" who showed up for our beginner's fitness workouts in Central Park in New York City, and especially my helpers from the Road Runner's Club, Bill Greenwald, Marcy Schwam and Ann DeGroff. Peter Roth graciously gave his time to help with the beginner's clinics, and took the authors' promotion pictures. The 300 members of my running club at the YMCA and my present club, the Greater New York AA, contributed in many ways—particularly Jerry Mahrer, Sam McConnell, Bill Horowitz, Don Dixon, Mike Cleary, Arno Niemand and our national caliber women's team members Lauri Pedrinan, Jane Killion, Ellie McGrath, Mary Beth Byrne, Mimi Beams, Mary Rodriguez, Nina Kuscsik and Toshika d'Elia. Let's all raise a special toast to the George Washington Bridge—and to Martin's saloon.

Jim Ferris, who uniquely combines a broad knowledge as a top competitor with the ability to instruct beginner runners, gave his time, comments and special skills to this book. His coaching guidance also greatly improved my personal race times while increasing my knowledge of this sport.

Five people have also been key figures in my addiction to running, and I want to thank them: Bill Coughlin; Carl Eilenberg; Al Stringham and Dr. Fred Grabo of Rome, New York; and Joe Henderson, an editor of *Runner's World*.

My fellow members of the Board of Directors of the fitness consulting firm, Robert H. Glover and Associates, Inc., all contributed significantly to the development of this book as friends, runners and advisors. They include John Eisner, Richard Jacobson, Stanley Newhouse and Richard Traum, Ph.D. The firm is located at 522 Fifth Avenue, New York, N.Y. 10036.

A very special thanks also goes to Alan Dodge, who typed much of the first drafts of this book, and put up with me as my assistant during the whole process. And, of course, a special word of praise to our editor, Martina D'Alton, who progressed from beginner runner to marathoner during the completion of this book.

And what book would be complete without thanking one's family: my parents, Mr. and Mrs. H. Ross Glover, and my grandparents, Mr. and Mrs. Carl Burger, for their support throughout my life.

## INTRODUCTION: DOWN THE ROAD TO FITNESS

We are in the middle of a revolution. Suddenly, in the mid-seventies, Americans by the tens of thousands are stripping off their clothes, pulling on shorts, lacing up shoes, and running. They run everywhere: in city parks; along rivers, lakes, and oceans; up and down mountains; in gyms and field-houses. They are running for their lives. They run because their friends are dropping dead from heart attacks. They run because they are fat, or scared or tense. They run because their lives are sedentary, made too easy by machines. As Dr. Joseph Arends says, "This is the Metalic Age. We have gold in our hearts, silver in our hair, and lead in our pants."

Now, we are getting the lead out. The National Jogging Association counts more than 10,000 dues-paying members. *Runner's World*, begun in 1966, has more than 100,000 subscribers. The Road Runner's Club of America, founded in 1957 by Browning Ross, now has more than 100 chapters across the country, with 50,000 members. Its most active chapter is the New York Road Runner's Club, sparked by its president, Fred Lebow. In three years during the mid-seventies, the New York RRC membership quadrupled in number; in Manhattan alone, the Road Runners and the West Side YMCA put more than 10,000 runners, most of them beginners, on the road to fitness.

The city now sports two of this nation's most spectacular running events: the women's "Mini-Marathon" in Central Park and the New York City Marathon.

Today, running is America's fastest growing sport. The National Jogging Association states that there are more than 10 million joggers in the United States. Their ranks are constantly being swelled by enthusiasts from other sports—like the nation's 29 million tennis and racquetball players—who are discovering that they must get into shape, and stay in shape, to play those sports. We are spending $2 billion a year for everything from running shoes and shorts to stationary bicycles, treadmills and health foods. In 1977, for example, Stow-Mills, the largest health food distributor in New England, was selling 12 tons of granola *every month.*

The surprise of this revolution is not only its numbers, but also its reasons. Most Americans begin running for the health benefits, and then discover that running is also relaxing, meditative, therapeutic. Many of them are running longer distances. A decade-long interest in jogging and bicycling has deepened into a fascination with races, from those of 5 miles to marathon length (26 miles, 385 yards), and beyond. In 1963, for example, 100 runners started the 7.8-mile Bay-to-Breakers run in San Francisco. By 1977, the number was 8100 official runners, with another 3500 running unofficially. The 1975 New York City Marathon had 500 runners. In 1977, more than 5000 men, women and children, ages ten to seventy-two, jogged to the starting line to begin the race by crossing the magnificent Verazzano-Narrows Bridge. In Boston that same year, this famous Marathon was so crowded with runners that at the gun it took 3 minutes and 45 seconds for all of them just to cross the *starting* line!

There are more than 50,000 marathon runners out there

jogging around the United States, and many of them are well over forty years old. For example, among the 1981 men and 107 women who ran the 1976 New York City Marathon, 352 were in their forties, 86 in their fifties, and 20 in their sixties. The oldest was seventy-one.

By the end of the 1970s, running for your health may very well be replaced by running for "euphoria." Americans are already learning that they can get "high" by running long distances. Those who run 30 or more minutes frequently report an altered state of consciousness, a meditative state that is almost Zenlike. One medical report says that people who exercise vigorously for more than 10 minutes on a regular basis release larger amounts of the hormone epinephrine, which doctors call "the chemical basis for happy feelings." (See chapter 16.)

Physicians are also using "running therapy." Dr. Thaddeus Kostrubala, a San Diego psychiatrist, began running with patients who weren't making progress in conventional therapy. His initial group included a paranoid, a mental depressive, a heroin addict, and a man who had tried to commit suicide by refusing to eat. "I am stunned by what I see happening to these people," Dr. Kostrubala reported to *Newsweek* in May 1977. "They are working, getting married, having children and still running. We are dealing here with something that changes personality."

Dr. Ron Lawrence, president of the American Medical Jogger's Association, describes the running experience this way: "I am convinced that running extends life. But even if it didn't add a single day to a person's life, it would be worth doing because running clearly enhances the quality of life. First, if you stick with it for a year, you're hooked. Running's addictive. Second, it changes your whole life-style. Nobody's ever the same again. Running produces tranquility. We know it changes a Type A [highly competitive] personality to a Type B. You get away from the rat race on a regular basis.

"You quit smoking in order to run long distances. Your consumption of alcohol drops for the same reason. You simply have more fun if smoking and drinking don't slow you down. Eating habits change because good nutrition is an integral part of aerobic exercise. Your total well-being improves. You sleep better but require less sleep. Your sex life is enhanced. Anxieties decrease, and you're better prepared to cope with stress. Work productivity improves. You get away from the TV and begin seeing a new world around you."

When Jack Shepherd, my co-author, entered my fitness office in September 1975, he looked like any other out-of-shape American. He had just finished writing *The Adams Chronicles*, a national best-seller, and was slightly overweight and very tense from months of sitting and typing. He talked nervously as he changed into shorts and sneakers for his fitness test. He wanted to begin a jogging program, he told me, because he thought he should have more exercise. He was, after all, thirty-seven years old; friends of his had already suffered and died from heart attacks.

I have heard this story thousands of times. Since 1971, I have started more than 5000 men and women running down the road to fitness. My students now range from joggers who are just beginning, to intermediate runners covering up to 5 miles a day three days a week, to national class women marathon runners. Almost all of us who begin running do so for one major reason: We think it's good for us. We've read and heard about its health benefits, especially to the heart and lungs.

Shepherd was no different. He looked fit, or almost fit, and ready to run a mile or more. In fact, he was dangerously out of shape. He couldn't pass any of my flexibility tests. When I took his resting heart rate, it was 108, far above the normal range of 60 to 80 beats per minute for men. His blood pressure was measured at 160/90, also above normal, and I couldn't even test him on the bicycle ergometer because his heart rate would shoot up too fast.

Shepherd became a man of distinction: He was the first person to flunk my fitness test! Worse, when he mentioned it to his wife and friends, they laughed. How can anyone flunk a fitness test for a beginner's class?

Yet Shepherd was the epitome of the average middle-aged American man (or woman). He wasn't aware of how out-of-shape he had gotten, but he knew he couldn't run the length of a city block, or climb a flight of stairs, without becoming breathless. He was the epitome of Dr. Thomas K. Cureton's warning, "The average middle-age man in this country is close to death. He is only one emotional shock or one sudden exertion away from a serious heart attack—this nation's leading cause of death."

Obviously, Shepherd is still with us—and, I might add, full of vigor and bite. What did we do? First, I sent him to his doctor, who gave him a stress test and a 24-hour out-patient, ambulatory electrocardiogram (EKG). A minor heart condition was discovered, and a medical conclusion similar to mine was reached: Shepherd was grossly out of shape. Start exercising!

In December 1975, he entered my beginner's fitness class at the Y. For the next eight weeks, Shepherd and the men and women in his class took my beginner's program detailed in chapter 2. At first, like many other sedentary Americans, Shepherd couldn't run for 20 consecutive minutes. So he ran 2 minutes, walked 2, ran 2, walked 2 during that time period.

After eight weeks, however, he was out of the gym and into Central Park, running a mile and then 2 miles non-stop. By the end of six months, he was up to 5 miles. His resting heart rate was down to 75 beats per minute; his blood pressure had also dropped to normal. Now, I'm determined to get Shepherd into the New York City Marathon. In 1976, 58 of my runners entered the marathon, and 56 finished. Of these runners, 10 were beginners who had started running less than eight months before they ran the 26 miles. In 1977 over 70 runners—including 50 novices and 25 women—from my team, the Greater New York AA, completed the event.

So, this book combines the knowledge and experiences of an out-of-shape, middle-age American who came back, with that of a high-school and college athlete who now runs several marathons a year and coaches world class runners. The early chapters are ordered somewhat in the pattern your running life will take: from beginner to competitor.

Don't over-estimate your level of fitness. Be honest with yourself. Shepherd knew he couldn't run a city block; he also knew when he was ready to run for 20 consecutive minutes. If you cannot run for 20 minutes, you're a beginner. Start there, and be patient. If you are a weekend athlete, you are probably not in shape either. In fact, you may be in danger: Too many of us believe that a round of golf or a few sets of tennis on Saturday or Sunday constitute fitness. They do not.

To be fit, you've got to run, walk, bicycle or swim vigorously at least three times a week. I've already heard all the excuses: I don't have time; I don't want to sweat; I can't stick to a schedule; I'm too old; I'm too busy; or, worst of all, running isn't fun!

I prefer running. My reasons as an adult are given in the next chapter. But I also know that I was hooked as a kid. In

1963, a junior in high school, I went out for track, ran the half mile, and won fifth place in the Livingston County (N.Y.) Championships. The next year I became a 2-mile runner and an instant "hero"—the "marathon man" of the team and a county champion. But in college, I injured both knees, and doctors told me I would never play sports again, I never realized how much I loved to run until I couldn't. So, I cheated: I played a little basketball and baseball in college, and later in Vietnam with the U.S. Army. But I missed running. When I started working as the physical fitness director of the Rome, (New York) YMCA in 1971, the Y didn't have any joggers at all. Running was just becoming the sport of the seventies.

In the 1960s, a movement led by Arthur Lydiard, Bill Bowerman and Dr. Kenneth Cooper promoted running as a health-promoting activity. A new term made the rounds: "aerobic fitness." Even so, runners were few and far between; whenever one passed another they would wave and smile. In some parts of the country, runners who ventured out in flimsy shorts were laughed at, or worse. A few had cigarettes tossed at them, or bottles. Some were chased by cars, or shot at.

In Rome, I was quickly challenged by Carl Eilenberg, a local radio announcer, to run/walk 20 miles in a Walkathon for YMCA Youth, which we co-chaired. Carl announced on the air that if we both didn't make it, we couldn't collect the pledge money. More than $1000 was "bet" against us. Eilenberg, a former fat man, and me, a cripple, didn't look like we could complete 100 yards, but we started and finished the ordeal. (My time remains a closely guarded secret.) I admit, however, that I was beaten by a forty-two-year-old jogger, but at least I was running again.

In 1972, I saw Frank Shorter win the Olympic Marathon on TV. I knew I had to start long-distance running again. But I didn't want to start it quite this way: I visited Mike Wiley, a former hurdler, in his Kansas University apartment, and we drank beer all night with a group of other runners. There was a marathon the next day, and as the beer went down the challenges went up. More beer, more challenges; when dawn shone I agreed (as I remember) to run. Anyway, a few hours later I found myself on the starting line, a little furry around the tongue. I actually finished—perhaps due to the "foresight" of carbohydrate (beer) loading—and returned to Rome determined to train for and complete the Boston Marathon.

That's when Al Stringham, a co-founder with me of the Roman Runners, introduced me to two important things: regular long runs, and *Runner's World* magazine. *Runner's World* became my coach; Joe Henderson, its editor, my inspiration; and Dr. George Sheehan, a cardiologist and its medical editor, my life saver. Dr. Sheehan's articles about podiatrist Richard Schuster's work with shoe inserts led to a great discovery: My knee pain didn't mean that I needed surgery. I merely needed proper shoe inserts. It worked, and I was off and running.

So were a lot of other Americans. In the early seventies, running and fitness classes were promoted to prevent heart attacks. A new term swept the country: "cardiovascular fitness." I started a runners club in Rome, a youth track program, group workouts—and cardiovascular-fitness programs. I was also sensing a change in my personality: As I ran more, reaching toward 10 miles a day, I was becoming less competitive and more contemplative. I was, as Dr. Lawrence said, seeing a new world around me.

In 1975, when I became Fitness Director of the largest YMCA (12,000 members) in America—New York City's West Side—I was faced with classes still involved with the sixties concept of fitness. "Calisthenics drills" with rapid movement were being taught and so were lots of muscle-strengthening exercises. Running meant a five-minute burst around the gym; relaxation and stretching exercises were ignored. Few women ventured into the classes.

Al Melleby, my supervisor at the Y, brought me in as a runner to emphasize the importance of running and fitness. I slowed everybody down, wrote a manual for the instructors, started fitness and stress testing. Within one-and-a-half years I had tested more than 1000 men and women, and gotten 2000 started in beginner's, intermediate, or advance running classes. Even Jack Shepherd joined.

In May 1977, I teamed with Norb Sander, M.D., a national class runner, to organize a sports-medicine facility, the City Island Fitness and Medical Center in New York City. By 1978, I had formed Robert H. Glover and Associates, Inc., a fitness consulting firm dealing with individuals, community agencies and corporations. These groups and our Greater New York AA runners began at a time when fitness fever had all but the most confirmed sedentary Americans on the road. More of us were running, or beginning to run, than ever before in the history of the country.

Even better, more women are running today than ever before. The number of women runners in the New York Road Runner's Club, for example, has jumped from 10 to more than 500 in three years. In 1972, 150 women ran in the Mini-Marathon. In 1977, more than 2000 entered. Most of these were steady joggers who loved the chance to run with (and against) a smaller number of national class women runners for the 6.2-mile distance.

Today, no one has an excuse not to exercise, and especially not to run. You're too old? If your doctor says you can run, do it! Running is the only sport that rewards you for growing older. Most foot races now include awards to runners in the forty-plus, fifty-plus, sixty-plus and seventy-plus age categories. A World Masters Championship and several noteworthy local races are held across the country for runners over forty years of age.

During one of my Saturday morning beginner's classes in Central Park, a gray-haired woman came up to me and said, "My doctor tells me that anyone over sixty-five shouldn't run. I'm sixty-four. Do I have to stop running when I'm sixty-five?"

I asked her how she felt. "Fine," she replied.

"Any medical problems?"

"No."

"Did you enjoy running this morning?" I asked.

"I loved it," she said with enthusiasm.

"How far did you go?"

"Two loops," she replied, indicating a route of about 3 miles.

I was delighted. "You're obviously too *young* not to run!"

Almost everyone can hit the road. Postcardiac men and women, under close supervision, ran in my YMCA classes. Other medically supervised programs, either in clinics, at Y's around the country, or under the supervision of private doctors, help men and women who have suffered heart attacks to run. In fact, the most convincing evidence that running protects against heart disease comes from the rehabilitation of heart attack victims. As we detail in chapter 11, men and women who have had heart attacks, stopped smoking, and started running at least three times a week, have one-sixth the number of second, often fatal, heart attacks as people who don't exercise at all. Now, we are even seeing recovered heart attack victims enter marathons. In Hawaii, for example, postcardiac patients run the Honolulu Marathon wearing black shirts with large red, broken hearts stitched on them.

I have blind friends who are runners, and others with cerebral palsy. Dick Traum, who wears an artificial right leg, began running with me in 1975. He entered the 1976 New York City Marathon, and completed the run full of vigor. In fact, he took a wrong turn, and ran an extra 2 miles, then announced to me: "Bob, I've just finished the Ultra Marathon." Now Dick occasionally runs with another amputee, Jack Terry, who ran with him in a Central Park YMCA race. Dick is also forming The National Amputee Runner's Club. Another group, "runners" confined to wheelchairs, covered the Boston Marathon route ahead of the others in a National Wheelchair Marathon Championship. Pushing a wheelchair instead of legs up and down those hills is aerobic.

Whole towns are out running. Over thirty-one cities have built 2-mile fitness trails that combine walking and jogging with twenty exercise stations to develop strength and agility. Signs along the way explain what exercises to perform with the equipment on hand—pull-ups, perhaps, or jumping logs. However, running is the basic exercise; the heart muscle takes precedence over the pectorals or biceps. Says one enthusiast, "No one ever died of weak arms."

These courses are commonplace in Europe—Switzerland alone has more than four hundred. "The exercises supplement jogging, adding interest and stimulation," says Dr. Ruth Alexander, head of the women's Physical Education Department at the University of Florida, where a trail runs around Lake Alice. "As we get older, we lose our flexibility faster than anything else. That's why the bending, twisting and squatting are excellent."

Industry is also joining in. Jess Bell of Bonne Bell Cosmetics built a track that includes a man-made hill outside his Cleveland plant, and encourages employees to run during their breaks and lunch hours. Some 50,000 other companies, including 300 of the Fortune 500, have planned and supervised exercise programs. In 1960, at El Segundo, California, Rockwell International started an ambitious program to have every employee, and his or her family, following a daily exercise routine. Xerox, which has stressed employee fitness since 1965, built a training school with "living-and-learning" accommodations for a thousand employees near Leesburg, Virginia, surrounded by two thousand rolling, wooded acres. And high above the stress and tension of Manhattan, in Rockefeller Center, Exxon's intensive program is supervised by a white-coated medical staff. Their fitness lab contains 10 exercise stations open to 300 executives who are encouraged to spend an hour three times a week keeping themselves in shape.

Over at *Forbes* magazine, employes who *don't* exercise are gently admonished with notes from their colleagues. Malcolm Forbes, fifty-seven and president of the company, believes "it gives the whole firm a sense of team spirit," and is right in there sweating on the rowing machine and stationary bicycle. These and other corporations are spending more than $2 billion a year on corporate physical fitness programs. They view fitness as a wise investment for preventing disease and disability among their employees. I started a fitness program for a corporation after its insurance company threatened to raise its premiums because thirteen of the corporation's fifteen top-level executives had high blood pressure and were overweight. Now they are jogging toward better health and more productivity.

Not long ago, an editor at Random House in New York, whose husband works for the Chase Manhattan Bank, noticed a difference in his behavior. He was calmer, more vigorous, and slept better. They began taking long walks together in Central Park—something they hadn't done since they were first married.

Their sex life, too, was returning to earlier enthusiasms. "I couldn't understand what was happening to him," she said, "so I asked him, and he told me that about six months earlier he had become eligible for Chase's executive fitness program, and he's been working out about three times a week. I don't know if the bank's getting any benefits from all this, but I am."

Corporations are not confining their involvement to running for health. They are also beginning to include competitive running in their programs. In 1977, the Road Runner's Club of New York initiated a very popular series of corporate races sponsored by Manufacturers Hanover Trust. Awards were broken down by type of company, and Central Park filled with four hundred runners—bankers jogging against bankers, Wall Street lawyers versus Wall Street lawyers.

Despite all this activity and enthusiasm, almost one American out of every two does not exercise at all. "Hypokinetic disease"—the disease of inactivity—is a fact of life for almost half of us, including our children. Few Americans exercise enough to run 100 yards at a slow pace without hard breathing and dangerous heart strain. Dr. Norb Sander says, "My patients need fitness more than they need medicine." They are victims of sedentary jobs, inertia—and technological "progress."

In the 1930s, Dr. Paul Dudley White publicly disowned his automobile, and started bicycling to work. People thought he was nuts. In the 1950s, he became President Eisenhower's physician, and when the President suffered his first heart attack, Dr. White had him back on the golf course within four weeks. Too few Americans are willing to get out of their cars, or elevators, or other machines of ease, and start exercising. The medical results are well documented: Increased inactivity and obesity have led to an epidemic of heart disease, deaths from heart attack, strokes, and related illnesses. Heart attack is the nation's number one killer, with 650,000 American victims in 1977. The number of deaths from cardiovascular disease, although dropping slightly in the mid-seventies, still claimed 979,180 people in 1976. Ulick O'Connor, the Irish poet, author and playwright, put it all into perspective, "When he popularized the motor car, Henry Ford could never have thought that he was unleashing bacilli that would strike down men in middle age like a medieval plague."

Too many of us are victims of the disease of inactivity. We are lazy and fat. When Yankee Stadium was remodeled in 1974, it contained 9000 fewer seats than the old "House that Ruth Built." Why? The seats had to be widened from 18 inches to 22 inches to contain the expanding American posterior!

So, we begin by running for our lives: to control our weight, lower our blood pressure, slow the aging process, help prevent heart disease. It is generally agreed that exercise programs improve strength, stamina, coordination, flexibility. Running also gives an overall sense of well-being. Fred Meyer, a vice president of the Tyler Corporation in Dallas, says that "running long distances builds perseverance, and helps me solve business problems." It also helps us tolerate stress, and it may even prolong life, and offer protection against heart disease.

Dr. Thomas Bassler of the American Medical Jogger's Association says running 6 miles a day and finishing at least one marathon is absolute protection against heart disease. He claims, "It is safe to say that a hobby marathoner who finishes a four-hour marathon has at least six years of coronary heart disease protection." At the other extreme, Dr. Meyer Friedman and Dr. Ray Rosenman, authors of *Type A Behavior and Your Heart*, argue that running is a form of "mass suicide," with no redeeming qualities—either physical or spiritual. You should know that Dr. Bassler is a marathon runner, and Drs. Friedman and Rosenman are not.

We discuss this issue more fully in chapter 12, but we are finding that more doctors are advising patients to run. A report in April 1977, from the Royal College of Physicians and the British Cardiac Society states that people who exercise vigorously are less likely to have coronary heart disease than those who don't. Recent research at the Jefferson Medical College in Philadelphia suggests that vigorous exercise may inhibit the growth of cancer.

Ultimately, it comes down to this: The people who claim running isn't healthy are usually nonrunners while those who claim it is are generally runners. Men and women already on the road to fitness know it feels good because they feel better and their lives are being enriched and invigorated.

If you're not a runner already, start exercising. But what do I mean by exercise? Simply stated, three basic things: Change your clothes, sweat, and shower. Let's agree from the start that we are going to sweat. You may even get to like it. You may recognize it for what it is: a healthy sign of an exercising body. The sweat will come from running, which is the basis of my exercise program. We are going to run slow, and far, but don't panic, because it will be easy. We will run because I agree with the doctors on the President's Council on Physical Fitness and Sports who rated fourteen popular forms of exercise and evaluated them in terms of health benefits. Jogging, bicycling and swimming came out first, second and third. I would also add vigorous walking. These are the rhythmic exercises that use the major muscles repeatedly. The other kinds are the power exercises, such as weight lifting and isometrics, which require short, rapid, forceful movements and put stress on the heart for short periods. The stress on the muscle bundles during contractions tends to impede circulation rather than aid it. On the other hand, jogging or running involves vigorous contraction and relaxation of the large muscles of the legs and trunk. Sustained for a period of time, this kind of exercise will raise your body temperature, increase your heart rate, and induce sweating. The rewards will be a greater ability to consume oxygen during strenuous exertion, a lower resting heart rate, less fatigue-inducing lactic acid produced by your skeletal muscles, reduced blood pressure and more efficient heart and lung action.

While the doctors research and debate the relative benefits of exercise, we are going to run. At first, if you are just beginning, you may find it rough going. Then, after a while, you will feel better—and better. You may even become addicted and want to run every day, especially if you discover meditative running and its euphoria. The way I see it, if I can get Jack Shepherd running and in shape, I can get anyone to run—even you.

# 1 THE RUN-EASY METHOD: A BASIC PROGRAM FOR ALL RUNNERS

How fast should I run? How often? How far should I go?

These are important questions to anyone starting a jogging program, or already getting back into shape. My exercise philosophy agrees with that of Dr. Ernst van Aaken who says, "Run slowly, run daily, drink moderately, and don't eat like a pig." I believe in running easy, running long, running aerobically. I call this the "Run-Easy Method."

Most books on running preach systems. The common theory is that we must be programmed to follow a rigid, systematic schedule that tells us in advance what we will do every day for eight to twelve weeks of robotlike existence. But I hate schedules. I find them too rigid and scientific. Running embodies a special freedom: a freedom from the computerized world, a return to nature. My plan for running revolves around people and such unscientific principles as feelings and body language. I believe that running should be easy, simple, fun. Running at an easy pace, you'll find that your body will gently move into a new life with a minimum of discomfort.

The National Jogging Association says, "Run Gently." Joe Henderson popularized the term "LSD" (Long Slow Distance) based on Dr. van Aaken's training methods. "Train, don't strain" was Bill Bowerman's Golden Rule. "Run Easy" is just another name for the same principle. We are all saying, "Throw away the stopwatch, and listen to your body instead."

Pace is the most important and difficult part of running to learn. Too often we are in a hurry. But we can't rush to get into shape and we shouldn't run in a hurry. Instead, running should relieve the pressures of our hurried pace. Of course, you can run so that time counts—the first 20 minutes for the beginner runner—but not distance. My point here is simply: Get out of the distance hang-up, where runners greet each other with "How far did ya run?" You can run for distance if you like, but if you combine distance with time the result is competition, the desire to hurry. It brings the hectic pace of your work-a-day life to the leisurely pace of running. I insist that you run easy. To do otherwise is to encounter not fitness, but often injury and frustration.

My Run-Easy Method involves three simple steps: Warm-up, Run, Cool-down. Everyone who exercises follows this same pattern, including veteran runners. As you progress, you may want to add exercises (listed in chapter 6), or practice yoga (chapter 16), or run for a longer time. I've found it best, however, to develop a good basic warm-up and cool-down program, and stick to it. This book offers more than 100 various exercises, so you shouldn't have any problem developing your own favorites.

Remember, the only person you compete against during your workouts is the old, "out-of-shape" you, and no one else. Let other runners brag about their running mileage or times. You should exercise at your own speed. When you run—and I'll emphasize this again—run at a pace that enables you to talk with someone. Consistency and endurance—not speed—are the key.

Run for fun. As your muscles firm and stretch, as you relax, eat and sleep better, meet new friends and discover that running can be graceful and fun, you'll soon understand what Joe Henderson meant when he wrote in *The Long-Run Solution*, "Running only to exercise the muscles is like eating only to exercise the jaws, or having sex only to train the pelvis."

## GETTING STARTED

There are two types of exercises, power and rhythmic. Power exercises like weight lifting and isometrics require short, rapid, forceful movements. They put stress on the heart for short periods, and the stress on your muscle bundles during contractions tends to impede circulation rather than aid it.

Rhythmic exercises like jogging, bicycling, swimming, brisk walking, stationary cycling—even vigorous dancing—use the major muscles repeatedly. I prefer jogging or running, which are cheap (total cost: shoes and shorts), aerobic and produce physiological changes leading toward fitness. Jogging or running involve vigorous contraction and relaxation of the large muscles of the legs and trunk. Sustained for a period of time, this exercise will raise your body temperature, increase your heart rate and induce sweating. The rewards will be a greater ability to consume oxygen during strenuous exertion, a lower resting heart rate, less lactic acid produced by your skeletal muscles (therefore less fatigue), reduced blood pressure and more efficient heart and lung action.

Therefore, I view the appropriate *type* of exercise as running or jogging. But, like Joe Namath, you may not be able to run; swimming, brisk walking, and the other rhythmic exercises are also acceptable, and are useful when you must recover strength after illness or maintain your fitness during injury.

But running is the heart of my program—and my life. It's cheap. It's enjoyable all year round and anywhere you travel. You will soon find that there is no better way to see, hear, smell or feel your community or vacation spot. If you run alone, you can meditate and solve problems. Or, you can run in a group, for fun. More and more runners are exercising with others. It's a terrific way to meet new friends and accomplish something at the same time.

Running gives the unstructured and undirected life discipline and purpose. You have a sense of direction, and goals. I solve many of my work problems while I run. Several chapters of this book were created during runs. Running, as we discuss in chapter 16, can also be therapeutic.

You can set whatever goals you wish. Getting into shape to run around the neighborhood, or to complete 5 miles, can be reason enough to start running. I know several women runners who began with one purpose in mind: running the Mini-Marathon in New York City, a distance of 6.2 miles.

Veteran runners already know the benefits of running, and may have set their goals, such as completing several marathons. But they can also be sloppy, injury-prone or lacking in specific running techniques. Even if you are in relatively good shape or are a competitive runner, the Run-Easy Method will help you form the basis for a proper running program that you can follow easily. It will add a variety of exercises, running techniques, and goals to your life. Further, veteran runners may find that they need to weed out bad habits.

## THE FIRST STEP

Determine what kind of runner you are. Are you a beginner, an intermediate or an advanced runner? Whichever you are, the Run-Easy Method will fit your level; its three basic steps, detailed here, are equally important no matter what your running ability.

If you cannot touch your toes, perform certain stretching exercises, or walk up several flights of stairs without becoming breathless, you are probably a beginner. Actually, I define a beginner as someone who cannot run easily for 20 consecutive minutes at a steady comfortable pace, and talk while running.

Don't be dismayed. Most American men and women are so badly out of shape that they cannot jog a city block without breathing heavily and straining their muscles, lungs and hearts. Right now, it's important to remember several things. Running is not a *macho* sport; you can declare yourself a beginner without shame. Also, you can admit that it took years of gluttony and piglike living to get out of shape, and it will take months to get back in. But getting back into shape with the Run-Easy Method will almost be a pleasure. I said *almost*.

Still not convinced? Dr. Kenneth Cooper suggests that you strip to your underwear and stand facing a full-length mirror. Do you like what you see? Okay, now stand sideways. Still look good?

Everyone who is beginning to run—whether or not you consider yourself a beginner—should get a medical check-up, and a fitness evaluation. Thousands of men and women merely pull on their expensive jogging suits and shoes, open their front doors, and fly. But they are soon bored, discouraged or injured. The most dangerous exercise you can do is to start out vigorously, and run once a week. The weekend jogger is a killer—and he himself is the victim.

Don't skip the medical check-up. You should be certain that you do not have an ailment that could be made worse by exercising. You should also begin this program slowly.

I will stress this again in the chapter on beginner runners. But this program will get the sedentary man and woman into minimal shape after eight weeks. It requires only two things: your commitment and a common-sense schedule. (I know, I said I hate schedules, but mine is painless.)

## FREQUENCY

Beginner runners will run three or four times a week. As you get into shape, you can run more frequently. Beginner competitors and advanced runners may exercise daily, sometimes twice daily. Even they must follow a hard-easy pattern. Track coach Bill Bowerman suggests (and so do I) the plan of alternating hard workouts with "active rest." The average jogger shouldn't put together several days of hard or long workouts. He or she should plan for rest days, slow-run or short-run days, and days off. For all but the most serious runners, I recommend a six-day running week with a planned day of rest. During those six days, alternate between long and short runs (or hard and easy).

To the beginner this may sound like a lot of time, and "lack of time" is the most common excuse not to run. However, I'm only asking you to put aside a minimum of three hours of an entire week when you first start. You, and others like you, may reply, "But I don't have the time." You do.

How long do you take for lunch? Two hours? Take one of them for your health. How many hours per week do you watch television? Take an hour (or more) from there. How much time do you spend napping, or staring out the window, or resting in your chair behind your desk, or idly thinking about what you might be doing? Take an hour or more from that wasted time. As you will see in detail in the next chapter, time is the one thing I know you've got. You can easily find 3 hours out of the 168 hours in every week.

## INTENSITY

You must exercise vigorously for at least 20 minutes. This does not include the warm-up or cool-down periods. The period of intense exercise—the run—should increase from 20 to 30 minutes or more as you become better conditioned. During this time, you must reach and maintain an aerobic level of exercise. That is, you must make your heart work hard. During the following fitness program, I'll detail what I mean.

Thinking you are already in good condition is dangerous. You must reach your level of intensity slowly. If you cannot run for 20 consecutive minutes, admit that you are a beginner. Make a personal commitment. Tell yourself that you are going to prepare your body to run, and run at a slow, easy pace for the next eight weeks.

Too many people begin to jog on their own. They don't bother with a warm-up or a cool-down. Even their running is based upon bad ideas and worse practice. I've actually seen people at the Y walk around the track and then sprint until they are breathless, then walk again, then sprint. They are not working at an aerobic rate, and they are inviting injury, or worse.

The weekend jogger who dashes out for a mile run once a week is also a beginner runner, and a foolhardy one. He—women usually aren't so bullheadedly competitive—doesn't think he needs to warm up and cool down. He especially doesn't want to get into a "sissy" beginner's program. But these runners—the determined but out-of-shape—particularly need a fitness program and cautionary guidelines.

So, after your doctor tells you that you may run, let's agree on several things: You are going to set aside three hours or more a week; you are going to exercise vigorously for at least 20 minutes; you are going to warm up, cool down, and run within your limits. And you are going to do this for the next eight to ten weeks.

## THE RUN-EASY METHOD

Okay, let's get started. Remember, Jack Shepherd was in dangerously bad shape when I got him into my beginner's fitness class. He has traveled down the road to fitness, and you can do it too. Be determined—but also be patient. Muscles and wind won't return in two weeks—but they will return.

The following program is for every runner, whatever his or her level. What varies according to conditioning is not the basic Run-Easy program, but its intensity and duration. Since beginners need special instructions not applicable to more advanced runners, I will repeat some of this program in the next chapter.

But the three phases—warm-up, run and cool-down—are the same for every runner. The time spent at each phase, and the number of exercises or minutes run, will vary according to your fitness level. But no runner—beginner, intermediate, or advanced—should ever skip any of the three parts.

### Part One: Warm-up
*Minimum time:* 15 minutes.
*Object:* relaxation and stretching.

The warm-up consists of relaxation, flexibility and strength exercises, and walking as a preparation to running. The warm-up is often overlooked, even by experienced joggers who love to dash out of their homes and do a few fast miles. That practice may be dangerous to your health.

If you think you can skip the warm-up, consider a recent California medical study of men ages twenty-five to fifty-two, who were already in good-to-excellent physical condition. They all had had stress tests and normal electrocardiograms (EKG) under maximum exertion. These men were asked to step on a moving treadmill, rolling at 9 miles per hour and inclined at a small grade, and begin running without any warm-up. When they did, two thirds of these well-conditioned men developed abnormal EKG's. The reason was inadequate coronary blood flow to the heart's myocardium. Later, when these same men were asked to warm-up for five minutes before running on the moving treadmill again, their EKGs were normal.

The study concluded that sudden exertion can cause heart attacks, even among men in good physical condition. But when the heart is given time to warm up, the coronary arteries dilate, allowing more blood to flow through them. In other similar studies, high blood pressure also resulted from exertion without proper warm-up.

The 15-minute warm-up is designed to get your heart rate up. But it is also important for relaxing and stretching tense muscles. Tensions that build in the body must be released, including those caused by running. (Hence, warm-up and cool-down contain similar exercises.)

Beginning your warm-up with relaxation exercises will help "break" muscle tension that frequently causes muscular strains, especially back pain. Such exercises also "warm up" muscles that are tense and difficult to stretch, and therefore should precede the stretching exercises.

This section also emphasizes stretching exercises that will lengthen the hamstring and calf muscles along the backs of your legs, and reduce stiffness and rigidity of the trunk. A muscle works best at its maximum length. It is more efficient—producing more power—than a shorter one. However, stretching a muscle properly means stretching it slowly. It cannot be done by bobbing or jerking motions, such as bouncing downward to touch your toes. This action may actually tighten the muscle instead of stretching it.

Physiologists divide stretching exercises into two types: ballistic and static. "Ballistic" exercises are the standard vigorous calisthenics that feature quick, repeated movements. Boot camp instructors thrive on these. "Static" exercises involve slow and rhythmic stretching, stopping and holding a position at the first point of discomfort.

Both types of exercises are effective. But static stretching exercises are much safer and aid in eliminating muscle soreness. Try it. When Arnold Spellun, a New York City lawyer, started jogging, he noticed stiffness down the backs of both legs every day after running. Jack Shepherd, visiting the Spelluns while working on this book, suggested "static" exercises both before and after running (Exercises 10 and 13). To the delight of both men, Spellun's leg stiffness went away immediately.

Dr. Clayton Myers, National YMCA Fitness Director, recommends that your warm-up include

- exercises that stretch muscles and put joints through their full range of motion, but that do not strain them against resistence;
- stretching that is rhythmic, with a natural flow from one exercise to the next, and that avoids sudden changes and breaks;
- variety to make the warm-up enjoyable and reinforce the simple concept that body motion is fun;
- exercises combining muscle stretching with increased activity of the heart and cardiovascular system;
- the use of every part of the body in natural motions.

The function of the warm-up, Dr. Myers states, "is to help meet the increased demand for oxygen by the heart, lungs, and active muscles. Specifically, the small blood vessels are opened up not only in the heart's coronary circulation but also in the peripheral capillary circulation of the legs and other areas of the body. The warm-up also stretches certain leg muscles exerted by jogging."

Part of the warm-up also includes calisthenics. Both men and women runners must strengthen their arms, legs and abdomens. This conditioning will improve posture, and aid in preventing injury. If you are out of shape your arms, legs and trunk probably cannot support vigorous activity. For runners, the anti-gravity muscles—the abdominals, quadriceps (thighs), and shins—need to be strengthened to balance the strength that running gives to the back and the backs of your legs.

The strengthening phase of the warm-up includes exercises for the anti-gravity muscles and the development of the upper body in both men and women for a firmer bust, stronger chest, flatter abdomen, better posture. These exercises reduce the possibility of injury and create a better running chasis. I particularly recommend sit-ups, push-ups, and special exercises for the quadriceps. Dr. Myers makes several other recommendations for this part of the warm-up:

- Avoid working on calisthenics without let-up. Exercise, then rest, then resume, then rest. The adult body will prolong and improve its efforts if rest periods are interspersed with the exercises.
- Avoid isometric exercises, which cause resistence to blood flow. Keep in motion, but don't convert any exercise, such as push-ups, into a trial against exhaustion. If the goal is a certain number of push-ups, break them into two or more sets rather than overexhaust the body.
- Avoid freely swinging the body against a fixed joint. If you can't touch your toes while the knees are locked, don't try

to do it by forcefully bouncing downward. The result
might be a strained back, tendon, ligament or hamstring
muscle.

- Include exercises for all major joint movements.
- Keep shifting forceful work from one muscle group to
another to avoid local fatigue. Do not do more than two
consecutive abdominal or two consecutive leg exercises.
Try something else in between.

To these, I would add a few other guidelines for this phase
of the program. Avoid full deep-knee squats. The old Airborne
squat-jumps are dangerous. Knee injuries may result. Thighs
should not be lower than a position parallel to the floor because
of the possibility of straining your knees, causing damage. Also,
do not perform exercises that cause hyperextension of the back.
These include exercises in which both legs and both arms are
raised simultaneously when lying on the stomach, or in which
the legs and head are raised while lying on your back. These
exercises can cause back injury, and should be avoided. Standing
upright and "bouncing" on the toes should be done only after
a good warm-up, and then only minimally. Bouncing puts pressure on the shins and may produce calf tightness. The following
exercises are designed to help you develop a good, basic warm-up
and cool-down program, and to avoid injury. During your exercises, give your muscles a chance to relax. Muscles should be
tightened and then let go; do not force the holding of a position
for too long. Rotate lying on your back and lying on your
stomach to alternate muscle group strain. Remember that muscle overload is necessary to gain strength, but you should perform such exercises gradually. Progressive strengthening exercises, such as sit-ups and push-ups, will help you develop, and
also avoid injury. Finally, progress at your own rate; do not try
to keep up with more advanced or fit runners.

**The Warm-up Exercises\*** Lie on the floor with your knees flexed. Relax for a moment. Do the following exercises in order during every workout.

1. *Belly Breathing* Lie on your back, knees flexed, eyes closed. (By knees flexed I mean bent, with feet flat and heels close to your bottom.) Take a deep breath and concentrate on letting your stomach rise as you breathe in. Let go. Do this about 10 times. To be certain that you are breathing properly place a book on your stomach. It should rise as you breathe in.

2. *Head Roll* On your back, knees flexed, eyes closed. Breathe normally. Roll your head slowly to one side, and let it relax and go limp. Return slowly to the center and roll it to the other side. Go limp. Repeat 3 full rolls or more—right to left and left to right being one roll.

3. *Shoulder Shrug* On your back, knees flexed, eyes closed. Relax. Take a deep breath, sliding your shoulders up towards your ears. Exhale, letting your shoulders drop limply to a normal position. Repeat 5 times or more.

4. *Leg Limbering* Still on your back, with your knees flexed, eyes still closed. Breathe comfortably. Slowly draw one knee up toward your chest as close as you can. Slowly lower the leg back to the flexed position, and then slowly let it slide forward and drop loosely. Return to the flexed position. Repeat with the other leg. Do this 3 times with each leg. Good for hamstring muscles.

5. *Double Knee Flex* Lie on your back, both knees flexed. Pull both knees up to your chest as far as you can without raising your hips. Lower your legs gradually to the flexed position. Do at least 3, up to 20. Good for abdominal muscles.

---

\* Most exercises are from Dr. Hans Kraus's book, *Backache, Stress and Tension*, and his program, "The Y's Way to a Healthy Back."

**6. Double Knee Roll**   On your back, both knees flexed, arms outstretched to your side, palms down. Roll both knees together to one side until the outside knee touches the floor. Keep both palms on the floor. At the same time, turn your head to the opposite direction, and hold. Remain in this position for a few seconds, then roll to the other side. Do one complete roll 3 times. Good for abdominal and back muscles.

**7. Cat Back**   Kneel, resting on your hands and knees. Breathing in, arch your back like a cat, tucking your head in, chin to chest. Reverse, bringing your head up, expelling your breath and forming a "U" with your spine. Repeat 3 times. Good for abdominal and back muscles.

**8. Pectoral Stretch**   Still on hands and knees. Slide both hands forward, bringing your elbows to the floor and then your arms. Keep your back and head straight, your thighs perpendicu-

**Double Knee Roll**

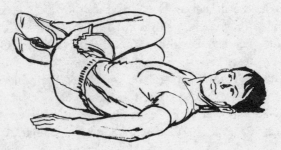

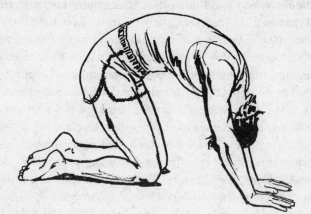

**Cat Back**

**Pectoral Stretch**

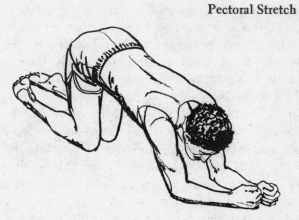

lar to the floor, hips up. Return to kneeling position, rest, then repeat 3 times. Good for shoulder and back muscles.

**9. *Push-ups*** Do as many push-ups as you can comfortably and with good form. Try 5, and work up to 15 or so. Keep your back straight, fanny high, with your body resting on your hands and toes. Lower yourself, touch only your chest to the floor, and raise up. If this is too difficult, use the modified form by resting on your hands and knees. Good for arms and chest.

***Rest*** Now, you should relax momentarily on your back. Take a minute. Spread your arms out wide. Open and close your hands. Take deep breaths. Slowly slide your arms along the floor until they are overhead, and your body is entirely stretched out. Heart rate should drop below 110–120 beats per minute.

**10. *Hamstring and Calf Muscle Stretch*** Lie on your back, both knees flexed. Let one leg slide forward and drop. Point your toe, and slowly raise the straightened leg up into the air as far as you can without bending the knee. Do not jerk or force it. Keep your hips on the floor. Slowly lower the leg to the floor, and let it relax. Now, cock the heel—pointing the toe toward the knee—and again raise the leg. You should feel the stretch in the calf muscle. Lower the leg slowly. Repeat with the other leg. Do both exercises with each leg 3 times. Good for calf and hamstring muscles.

**11. *Sitting Stretch*** Sit up, with legs apart, hands together and arms outstretched. Slide your fingers down one leg as far as possible, and hold. Keep the back of your knee flat against the ground. If you can reach your toes, pull on them gently. Hold for a few seconds, and return to a sitting position. Then repeat on the other leg. Do 3 sets. Then put your feet together and slide hands down legs. Reach as far as you can, and hold for a few seconds. Do not jerk or force the stretch. Good for hamstring muscles.

**12.** *Sit-ups*  Lie on your back, knees flexed. Hook your toes under the sofa, bed or other stable object, or have someone hold your feet. Put your hands behind your head, "roll up" smoothly to a sitting position with your head close to your knees. Breathe out as you roll up. Now, roll back smoothly, breathing in. Do this slowly, carefully; do not arch your back or strain for one extra sit-up. Start with 5 and work gradually up to as many as you can comfortably do with good form. Good for abdominal muscles.

A special word is needed about sit-ups. One of the major causes of back pain is not "weak back muscles," but weak stomach muscles. If your abdominal muscles can't properly carry their workload, then your back muscles may overstress, resulting in back pain.

Sit-ups, properly done, are an excellent way to keep abdominal muscles in tone. Yet most Americans do not perform them correctly. Our coaches and drill instructors have for years emphasized very fast, multi-repetition, straight-legged sit-ups that are not only incorrect, but also harmful to your back. Straight-legged sit-ups use both the abdominal and hip-flexor muscles. Many people can do them but cannot do sit-ups with knees bent. Their stronger leg muscles compensate for their weak abdominal muscles.

Always do sit-ups with your knees bent. That takes the pressure off your lower back and maximizes the use of your abdominal muscles. Sit-ups should not be done in a fast or jerky motion. Arching the back or bouncing off the floor for high-speed sit-ups puts tremendous strain on your back. Instead, "roll up" smoothly, as suggested above, breathing out as you come up. Roll slowly down. "Gutting it out" for a few fast sit-ups, or a few extra, is inadvisable. The result may be a strained back. Instead of pushing for a few more sit-ups, do some other abdominal exercises (see chapter 6) and return for another set of sit-ups later.

The stomach muscles should be relaxed between each sit-up, even for a brief second. A long series of abdominal work may be dangerous; as your muscles get tired, you tend to arch your back or jerk yourself up to compensate. The result may be a back injury. Space your abdominal exercises throughout your workout. More important, do only as many sit-ups in one set as you can with proper form. Gradually add more as you become stronger.

Some beginners cannot do sit-ups with their hands behind their heads. If this is the case, you can work into proper sit-up form by a series of progressive steps. Try each step until it becomes too easy, and then move to the next. First, lie on your back, raise your knees with your feet flat on the floor. With your arms at your sides, raise your head, chest and arms off the ground in a half sit-up. Do several of these. The next step requires that you keep your arms at your sides but roll slowly into a full sit-up. After you can do these easily, try folding your arms across your chest, and rolling slowly into a full sit-up. After doing the above for several weeks, place your hands behind your head, elbows extended, and roll into a full sit-up. This is the proper form. Remember to keep your knees bent, roll into the sitting position without jerking, and breathe out as you come up.

**Rest**    After sit-ups, relax a moment. But as you get stronger, you may want to "rest" by curling up into the bicycle position—feet extended high into the air, hands on hips—and pedal a while.

**13.** *Standing Hamstring and Calf Muscle Stretch*   Stand about three feet from a wall, tree, or lamp-post. Put your hands on the wall, and lean. Keep your hips and back straight, heels firmly on the ground. Now, slowly allow your straight body to lean close to the wall. Drop your forearms against the wall, so you are touching it from elbow to hands. Back straight, heels flat, tuck your hips in toward the wall. Then, straighten arms

**Standing Hamstring and
Calf Muscle Stretch**

and push your body back to a standing position. Repeat 3 times. Excellent for hamstring and calf muscles.

Next, stand close to the wall, feet together, hands on the wall. Bend at the knees, keeping your feet flat on the ground. You will feel your Achilles' tendon (behind your heels) stretch.

**14. *Front and Back Stretch*** Stand. Hands on hips. Slowly bend forward from the waist, and then slowly bend backward. Keep your back straight. You may want to bring your elbows forward as you bend forward, and back as you bend back.

Next, place your hands at your sides, palms inward. Slowly slide the left hand down the left leg as you bend leftward. Simultaneously, raise your right hand overhead, arm straight. Twist your head to the right and look at the palm of your right hand. Repeat on the other side. Do 3 times each. Good for back, abdominal and hamstring muscles.

**15. *Backovers*** Lie on your back, knees flexed, arms at your sides, palms down by your thighs. Slowly raise your hips and curl your back, raising your legs—knees leading—toward the floor by your ears. Do not force. Hold the position for 20 or 30 seconds. This is a variation of the yoga Plough, or Halasana (see page 342).

If you are able, lie on the floor, legs stretched out in front. Now, slowly raise the legs and the lumbar part of your back, and bring the legs behind your head until the toes touch the floor. Hold for 10 to 30 seconds. If you wish, stretch your arms, palms up, over your head on the floor, for additional stretching. Good for back and hamstring muscles. If you have any back trouble or your muscles are out of shape, you should be cautious while trying this exercise.

**16. *Leg-up Stretch*** Stand up, place one foot on a table, the back of a chair, a railing or the third or fourth stair. With both

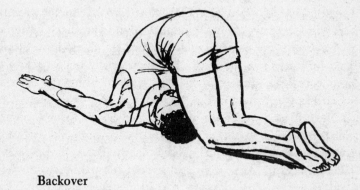

**Backover**

hands, slowly reach down as far as comfortably possible toward the foot. Keep the leg straight. If you reach the toes, pull gently. Hold the position for a few seconds. Do not jerk or force the stretch. Repeat with each leg three times. Good for hamstring and back muscles. If you have back trouble or your muscles are way out of shape, be careful performing this exercise.

Before starting out, take a moment to perform a final exercise to stretch your quadriceps. With one hand holding a chair or lamp post or railing for support, reach back with the other and—by raising your foot behind you—grab your toes. Pull upward. Do each leg 3 times. Or, if you prefer, lie on your stomach, and reach both hands back and behind you to pull on both toes at the same time.

Begin walking along your jogging route

**Part Two: The Aerobic (Run) Phase**

*Time:* At least 20 minutes.

*Object:* Vigorous exercise.

Now you are ready to run. Beginner runners will find a detailed, progressive program in the next chapter. But every runner, whatever his or her level, must understand that running is the core of this program. We are all runners—some of us run longer or farther than others.

As you have been moving from relaxation to stretching to calisthenics, you have been building up body heat. Your muscles have been demanding more oxygen and, to meet that demand, your blood vessels have been dilating, your heart and lungs working harder and harder (see chapter 12). You're almost ready to go. Now, you should move from walking to running; it is important to begin this phase with a properly relaxed and stretched body. The transition from calisthenics to aerobics is achieved by moving from warm-up exercises to a brisk walk to a slow jog and then settling into your running pace.

Here, as I mentioned, runners do separate into categories depending upon their fitness. Beginners will want to walk, run, walk, run, walk. They should follow a simple pattern: Run until you are ready to walk, walk until you are ready to run again. The idea, detailed in the next chapter, is to keep moving by walking or running for 20 minutes.

To be minimally fit, you must perform at least 20 minutes of aerobic exercise at least three times a week. What do I mean by "aerobic exercise"? This is the pulse-rated system of exercise, developed by exercise physiologists, which is supported by the American Heart Association and leading fitness experts. Beginners, moderately-fit intermediates, or conditioned runners will all exercise their hearts aerobically, but at different rates depending upon age and level of fitness.

The aerobic theory was developed by Dr. Kenneth Cooper in the 1960s. Aerobics means "promoting the supply and use of oxygen." Dr. Cooper defined as aerobic such exercises as walking, jogging, bicycling and swimming. These activities, done at a vigorous level over specific times, burn calories and strengthen your cardiovascular system. The main principle of aerobics is that your body must exercise at a rate that demands large amounts of oxygen for a sustained period of time, preferably at least 20 to 45 minutes three times a week.

Weight lifting or isometrics are not aerobic. Tennis, handball, squash, touch football and other sports are aerobic to some degree, but allow only for bursts of activity rather than sustained effort. Skating, cross-country skiing, hockey, soccer and hiking provide enough stress for cardiovascular response. In contrast, softball, bowling, doubles tennis and golf do not.

Jumping rope may be aerobic, but it is also dangerous. It is hard on your legs, and takes skill to do well. But worst of all, unless you warm up properly, jumping rope will accelerate your heart rate too quickly, and heart attack is a real possibility for previously sedentary men and women. Still, rope jumping offers good maintenance work for runners while traveling.

The basis for aerobics is important. The more oxygen we supply to our bodies, and the more efficiently the body can utilize this oxygen, the more physically fit we become. We breathe in oxygen from the atmosphere, and our lungs supply the blood with oxygen. Our heart pumps this life-supporting oxygen-enriched blood to the body tissues, where it combines with the fuel sources to produce energy. The blood then carries carbon dioxide and other waste products to the lungs for release back into the atmosphere.

If the body does very little work, then it becomes "deconditioned" and cannot perform this cycle well. As Dr. Thomas

Cureton, Ph.D., who trained my early mentor, Al Melleby, says, "The human body is the only machine that breaks down when not used. Moreover, it's also the only mechanism that functions better and more healthfully the more it is put to use." By stressing the body with physical exercise, we improve the efficiency of the oxygen-transport system; the lungs become stronger; the heart beats less and pumps with more strength; the blood carries more oxygen; the blood vessels increase in number; the peripheral circulating system increases its efficiency; the cells "pick up" oxygen more easily.

Dr. Cooper and I agree that aerobic exercises increase our oxygen intake and that we should exercise at least 20 to 45 minutes three times a week. To arrive at aerobic fitness, we should bicycle 30 miles a week, or walk 15 miles, or swim 1½ miles per week, or—and this is really the simplest—run a total of 6 miles a week.

But how fast should we run? Dr. Cooper awards points for increasing speeds over a fixed distance of only a mile or so. This is where we disagree.

In my Run-Easy Method, I believe aerobic exercises should be based on maintaining a "steady state" heart rate for at least 20 minutes. Runners should follow two simple guidelines in governing their pace: First, they should run at a even pace during which their heart rate levels off at a "steady state" well within their training range; second, they should run at a pace that allows them to pass the "talk test." That is, you should be able to carry on a conversation while running; your pace should not leave you breathless. If it does, you are working harder than your muscles can adapt to the new stress of running. Three things may happen, all bad: your muscles may tighten, leaving you open to injury; your running may become an unpleasant struggle; you may become anti-social. After all, if you can't talk, how are you going to visit with all those friends jogging along with you?

**Heart Rate**  As you run, you will have to keep in touch with your heart. Most veteran runners can easily tell what their heart rate is while at rest, during warm-up, and while running. But a beginner will need to learn to check his or her heart rate at rest, during the warm-up, and several times during the run. (After eight weeks or so, this will become second-nature and you may not need to make these frequent checks.) Keeping in touch with your heart, for a beginner means taking your pulse. Pulse-rate is the number of heart beats per minute. There are four pulse-rate checks important to developing a safe training guide for exercise.

1. *Resting Heart Rate*  The average resting heart rate for men is 60 to 80 beats per minute; for women, 70 to 90. A very fit person's heart rate may be at 60 or below; marathon runners "normally" have heart rates in the 40- to 50-beat range. An individual's resting heart rate will drop after a few weeks of consistent aerobic exercise.

Check your rate in the morning. One easy way is to press the index and middle fingers of one hand against the upturned wrist of the other, about in the middle. Or, placing your thumb against your chin, touch the carotid artery on either side of your Adam's apple with the tips of your first two fingers. Don't press too hard! When you feel a pulse beat, count the number for 10 seconds, and multiply by 6. That's your resting heart beat. If, once you have established your normal resting heart rate, you find it is higher than usual one morning, you may be over-training and should cut back in your program. In the event of an emergency, experienced runners should quickly explain their low heart rate to attending physicians. Dogtags worn around the neck with your name, blood type and heart rate may be a good idea.

**2. *Maximum Heart Rate*** This is the point at which the heart "peaks" out. It can't satisfy the body's demand for oxygen and cannot beat any faster. Maximum heart rate is at or near the level of exhaustion. Physiologists have devised a method to estimate your maximum heart rate: Subtract your age from 220. *This is not a goal.* It is merely a figure from which we can obtain your training heart rate.

**3. *Training (Exercise) Heart Rate*** This is the aerobic heart rate, the rate that provides sufficient training effect for your cardiovascular system. This "target zone" of safe, beneficial training falls between two numbers, the target rate of 70 percent of your maximum heart rate and the cut-off figure of 85 percent of maximum heart rate. (The 85 percent figure is the approximate border between aerobic and anaerobic states.) It really isn't as complicated as it may seem.

First, find your heart rate at exhaustion by subtracting your age from 220. Your target, aerobic heart rate is 70 percent of this number, and your cut-off (slow-down) rate is 85 percent. To save you some hard math, we've included a heart rate chart.

The pulse rates are based upon a predicted maximum, and thus some error is possible. One runner may be able to exceed his or her cut-off rate without "breathing hard," or he or she may feel tired at a lower level. The "talk test" is a good monitoring device. If you are running so fast that you cannot converse with someone, slow down! Exercise should be fun and beneficial, not exhausting.

During your run, if you are a beginner, occasionally stop and take your pulse. Take it within 10 seconds after you stop to get

The following chart designates heart rate targets for various age groups:

| Age | Target HR (70%) | Cut-off HR (85%) |
|---|---|---|
| 20–25 | 140 | 167 |
| 26–30 | 134 | 163 |
| 31–35 | 131 | 159 |
| 36–40 | 127 | 155 |
| 41–45 | 124 | 150 |
| 46–50 | 120 | 146 |
| 51–55 | 117 | 142 |
| 56–60 | 113 | 138 |
| 61–65 | 110 | 133 |
| 66–70 | 106 | 129 |

Training Range

an accurate count. Keep moving a little if you can. (If you're running on an indoor track, get off to let others pass.) Then, continue your exercise. If you are over the target zone, walk. If you are under it (the 70-percent figure) increase your pace a little.

**4. Recovery Heart Rate** The cool-down, as I will describe, is essential after all exercise. A leisurely 5-minute walk after your run should bring your pulse down below 120 beats per minute; below 110 for those over fifty. That's a goal; if your pulse doesn't drop that much during the 5-minute walk, keep walking. After an additional 5 minutes of stretching and relaxing exercises (described in a moment) your pulse should be within 20 beats of your pre-exercise resting heart rate.

"Listen to your body" is a key to training for all skill levels. So, check your heart rate periodically as you run, but mainly go by how you feel. If your heart rate is slightly above range, but you feel okay and can talk comfortably, then you are probably one of those few who don't fit the estimated heart-rate chart. But don't look for an excuse to push up your heart rate. I prefer to keep beginners at 70 percent of the predicted maximum heart rate to be extra safe.

My co-author, Jack Shepherd, took almost a year to reach this level. He was so out of shape at first that he could hardly run 2 minutes, walk 2 minutes for the 20-minute period. Worse, when he ran, his exercise heart rate exceeded the cut-off. He should have been between 127 and 155 beats per minute; instead, after running for only 2 minutes, Shepherd found his heart rate often at 165 to 170. He walked until it returned inside his target range, and then ran again. Sure enough, during the first six weeks, his heart rate would frequently exceed the cut-off limit.

When I ran alongside him, I'd ask Shepherd how he felt. "Oh fine," he always replied. And he did. But he never told me his heart rate was exceeding his cut-off level. If he had, I would have made him slow down—and he wanted to run more than anything else.

As it turned out, after running for more than two years, Shepherd really has to work to get his heart rate into his target exercise zone. He has to work harder to get the same benefits, but he is also in much better shape and more able to put out the extra effort. Best of all, his resting heart rate, which was often 90 or more before he began running, is now below 65. His heart is beating less, and pumping more efficiently.

Now you are warmed-up, stretched, and your heart is beating faster. To make the transition to aerobic running, start walking briskly. As you walk fast, stretch your legs and arms ahead of you as far as you can; reach out with them.

Now jog slowly. Be sure that you run lightly on your heels, not your toes. Run heel/toe, much the same as walking. Running on your toes may cause shin splints or calf pain. You will soon learn to "rock" on your heels—hitting the ground heel first, then toes. This may feel strange at first, but it will soon become very comfortable. It will also allow you to run longer distances. Running on your toes is only good for fast sports where pivoting is essential. For more details about proper running style, see chapter 5.

Jogging slowly, if you are not winded, you should find a comfortable pace. You *must* be able to talk to your running partner as you jog along, or hum a tune if you are alone. If you cannot talk, slow down, or walk—but walk briskly enough to keep near your training heart rate range. The basic rule is: Walk until you are ready to run, run until you feel the need to walk.

Beginner runners can break down the 20 minutes of exercise with a variety of tricks; they should also take their pulse rate frequently during this time. Both these things will be discussed in detail in the next chapter. Intermediate runners may be able to run continuously for the 20-minute period. That's fine, as long as you can talk while you run, and as long as your heart rate doesn't exceed your target zone.

After 20 minutes, you have completed the aerobics phase of the program. Keep several things in mind. Your run should begin at a moderate pace and, if you are an intermediate or better, increase until you find a comfortable running pace. You should exercise so that your heart rate remains within your target zone for the 20 minutes. You should be comfortable, but also aerobic. Most important, keep a steady pace throughout—even if you are walking, running, walking. Keep moving. Don't finish with a sprint. Avoid rapid running with high knee lift. Both activities greatly increase your oxygen debt and heart rate, which is dangerous for beginners and intermediates. Finish your run with consistency and ease. You should complete the run exhilarated, not exhausted.

Running backwards and sideways can cause injuries and should be avoided. Also, if you run indoors, no more than two thirds of the running time should be in one direction. Running in a gym places a severe strain on the inside leg. The changing of direction will reduce possible foot and leg injuries, as well as break your routine.

Finally, "train, don't strain." Walk briskly when not running, and don't become fatigued.

### Part Three: The Cool-Down Phase
*Time:* 10 minutes minimum.
*Object:* relaxation and stretching.

This is the last, but equally important, step of the three-phase Run-Easy Method. It is the easiest to omit. But when runners skip the cool-down, they frequently get injured because they haven't stretched and relaxed their muscles after a run. Inexperienced joggers tend to dash out of their homes, run, and dash back, heading straight for the refrigerator and a cold beer. The only thing I approve of is the cold beer.

Generally, the cool-down is the warm-up in reverse. After running, slowly jog and then walk for perhaps 5 minutes. Follow this by slow, rhythmic stretching exercises and relaxation. The purpose of the cool-down is to return the body to its pre-exercise level, insuring the return of the blood flow to the heart from the extremities, and preventing muscle tightness. It is also essential to get your heart rate slowed and returned to normal. All horses are walked after vigorous exercise for these same reasons. It makes horse sense for you to do the same.

Six to ten minutes after you stop running, check your heart rate. The pulse should be within 20 beats of the pre-exercise heart rate—approximately 100 or less. If your pulse is above this, continue a slow cooling off by walking easily and relaxing.

Next, pause. Repeat some of the exercises from the warm-up, in this order:

**1.** *Leg-up Stretch* Relax. Slowly stretch those muscles so that they will be loose tomorrow.

**2.** *Standing Hamstring and Calf Muscle* This is one of the most overlooked exercises after running. The muscles in the backs of your legs are tight from running; stretch them out. Don't forget the Achilles' tendon exercises; you'll feel it tomorrow if you do.

**3.** *Backovers* Stretch the muscles of your back. As you run, muscles along the backs of your legs and your spine are strengthened. They now need to be stretched and loosened.

**4.** *Sitting Stretch* Pull slowly on these tightened muscles, and enjoy the chance to sit down.

**5.** *Leg Limbering.*

**6.** *Shoulder Shrug* This may be done standing or, if you prefer, on your back.

**7.** *Head Roll.*

**8.** *Belly Breathing.*

Every runner—beginner to advanced—should do these exercises while cooling down. The idea is to stretch your hard-working muscles, and to relax you and your body to avoid injury or stiffness.

On your back, flex your knees. Let one leg slide slowly forward, and drop to the floor. Raise the leg 10 inches off the floor and tighten. Hold for 10 seconds. Drop it, relax, return the leg to its flexed position. Repeat with your other leg.

Now, push the small of your back into the floor. Hold for 10 seconds, then let go. Raise one arm high into the air, and tighten the fist. Hold for 10 seconds, then let it relax. Repeat with the other arm and fist.

Tighten the muscles in your face. Really make a contortion. Hold for 10 seconds, then relax.

Repeat the belly breathing exercises. Now, lie with your knees flexed, eyes closed. Allow your body to go limp. Think good, clean thoughts. Tell yourself that you feel very heavy, very loose. (I said *clean* thoughts!) Rest for 30 seconds to one minute.

Slowly, get up, rising to your hands, then knees, then one leg, then both legs but bent over, then slowly erect. Check your pulse. It should be within 20 beats of your pre-run exercise heart rate.

Now go have that beer (or orange juice). You've earned it.

As you begin the Run-Easy Method, here are some ground rules to keep in mind:

- Once you start, keep at it. Take an hour every other day. Start with gentle exercises and move slowly into the full program.
- Make your exercise hour "sacred" and free from interference. Pick the best time of day for you and stick to it. Never stop exercising or not begin because you are feeling too harried or too busy. That's when you need exercise most.
- Exercise one hour at a time. Build slowly and do not rush. Perform all exercises slowly, without jerking. Do not rush

through them, but make the pattern and performance of exercises also relaxing. Vary your exercises. Try new running routes. Join a runner's club.

How long should your workouts be? Here is a helpful chart:

| Workout Phases | Beginner | Intermediate | Advanced |
|---|---|---|---|
| Warm-up | 15 minutes | 20 | 20 |
| Run | 20 minutes (minimum) | 30 | 30–60 |
| Cool-down | 10 minutes | 10 | 10 |
| Totals: | 45 minutes | 60 | 90 |

Right now, you may feel that you cannot ever get into shape, or run five miles, or complete a marathon. You say you don't have the discipline, or the time. Or, if you're running a little already, you may feel you've gone as far (and as fast) as you can go. Maybe you've been piglike. Take heart from the following story:

Dr. Max Sanders, an exercise physiologist at the University of California, San Diego, is studying the value of exercise on the human heart. His laboratory animals are pigs, whose heart structure closely resembles that of humans. At first, Dr. Sanders used dogs. "But you take the average dog on the street," he says, "and put him on a treadmill, and he can run for two straight hours at a reasonable rate. That's far longer than any sedentary human—or pig—could do. When we started working with the pigs, they could run for only a few minutes at a time."

Now, Dr. Sanders has half his pigs jogging, and half "just standing around all day, like most people." The jogging pigs are divided into two groups: those who are healthy and those with heart damage. Already the jogging pigs are running 5 miles a day. And, Dr. Sanders notes, a well-conditioned pig can run a mile in less than eight minutes.

The way I figure it, if a hog can get into shape, anybody can.

# 2 BEGINNER AND INTERMEDIATE RUNNERS

"I don't have time."

"I've never been much of an athlete."

"I don't even know how to run."

"Running is so boring. I feel like a gerbil on a treadmill."

I've heard them all. In fact, at one time or other, Shepherd made all of those excuses. But let's start. Remember the Chinese proverb: "A journey of a thousand miles begins with one step." That first step is to agree that you are a beginner runner, ready, and somewhat willing, to get into shape. As I mentioned in the previous chapter, a beginner runner is someone who cannot run for 20 consecutive minutes at a steady comfortable pace. If you are running at least 30 minutes non-stop at a comfortable pace at least three—preferably five or more—times a week, you have reached that gray stage between beginner and advanced runner that I call intermediate. Most likely you fall in the middle somewhere—you can run, but not too far or too long.

Once you admit that you are beginning, or almost beginning, to run, that simple confession will probably make you feel better already. Next, remember to have a physical. Any strenuous exercise program should be approved by a physician, and you should start on a small scale and work up gradually. You are not going to overcome years of sloth in a few sweaty weeks, but you can make slow and steady progress toward your goals.

You should have a yearly medical check-up anyway, and can combine it with the start of this program. Health agencies have a variety of requirements for entering beginner fitness programs. The following points are emphasized by Dr. David Thomashaw and Dr. Norb Sander, who screen beginner runners at the City Island Fitness and Medical Center in New York City.

- Any healthy person under thirty-five who does not have high coronary risk factors should still get a physical examination before starting any exercise program.
- If you are over thirty-five, or under thirty-five with at least one major risk factor (smoking more than one pack of cigarettes a day, hypertension, hyperlipidemia, obesity, diabetes), your physical exam should include blood tests and a stress electrocardiogram.
- If you have a history of heart disease, a medically-supervised cardiac exercise program would be best for you.

Beware: Some doctors don't understand the benefits of regular exercise. They may not allow you to run. If they don't give you a good reason, or—worse—won't explain their judgment to you, find another doctor. I only go to doctors who are also runners.

After you've seen your doctor, read this chapter carefully (and chapter 1). Also, try to find someone who can give you a thorough fitness test. Many corporate fitness programs are excellent; they check out their executives and give them individual fitness programs to be performed during the first eight to ten weeks. Before starting my fitness programs, I screen each participant. I also hear objections all the time: "I don't need these tests. My doctor says I'm in excellent shape." That means your heart's pumping and you're breathing. But how fit are you? Do you know how to exercise properly? Are you flexible?

I also counsel beginner and advanced runners by individual appointment about shoes and comfortable, not necessarily fashionable, running clothes, and I make an analysis of their running form.

Obviously, not everyone has these services nearby. What should you do? First, follow the guidelines about the medical check-up. Then, read and follow the program for the Run-Easy Method. Also, check the chapters on shoes, clothes, stress, running style or anything else that pertains to your questions or condition. Next, find an experienced runner—a good bet would be someone in your local Road Runner's Club (see Appendix) or jogging association—who will watch you run to correct obvious faults. I also encourage beginners to take advantage of supervised classes offered at their local YMCAs or fitness centers. A good instructor will hold you back when your enthusiasm pushes you faster than your physical limits, or encourage you when you become discouraged during the first few weeks. The group support of a class full of similarly fit runners is also buoying.

The next step is to make a personal commitment. Tell yourself that you are going to prepare your body to run, and run at a slow pace for the next eight weeks or more. Too many people begin jogging on their own. They don't warm-up or cool-down, and their running is based on bad ideas and worse practice. The weekend jogger, as I've said, is a danger to himself.

Commit yourself to getting into good shape. I am only asking you to set aside three hours a week at the start. But you may complain, "I don't have the time." You do. In fact, you can easily find 3 hours out of the 168 hours every week. Here's how:

1. Make a firm commitment that you will set aside one hour every other day for exercise.

That's roughly 1 hour from every 48. You're sleeping 16 hours out of those 48, and working 16 hours. That still leaves 16 hours for other things, and one of those hours could be set aside for exercise. Looked at on a weekly basis, 3 hours out of 168 hours in every week takes only 1/56th of your time for exercise. Best of all, what you do with the remaining 55/56ths will be enhanced and invigorated by what you do with that other 1/56th.

2. Make a schedule. Even though I hate them, in the beginning they can be a help. Block in your work hours and sleep hours. Allow time for eating and commuting to work. Now stop. Your next priority is to find those 3 hours of exercise. Block out 3 hours—one every other day, or every 48 hours—for your exercise program. Find the time that's best for you. Some runners prefer the early morning, when the day is fresh. It's great —they tell us—to wake up and start running. Joe Henderson, a morning runner, reports that he can actually cover several miles before he knows what he's done. Sudden houseguests or business meetings won't interrupt you, and watching the sunrise can be lovely.

Others prefer midday. Noontime runs are favorites of business men and women, especially in cities with organized group workouts (see chapter 17). I frequently hold noontime meetings on the run. Why not burn calories and ideas at the same time instead of stuffing booze and food into yourself? Many runners are substituting a run for those large and unnecessary lunches that make you sleepy all afternoon. You'll find that a run will invigorate you, and low-calorie foods like yogurt, fruit salads and juices taste terrific after a workout. You're beating caloric counts at both ends.

Shepherd claims that his joints won't turn until mid-afternoon. He runs in the cool of the evening. Most runners prefer this time, when they can release the tensions of the day, and separate the work world from the leisure or home world. It is cooler in the early evening, and in winter a run started at sunset sometimes ends up in moonlight.

Your schedule should be flexible. Yet you will also have to find a time that fits your life-style, and *stick to it!* Be firm; I find more and more nonrunners accept the fact that a run is valuable time well spent, and will rearrange meetings to fit a jogger's schedule. An increasing number of companies also consider exercise time valuable to them, and to you.

Set a priority. I usually run at noon, four times a week, and then in the evening with our group. I also run every Saturday and Sunday morning. All of my business meetings and social outings are scheduled around these times. Sometimes it's difficult for people to understand why I can't meet them for lunch simply because I'm scheduled to run. But they are changing, and you must learn to please yourself before you are going to please others.

Make a schedule: Monday, Wednesday, Friday; sunrise, noon or evening. Put it in your appointment book. Make a date with yourself. Bill Horowitz, my teammate and dentist who took up running at age forty, says, "I schedule an appointment for myself each day just as my patients schedule themselves to see me. I run when scheduled, come 'Hell or high water.'" Dr. Norb Sander used to run home from the hospital—about 15 miles. He saved time and gas, and got home earlier to play with the kids. Even the beginner runner can jog to and from work if it's only a few miles. You can alternate running and walking, and it's a great way to guarantee that you'll finish! If you're fastidious about sweat, bring a washcloth and towel and wipe off in the restroom. If your company provides showers, you've no excuse not to run!

## THE BEGINNER'S PROGRAM

Basically, the program for beginner runners is identical to that for all runners. Only the approach, level of intensity, and the method of beginning to run differ sharply. It is important that the beginner runner, or the intermediate training at a slightly more strenuous pace, be introduced to the exercises and to running at a graduated pace.

First, you should try to begin your workout at the same time every day. Habit is the best reinforcer. You should take your resting heart rate several times during the days before you begin training so that you can check your workout against it. You should know what your maximum heart rate is (220 minus your age); never exceed 85 percent of that number. Finally, you should also know your training heart rate; this is actually two numbers, a lower and upper range, that you can obtain from the chart on page 43.

Now, with all those numbers in your head, and your heart pounding, let's start. It's very simple. Put on your running shorts and shirt, a good pair of white socks and excellent running shoes (see chapter 10). Don't you look grand! I'm sorry, but now you must lie down on the dirty floor of a gym, on the grass, in a park, or perhaps on your living room or bedroom floor. If you're home, check for things under the furniture as you warm up; this program will do wonders for the house cleaning.

### Part One: Warm-up

Lie on the floor, knees flexed. Close your eyes. Relax with some deep breaths, slide your arms along the floor to a point above your head, and slide them back. Open your eyes. Do the following exercises in order at every workout. Each exercise has been described fully in chapter 1 (pages 29–37).

1. Belly Breathing
2. Head Roll
3. Shoulder Shrug
4. Leg Limbering
5. Double Knee Flex
6. Double Knee Roll
7. Cat Back
8. Pectoral Stretch
9. Push-ups
10. Hamstring and Calf Muscle Stretch
11. Sitting Stretch
12. Sit-ups
13. Standing Hamstring and Calf Muscle Stretch
14. Front and Back Stretch
15. Backovers
16. Leg-up Stretch

Don't forget to also stretch your quadriceps by pulling your toes and foot up and behind you. (See chapter 1.)

### Part Two: The Run

Begin walking slowly along your jogging route. As you walk, stretch your legs and arms ahead of you as far as you can. At first, this will be a walk-run workout. If you are further along, run until you feel winded (*not breathless*), then walk, and then run again.

Now, jog slowly. Be sure you run on your heels, not your toes. "Rock" on your heels much the same as when you walk. Hold your hands about waist high, elbows out, forearms parallel to the ground. (See chapter 5.) Do not clench your fists. Try making a circle with your thumb and forefinger, or try running with your hands slightly open; feel the wind.

Find a comfortable pace. Jog slowly and settle into it, but remember that you *must* be able to talk to your running partner, or hum, as you jog along. If you cannot talk, slow down or walk. Remember, also, that you can probably walk a mile or two already. When you begin, go for a walk with a little running thrown in. Gradually, replace that walking with running. Do this by walking until you want to run, running until you want to walk.

Most beginners will not be able to run more than part of the 20-minute run phase. There are ways of breaking down the 20-minute walk-run workout to create little goals for yourself. At first, try running 2 minutes and then walking 2 minutes for the 20-minute period. Then stretch yourself, when you feel ready, to running 4 minutes or 5, walking 2. Next, try 8/2, 8/2 for the 20 minutes. Then run with only a 2-minute walk in the middle. Finally, eliminate the 2-minute walk.

But at first, run 2 minutes. Then, while walking, take your pulse to be sure that it is within the target exercise zone. If it is too high, walk until it gets well within your range. If it is too low, keep running. Some runners find that their pulse takes a long time to decrease; they may have to keep walking longer than the 2 minutes to get it back into their safe exercise range. If you have this experience, walk more than you run. In fact, some beginners must start this program walking the entire 20 minutes before they can run. If this is the case, try a little running for 2 minutes at the beginning, 2 again in the middle and 2 at the end. But keep in touch with your heart.

During the first few weeks, take your pulse regularly as you run-walk. You'll probably notice that as you need to walk less, your pulse will also stay within your target range more. You'll be getting in shape.

Intermediate runners should also take their pulse during their runs. Most intermediate runners can run 20 consecutive minutes —my definition of such a runner—and may find it a bother to walk and find their pulse. Do it as you begin this program so that you'll be sure you are exercising safely and within your heart's exercise range. Also, remember to run at a pace that enables you to talk.

**Part Three: Cool-down**

After your run (and walk), be sure to cool down. Walk after running for 5 minutes. This may mean walking along your running path, or walking slowly back to your house or apartment. *Slowly*, that's the key word. Now is the time to take it easy. Next, pause. Repeat some of the exercises from the warm-up, in this order:

Leg-Stretch

Standing Hamstring and Calf Muscle

Backovers

Sitting Stretch

Leg Limbering

Shoulder Shrug

Head Roll

Belly Breathing

All are valuable to relax you after running. If you are working out on a hard surface, the shrugs and rolls will ease tension you may feel from having pounded the gym floor or pavement.

Every runner, beginner to advanced, must do these exercises during cool-down. Hard-working muscles should be stretched, blood returned from extremities, your body relaxed to avoid injury or stiffness.

Lie on your back for a while. Stare at the ceiling or sky. Repeat the relaxing procedures in chapter 1:

Pull your knees up. Then, let one leg slide slowly forward and lie flat. Raise the leg 10 inches off the ground, tighten, hold for 10 seconds. Drop it, relax, return the leg to its flexed position. Repeat with your other leg.

Push the small of your back into the floor. Hold. Let go. Repeat several times. Raise one arm high into the air and tighten the fist. Hold for 10 seconds, then relax. Repeat with your other arm and fist.

Tighten the muscles in your face. Hold for 10 seconds, if you can, and relax.

Lie with your knees flexed, eyes closed. Allow your body to completely relax. (There are some good meditation ideas in chapters 6 and 16 for this.) Rest for 30 seconds to a minute.

The purpose of this brief relaxation period is to make your body loose and stretched. You may find, both for variety and fun, that some yoga exercises can be inserted here (see p. 341).

Slowly get up, rising to your hands, knees, one leg, then the other, and then erect. Check your pulse for the last time during the workout. It should be within 20 beats of your pre-run exercise rate or below 100.

After eight weeks, you will find it easier to run. If you follow the Run-Easy Method, you should also discover that you are able to stretch and relax better, that your lungs and heart are already beginning to work without agony during your runs, and that you want to run more. You've survived the start-up program.

Now the struggle becomes one of continuing. As your body gets into shape, the challenge of running may start to fade. You may have progressed to the point of being a confirmed, non-competitive fun runner, or you may be on the edge of becoming a beginner competitor. You have reached that area between beginner and advanced runner that I call intermediate.

An intermediate runner fights growing boredom, and overconfidence. He or she is hard to teach, stubborn, sometimes frozen into a set of exercises and a pattern of running that cannot be changed. Too often, this is the time when runners get hurt. It can happen to you. You are getting into condition, you know the warm-up and cool-down exercises, the distances are coming easier. You may start skipping the full range of warm-up and cool-down exercises to save time; who needs something so elementary, you might say. The intermediate sometimes forgets the lessons of the beginner. He or she may not remember how good the relaxation exercises felt, or how important stretching is. An intermediate runner needs to reread these two chapters, and relearn the fundamentals. After you progress to the intermediate stage, you might want to pretend that you are a beginner, and go back over the exercises you learned during your first week. You'll relearn some vital steps, and surprise yourself about how far you've progressed.

You may become an intermediate runner, and then stop running. You may have a long illness, or an extended period of pressing work when your schedule—created with such conviction—is lost. These pauses can be valuable because they will force you to return to a beginner level for a few weeks. Jack Shepherd, after moving to Vermont, stopped running for almost three full weeks. He got back to his 5 miles a day in gradual steps. First, he reviewed all of his beginner exercises. Then he ran a mile, and was shocked by the long-forgotten stiffness in his legs and back. Every other day he added a little distance—but not too much too soon. By the end of a week, he was easily running 3 miles, and within ten days he was back to 5 miles. In the interim, he had rediscovered his basic exercises and relearned the fun of adding mileage.

There is another kind of intermediate runner who worries me a great deal. He (sometimes she) is the athlete who has let five years or more of inactivity slide by and decides to "get back into shape." This vow usually implies getting into shape in a short time. The husband of an editor in a New York City publishing house was once a college soccer star. At thirty-two, he thought he'd try again. He wasn't fat, didn't smoke, and played tennis occasionally, when he had the time. He was offered the chance to play soccer with a pick-up group in Central Park, and grabbed it. The first Sunday was marvelous: He zoomed all over the field thumping the ball and reliving his adolescence. Monday, however, was hell. So were Tuesday through Thursday. Within a month, he played again. He pulled a hamstring. Two months later, he ventured out upon the field, lasted less than half an hour, and became a permanent fixture at goalie.

Would this man be a beginner jogger? No, you might say. But I argue that he is—although he'd never admit it. He may have a tremendous reservoir of strength and stamina at thirty-two, but his muscles and feet, his knees, heart and lungs, will ache as much as anyone's. He's been too inactive too long. He should start all over. He should start with a common-sense progressive "reshaping" along the same pattern as the beginner, but perhaps moving ahead at a faster pace. Instead of eight weeks, perhaps he will reach the 20-minute run goal within six or five weeks, or less.

The intermediate level is where most runners arrive—filled with gratitude—and where they stay. They run forever at this level of fitness. That's fine. Remember, the purpose of this sport isn't merely to increase health, but mostly to have *fun*.

At this new level, you will notice that changes have occurred. If you run about 3 miles every other day, you may find your weight, muscle tone and breathing much improved. You may want to run more, perhaps every day. You may begin exploring new parts of town during your runs. On business trips, you may look up other runners or running clubs, and run fresh paths with new vistas.

Jack Shepherd is an intermediate runner now. When he was running 5 miles every other day, he noticed that some days were far better than others. His rule was that one run out of three was awful; one out of three good, and one out of three terrific. Then, during one of his terrific runs, he discovered that he had covered the 5 miles without once thinking about his running, the pain, or the distance. He had been "running inside his head"—and decided to write that chapter of this book. He found that running new routes let him forget about time and distance, and concentrate upon discovery and beauty.

Here are some tips for the beginner and intermediate runner:

- Persist. It may not be fun at all, it may hurt. Your body will scream, "Why me?" But most runners will tell you that the first mile or two are the worst, even if it's a marathon distance you plan to cover.
- Set that schedule. Three times a week. Put it on your calendar.
- Keep a diary. Record your mileage daily, weekly, monthly and yearly. This record will motivate you and make you consistent. You may also want to record the time of day, weather, friends who ran with you and the stories they told, and how you felt.
- Go to a race. Run with others. Hang around runners. Join a running club that does not stress competition, but enjoyment.
- Be patient. You won't notice results right away. But you will notice them. Give yourself a chance.
- Reinforce your commitment. Buy a new pair of good running shoes. (See chapter 10.) Join a fitness class.
- Prepare your body for every workout by properly warming up, and cooling down.

Once you're underway, get a friend to start. The two of you will support each other when the weather turns bad, or when excuses blow in the wind. Beware of the "quitter's disease" which discourages many men and women. You may find yourself obsessed with forcing out that extra mile "at all costs." Avoid that, or running will become just another duty, like mowing the lawn. Soon you'll hate it and find any excuse to give it up.

Beginners, after the first four week, should set two goals— finishing four more weeks and searching for that feeling of "I want to run." Slow down. Allow yourself, after eight weeks, to go for a 30-minute run at a leisurely pace. Take it easy. You may be surprised. By spending an hour, running longer, you will overcome any dislike you may have of running itself. It may sound strange, but try it.

As an intermediate, seek variety. Try new running paths, yoga exercises, running clubs. If you're running 30 minutes more than three times a week, you're close to being an "addicted" runner. Here are some tips to help you stick with it:

- Join the "100 Mile Club' at your Y, and post your mileage faithfully. Or, form your own club.
- Subscribe to one of the runner's magazines, such as *Runner's World* or *Running Times*. Read books about running. They get me all jazzed up, and when they come into my office I push my work aside and read them cover to cover.
- Splurge a bit. Buy yourself a new shirt or warm-up suit.
- Take a day off. Just say "To hell with it." You'll return raring to go.
- When you're running 30 minutes or more during a single workout, enter some races, just for the fun of it. They will show you how fit you've become.
- Look for variety. Run a different route. Run your old course in the opposite direction. Explore a trail through the woods. Run with new people. Have someone ride along on a bike and chat with you.
- Join a running club, or start one of your own. Many runners have regular companions for their daily rounds. The

pressure of having to make the appointment and not let your partner down keeps you going.

- Run with people who talk a lot, tell good jokes and are jovial. My Wednesday night runs to the George Washington bridge are crowded, and you can hear the yakkety-yakking several blocks off.
- Show off! Run through your home town, past your friend's house, your old high school. Fantasize about how good you look, how proud you are of your running accomplishments. My pace always quickens and my form improves when I run down Main Street back home, or past a group of friends in Central Park. Shepherd, when he gets bored, pretends that he's in Madison Square Garden, racing against the Russian Master's champion. He swears that on good runs near his home in Vermont, he can hear the crowds chanting his name and the roar as he overtakes the red-shirted but fading leader just before the old farmhouse that marks the end of his 5-mile run. (He didn't look crazy when we started this book.)
- Convert others. Nothing compares with spreading the revolution. The enthusiasm of a new runner really catches people. You'll find you'll want to get others started.
- Party! More runners keep going so they can be invited to the great running parties. These parties are full of healthy, lively people, who claim that they keep in condition just so they can carry the beer safely back to the table. In fact, there's this race in Boston (not the marathon) . . . but that's in chapter 17. Anyway, it's great to go to parties where no one smokes.

The chart on page 49 setting up times for each of the three phases of the Run-Easy Method is a guideline. Now is a good time to start experimenting: Try new exercises from chapter 6, increase your sit-ups and push-ups, or add some yoga stretching from chapter 15. As you advance, you should add exercises to insure increased flexibility and strength. But most important, you should now begin to set running goals, and to look at yourself not as just another work-a-day person, but as a running person. You've added a whole new dimension to your life!

# 3 THE BEGINNER COMPETITOR AND BEYOND

Racing isn't for everyone. But I think every runner should try competition of one sort or another. For one thing, the era of the "fun racer"—the average runner—has emerged. The competition is not to win, but to better personal goals. After all, in most races today there are hundreds, perhaps thousands of entrants, but only a few top athletes.

The rest of us battle not against them, but against ourselves. And we win by meeting realistic goals, such as simply finishing the race. Leslie Buckland, a New York road runner, was so moved by "winning" the 1976 New York City Marathon that he produced a motivational film about it for salesmen, titled "Any Number Can Win." In it a competitive salesman-runner notes elatedly, "I won! Some other guy named Rodgers thinks he won. But I did. He was in a different race."

Nina Kuscsik doesn't think of racing as competition but as running together with other people "to show off what you can do." For the beginner competitor, the main thing is to get out there, pin your number on correctly, start slow and finish. Many more runners are entering races every year. They see their best times improve, they feel better physically, they stay in competitive form, then enjoy the special camaraderie that goes on before, after, and sometimes during a race.

I love converting good runners to good racers. Why? It can be the best test of your fitness and discipline, even though it also contradicts much of the advice given earlier to the beginner runner. It can cause both physical and mental breakdowns in fitness. It can lead to frustration. It works against the theories of "talk test" and "be sociable." Only a fool wants to destroy himself during a race. But we are all fools to varying degrees. The race excites because it makes us play the edges, realize boundaries, follow common sense. We overcome pain, and that's exhilarating. And we discover an honest flirtation with danger that must be respected.

We suffer individual hardships together in races. We respect a whole range of competitors. We test ourselves against ourselves and against the elements and, if we wish, against each other. In return, we understand ourselves and respect each other. The competitive runner wins by sharing his or her unique personal experience.

In a 5-mile cross-country race in May 1977, Tom Childers, a national class runner with the Atlanta Track Club, took a wrong turn late in the race on the tough Van Cortlandt Park course in New York City. Tony Colon, the Puerto Rican Olympian, who was in second place, yelled at Tom and corrected him. Childers beat Colon, who suffered his first defeat on this course, which is virtually in his backyard. In the 1977 Boston Marathon, the favored Bill Rodgers of Boston and fellow Olympian Jerome Drayton of Canada were battling neck and neck at 10 miles on a hot day. Bill's wife Ellen handed him water; he drank half and then handed it to Drayton. Shortly after that point Drayton made his move to clinch his victory. Nationally known runner-writer-doctor Joan Ullyot was being shadowed in the same race by the Greater New York AA's new national class marathoner, Lauri Pedrinan. At one point, Joan grabbed a handful of ice, cooled herself, and turned and offered some to Lauri.

Once, while I was lecturing, someone asked me if I really enjoyed the actual race itself. For the first time I realized how much I *hate* the race. This unique love-hate relationship with running begins weeks, even months before a big race, when my optimism is high. As race day approaches I get pessimistic and invariably develop all sorts of aches, pains and other excuses. The last few hours before the race are very bad ones for me. My confidence fades. But during the race, almost at the starter's gun, a new surge of confidence pumps my blood and drives me onward! How do I feel during the race? I hate it. I want to quit over and over. But I love it, too. The challenge of defeating fatigue, of reaching beyond my potential keeps me going forward. When I finish, I hate it. I invariably throw up. I often rival Doc Sheehan for moaning and groaning and praying to be saved from the grasp of the Demon Pain. Fortunately, all this fades with my first postrace beer. After the second, I'm ready to say I loved the race. Then analyzing it, I know I could have run faster "if I had made my move sooner." Or, another favorite line told to the person you beat in a stretch run, "I was only using the race as a workout." The sense of accomplishment, the telling of stories—"Wow, what did you think of that bleep-bleeping hill?"—binds the young and old, fast and slow. I hate races. I love races.

Despite this, competitive running is fun. I tell myself that a lot. And converting new runners to competitive running is even more fun—who else can I beat as I grow old? It's a chance to run with dozens or maybe thousands of other runners over the same course. If you finish well—in some races if you finish at all—you will be awarded a medal or certificate, and that will give your self-confidence a real boost.

If you are running at the intermediate level or better, you're ready. Surprisingly, many beginner runners are also ready to run in short (5-mile) races. In fact, almost anyone who has been running for eight weeks is good enough to race. Today, the "fun racers" in the back of the pack far outnumber the highly competitive front runners. Let them blow out the course while you concentrate on finishing. In New York's Road Runner's Club races, Marion Epstein, perpetually fifty-nine years old, often finishes miles behind the other runners. But the officials wait patiently for her to finish in her typical manner: smiling and blowing kisses.

## TRAINING FOR YOUR FIRST RACE

The first step is to train your mind. Convince yourself to train regularly, and to follow the fundamental guidelines of the Run-Easy Method.

Next, develop a base of endurance for racing. Pace yourself during your workouts to get a feeling of running at a steady clip. Most people pick a race of 3 to 6 miles for their first run. Let's use a 6-mile race as an example of how to train for your first race.

The general rule of thumb is that you should run at least twice the distance of the race itself *weekly* for several weeks before the race. For a 6-mile race you should build up to 12 miles a week; never increase the mileage by more than 10 percent per week. For best results break down the mileage into long and average runs, all at a conversational pace.

Look what Mary Rodriguez, a fifty-five-year-old secretary, was able to do. She started running for her health, after attending Road Runner's Club of New York beginner's running clinic in March 1977. Inspired, she ran for the first time and couldn't make it around a quarter-mile track. She showed up at a

Saturday morning workout in Central Park, and walked-jogged-walked with me for an entire one-and-two-thirds loop of the reservoir. Three weeks later she completed an entire loop, and her husband greeted her with a smile and kiss at the finish.

Mary then decided to aim for the women's Mini-Marathon in June, in New York. She worked out three times a week running 2 miles on a track, and on Sundays, she jogged 2 miles in a local park. On Saturdays she was all mine! She and I jogged and bantered, and she completed two loops of the reservoir (about 3.5 miles). After this test, she was ready for the hilly roads of Central Park. We ran with a group of twenty men and women who had followed a similar program for their first 4-mile run. Chatting all the way, they hardly noticed the hills, and all finished enthusiastically. The next Saturday, Mary Rodriguez ran 5 miles. The week before the Mini, she and several others like her ran the entire 6-mile course comfortably. On June 4, just seventy days after her first run, Mary started the 6.2 mile race, and finished in 1 hour, 13 minutes. She had progressed from a fifty-five-year-old woman who hadn't exercised in thirty-five years to a smiling, energetic "fun racer" in ten weeks! As she says, "Stick with it. It's worth it."

## THE FIRST RACE

Your best bet for a first race is a local "fun run." These are usually runs of 2 to 6 miles for which no awards are given or places recorded. Competition is minimized. Your next best bet for a first race is to run it with a friend who is willing to chat with you all the way, holding you back at the start when you're tempted to pass people, and supporting you at the end when you feel like quitting. Whatever you do, the key word is *finish*. Set a modest goal—preferably when you start your training for the race—and run well within your limits.

It is also important to realize that you can walk during a race if you have to. You may need a slight breather or perhaps the hills may be too much for you. Your goal, of course, is to run and finish the race nonstop with comfort.

### Food and Drink
Beginners should not worry about pre-race diets. On race day, don't eat anything unusual, and nothing at all within a few hours of the race. Do drink liquids, and drink them while you are running. (See chapter 14.)

### Equipment
Beginner competitors tend to wear too much clothing, or race in new shoes. Your body will heat up during a race, and even clothing that is comfortable for a training run may become uncomfortable in the heat of competition. (See chapter 9.)

Tennis shoes are out for training and racing. New shoes should be broken in gradually or they'll cause blisters. Just before the 1977 Mini-Marathon, a young girl came to me almost in tears. She had saved her money to buy a new pair of running shoes for her first big race, but couldn't find any in her size. Since the race was only a week away, I told her to wear her old running shoes. They were in good repair, just a little dirty. She did, and ran the race in comfort; nobody noticed in a crowd of 4000 feet that she wasn't wearing brand new shoes.

### Race Day
Here you are. The morning of your first race may find your heart pounding. Pre-race nerves strike the fast and the slow. You may take your leisure in the bathroom, eat toast, and drink orange juice (if that's your style) and read the paper. Carefully

pack your bag: Vaseline, an extra pair of shoelaces, shoes, shorts, shirt, jock or bra, an extra shirt to wear after the race, tape, liniment, warm-ups, postrace first-aid equipment, toilet paper, a hat in case its cold, a hat in case it's sunny, gloves in case it's cold, lock and towel.

Arrive at least an hour before race time so you can check in, warm up, and of course chat with other runners. You should always pre-register by mail so you can get right into line and pick up your number and perhaps a free T-shirt. If you don't pre-register, you often must stand in line longer, fill out forms at the last minute, pay a higher entry fee and get yelled at by tired officials. Warning: Not all races accept entries on race day. Better check in advance.

Proceed to the dressing area. Since you arrived early, you get a locker and have ample time to dress and apply your Vaseline, liniment, etc. Pin your number to the lower third of the *front* of your shirt, so the officials can see it as you finish. Fold or cut it so that the extra space at the edges is not in your way. Pin the number on each edge to make sure it is secure. I always bring extra pins in case they don't have enough. Also, memorize your number in case it gets destroyed by rain or splashing water.

Spend the next half-hour or more stretching, walking, and talking, and preparing your mind and body for the race. Tense runners arrive at the last minute to find you stretched and relaxed. Periodically jog for a few yards, and then stretch and relax. Half an hour before race time, take one last trip to the john, and be thankful you brought toilet paper. They've probably already run out. Proceed to the drinking fountain, and jog to the starting line.

Ten minutes before the start, peel off your sweats and place them in your easily recognized tagged bag. Carefully place the bag with the others. Very subtly jog behind the bushes for one last visit. Tie your shoes in a double knot. Line up toward the back of the pack to insure against getting trampled by the speedsters, or getting "pushed" into a fast early pace. Standing there among the crowd of runners, you may suddenly feel all alone, insecure, intimidated.

### You're Off

The crack of the gun propels you along with the flowing mass of runners down the road. "Why did I let Bob Glover start me on this madness?" you scream. But you're off. You fight adrenalin and hold back. Maintain a comfortable, slightly slow pace. Find a group of runners going at your pace, and join them. All will pull each other very easily for the first 3 miles. Then you hit a tough hill, or just run out of gas and feel the urge to quit. If you're running with a friend, encourage each other. Nina Kuscsik says, "You have a choice. You can quit or keep going. Just the knowledge that you can always quit sometime, is often enough to keep you going to the finish line."

Keep plugging away. If you feel very tired, slow down or walk a while, but keep moving. Mental fatigue is tougher, but you can overcome that, too, with conditioning during your workouts. You've worked too hard to quit so easily. I'm a veteran racer who is on the edge of quitting dozens of times in every one of my races. But in fifteen years I've run in more than three hundred races, and dropped out of only two of them. Once I had the flu, and another time a foot injury. If you become physically tired, slow your pace, walk, even walk slowly.

Nearing the finish line brings a new life, new confidence. The taste of personal victory overwhelms you; you drive toward the finish with a controlled spirit and uncontrolled smile. You finish out of breath and momentarily bend forward, hands resting on your knees as you catch your breath. Then you walk for a few minutes, stretch and relax. Now comes the fun: You brag to everyone in sight about how great you felt in your first race. Secretly, you'll begin plotting strategy for improving your time in the next race. After you stretch and shower, you can cheer the top runners as they receive their trophies, and know that you, too, are a winner.

Most competitors remember that first race vividly, and each of their tales is instructive and often inspiring. Ellie McGrath is a New York writer and runner; her story sounds best in her own words:

I had started jogging in October 1975, to lose a little flab. Gradually I worked up to a 6-mile loop around Central Park, and was relieved just to finish. Then I joined a YMCA where I saw flyers for a 4-mile race for women only. I thought it would be fun to see how fast I could run.

So, two weeks before the race I traded in my white canvas sneakers for a pair of Onitsuka Tigers. I'll never forget how good it felt the first time I ran in them. After canvas sneakers, it was like running on air. Relaxed by this newfound comfort and egged on by the idea that I had "tigers" on my feet, I started getting psyched about running in a race. I had never engaged in any kind of physical contest; my closest experience to competition had been trying to ride a bicycle faster than my best friend.

The morning of the race was sunny, but cold. Should I wear warm-ups? A sweatshirt? I took a chance and wore just shorts and a jersey. My intuition was good because most of the other women were running in lightweight clothes. I was intimidated by the other starters, some wearing team colors and T-shirts, their jackets emblazoned with team names such as Golden Spikes.

But with the eagerness of a rank amateur, I elbowed my way to the front of the crowd. When the starting gun went off right over my head, I froze. The bang frightened me almost as much as the thundering hoofs around me. Then I bolted.

During the 28 minutes and 45 seconds it took me to finish the course, I learned several things. If you start too fast, you get really tired. If you underestimate the hills on the west side of the park, you'll be sorry. If you stop worrying about all the runners in front of you and think instead of all of them behind you, you'll enjoy the race a lot more. Having committed the first two mistakes, the last tactic was the one that got me around the course.

Crossing the finish line was a tremendous thrill. There was my boss, really amused by the whole thing, holding a congratulatory can of Diet Pepsi for me. Beside her was my boyfriend, bewildered, holding my parka. I picked up my medal for finishing, and went home to indulge myself with a hot bath, a chicken salad sandwich, and a magnum of champagne.

After her first year of running competitively, Ellie McGrath had finished three 12-mile races, one 10-mile race, two 6-mile races, one 15.6-mile race, the Yonkers (N.Y.) Marathon and in the New York City Marathon scored points for our team's first place performance.

## GOALS: BEYOND THE BEGINNER

After a few races, you may want to increase your goals. Gradually add to your training mileage and the intensity of your workouts. Set reasonable but challenging objectives. Don't neglect the fundamentals discussed in earlier chapters.

Try for three goals:

1. The safest, least competitive goal is to extend the distance of your longest race. If you have run 6 miles, enter a race for 10, then 15 then perhaps a marathon. Finishing will continue to be a reward; only now the distance will be tougher.

2. Another goal is to improve your time over the same distance, then improve your time over a variety of distances. You'll soon hear other runners talk about setting "PRs" (per-

sonal records). Keep a diary; record your time and place for all races, and keep a record of your best time for each distance.

3. Aim for a certain place in the race, like the top 10 or even the top 1000. Or, aim for finishing within a certain percentage of the field. Percentages sometimes sound better to you and your friends. I remember being thrilled by placing in the top half of the field in my first Boston Marathon. When people asked me how I had done at Boston, and I said, "I finished 1012," they'd reply, "Oh, what happened to you?" Instead, by telling them I finished in the top half of a quality field they gave me the reply I sought: "Fantastic!"

Your individual goals should meet your individual needs at the time. For most of us, that means goals based on individual improvement. Let the elite run against each other.

## THE RACER'S EDGE: BE PREPARED

To meet goals, be prepared for your race. Physical preparation comes first. You must have a base of endurance. Build up for the race, but also keep fit year round by properly spacing less important races. Enter race day with a well-conditioned and well-rested body. "Heat train" before summer races, "hill train" before attacking uphill struggles. Run cross-country workouts before attacking a rugged and hilly course through the woods. Before a marathon, run long distances to condition you physically and mentally for those last long miles. (See chapter 4.)

Prior to a run, you may want to do some fast intervals of 220–440 yards to condition yourself to running in oxygen debt, and to practice the mechanics of sprinting. Your weight should be down when coming into a race. Proper diet and exercise will gradually get you into "fighting weight" in time for the big effort. An extra five to ten pounds is a lot of extra weight, and will make a major difference in your time.

## TRAINING: BEYOND THE BEGINNER COMPETITOR

How often should you train? How hard? What methods should you use?

Dr. George Sheehan finds that his aging body performs better on race day if he trains every other day. Most world class runners work out twice a day, and take a long run one day a week. I know runners who haven't missed a day in ten years, and others who take off a full two weeks twice a year. I've been beaten by both. Generally, I run six days a week, and rest a day.

Kenny Moore, fourth place finisher in the 1972 Olympic Marathon, wrote in *Road Racers and Their Training:*

"The basis for all training is that an organism exposed to stress will adjust if allowed to recover. But if it never rests, it just stays tired. I'm not in this to do work. I'm trying to improve. So I'm after the optimum formula of work, rest and racing, not the most difficult I can stand. I've found a dosage of one hard day and two easy brings improvement as quickly as any. It's something every runner must work out for himself."

The idea is to place enough stress on your body for training, but not enough to risk injury. Hans Hartmann has been running only two years. He rarely runs more than 40 miles a week. If he does, he gets tired and his legs rebel. Yet he won the master's division in the 1976 Baltimore Marathon and the 1977 Earth Day Marathon. On the other hand, I run 100 miles a week when I'm serious, and 70 miles when I'm merely maintaining a fitness level.

Ken Young has developed a "collapse point" theory. According to this, the point at which you break down in a race will be about one-twentieth of your total mileage for your past two months of training. Therefore, you should average about one-third of the race distance per day for the final six to eight weeks before a race. His recommended minimum for long distance races:

| Race Distance | Daily Average |
|---|---|
| 10 km / 6 miles | 2+ miles |
| 15 km / 10 miles | 3½ miles |
| 20 km / half-marathon | 4½ miles |
| 25 km / 15 miles | 5+ miles |
| 30 km / 20 miles | 7 miles |
| Marathon | 9 miles |

How fast should you train? What system should you use? Here we run into controversy.

The beginner racer should train only at a conversational pace at first. You've got to get to the finish line before you can worry about your time. You don't need speed work until you can run faster than your normal workout pace for one-half the race distance.

There are several types of training: LSD, fast running, "fartlek," hill training, intervals. They may be placed into two categories—steady and interrupted.

### LSD

"Long, slow distance" is the type of running we emphasized in the Run-Easy Method. According to "the father of LSD," Dr. Ernst van Aaken, slow training should account for 95 percent or more of the runner's work. Dr. van Aaken feels you should run at a pulse rate of 130–150, and be able to breathe and converse comfortably. LSD builds endurance, and it's fun. Dr. van Aaken noted at a New York Road Runner's Club clinic that man lacks not speed, but endurance, and LSD provides the runner with the stamina necessary to carry his or her natural speed over long distances.

Most coaches, however, feel that LSD should be combined with faster training. Arthur Lydiard feels the LSD should be interspersed with regular time trials. These would approximate race distances, and the runner would run a controlled pace roughly 15 to 30 seconds per mile slower than maximum. Lydiard also has his athletes run a little faster, "sticking close to their own aerobic-anaerobic border during long runs."

The key here is to run in a way that feels best for you. As you develop, you may want to use some of these more advanced training methods.

### Fast Running

This may be done as time trials over the race distance, or actual races used as training runs, or fast, overdistance work. Usually, this type of training is done at a relaxed, controlled pace, 5 to 10 percent below an all-out pace per mile for the race distance. However, it can produce fatigue and injury, and you can leave your best run on the training rather than the race course. So be careful, and hold back a little. This training should be specific to the runner's need. It simulates the racing conditions, and allows you to adapt mentally and physically—provided that your base of endurance is sufficient. The benefits are intensity, staying power, confidence, mental toughness. I feel that once a week a well-conditioned runner should either race or have a fast run of 6 to 10 miles with 90 percent effort.

### "Fartlek"

This is the Swedish term for "speed play." Free-style running is done over an indefinite distance for an indefinite time. Some segments of the run are performed at a faster pace than others, depending on the disposition of the athlete. This is my favorite type of training, especially for hilly, wooded trails. I change the pace repeatedly, charge the hills and stretch out on the downward slope. I accelerate, sprint, stride, stretch.

For the average runner, "fartlek" can be a playful period. It can also be fun as well as work for the serious racer. The latter should make half the workout hard going, but with adequate rest between bursts.

"Fartlek" is a good alternative to boring workouts. It is usually done on trails or grass, and combines all speeds from walking to jogging to sprinting. It helps develop speed and endurance at the same time. Gösta Holmer, who developed this training method, says that it gives "the feeling of self-creation of individuality." Perhaps. It is also an excellent way to sharpen up before a race, add interest to workouts, and get both aerobic and anaerobic benefits in the same session. Let your instincts tell you when to speed up and slow down—and enjoy this training method.

### Hill Training

This is run for several reasons. Downhill running increases the length of your stride and allows you to adjust to a faster speed than on a flat surface. It therefore helps improve running techniques.

Uphill running strengthens the leg muscles, especially the neglected quadriceps. Lydiard notes, "You need stronger quads to keep the knees up. I never saw anyone in the world move their legs faster than their arms." He described a typical hill training session that would take 20 to 60 minutes, depending upon your age and fitness level.

Step 1: Find a steep hill, and run up it easily until you're very tired. Let your body tell you when you've had enough.

Step 2: Find a shorter hill. Sprint up, pushing off the ankles, bouncing up the hill with a springing action (only after proper conditioning) to strengthen and improve the flexibility of the ankles.

Step 3: Run up the hill with long strides, high knee-lift, pumping arms. Jog at the top, and stride down fast. Do several quick wind sprints at the bottom (perhaps three times 220 or six times 50 yards). Repeat 2 to 6 times.

These workouts are always preceded and followed by slow jogging. Of course, slow, easy runs over hills also help strengthen the runner. Uphill climbs send pulse and breathing rates up and build muscle strength and confidence for conquering hills on race day. It is speed work in disguise.

It is important to start hill training with caution. Go into it gradually. Progressively increase your effort as you move from workout to workout, and always wear good training shoes.

### Interval Training

Usually this work is done on a track, with a stopwatch. It can be done elsewhere, however, and the clock isn't necessary. Intervals are a series of repeated efforts in which a predetermined distance is run at race pace or faster, alternated with measured recovery periods of easier running. It may be used for endurance work, pace work or speed sharpening. The stop-start technique allows the runner to go farther and faster than on a steady run. The variables are the distance run—between 50 yards and 1½ miles—recovery time and type—a predetermined number of seconds, recovery pulse level, or walk-jog recovery distance—the number of intervals performed, and the intensity.

Dr. Woldemar Gerschler and Dr. Herbert Reindel of Germany pioneered the interval system in the 1930s and argue that runners gain endurance by repeatedly running short distances at high speed, and taking short breaks with incomplete recovery. They developed a formula, "the Gerschler-Reindel Law," to determine the intensity of the interval. The running effort should send the heart rate up to 180 beats per minute. Then, the heart is allowed 90 seconds to return to 120–125 beats per minute. If this requires more time, then the effort demanded has either been too great or the distance too long. When the pulse returns to 120–125 beats per minute, the runner should start running again, even though it may take less than 90 seconds for the heart to recover.

Intervals help the runner to increase the body's ability to run with oxygen debt, and to learn to run hard in a state of fatigue, gaining the discipline to run a fast pace with endurance.

The usual interval distances are 100, 220, and 440 yards. Distance runners may also run longer intervals. I often do both. Once a week, I'll run eight 440-yard bursts and four 220 yards with a recovery jog of half or the full distance between each burst. Once a week I'll also run four 1-mile or eight ½-mile intervals at race pace in preparation for a 5-mile race, with a half-distance interval jog. I won't start the interval, however, until my pulse is below 125. The key to intervals is to keep the heart rate in the training range of approximately 120 to 180, and to pace the intervals evenly. Since all the intervals should be done at the same pace, the effort for the first few should be controlled, while the last few should be difficult.

Another good interval workout is the one I often do with Dr. Norb Sander along a dirt trail through the woods. Start with a 1- or 2-mile jog in one direction and back. Then start interval runs at whatever pace you desire. The first set is 1 minute out by your wristwatch; turn around and come back. Take a 2-minute rest between intervals and progress up to 5 minutes out and 5 minutes back—a brisk 10-minute continuous run. Then we reverse the workout beginning with the 5-minute run and ending with a slow jog. Runners of all abilities can do this workout together. In fact the runner trailing on the way out is the leader on the way back, and the faster runner can push himself to catch the slower runner.

Lydiard feels that American high-school and college runners do too much interval work, and that different workouts should be combined in a planned program for the advanced runner. Begin with the base period of six weeks to two months of endurance running, followed by four to six weeks of hill training (three hill workouts a week alternated with easy run days), and three to four weeks of "sharpening" on the track.

What plan is best for you? I feel that you should do most of your running at a comfortable pace. Most of us "run" rather than "train." We want to be fit enough to enjoy our races and see improvement, but not at the expense of losing the fun of the sport. However, you should also do some running at a pace that is slightly faster or equal to your racing pace to condition yourself and instill a rhythm necessary to racing. Therefore, I feel that the primary consideration for choosing your type of training and schedule should include:

1. Keeping up your energy level, health and stamina.
2. Maintaining a high interest level.
3. Avoiding overdoing it, and getting sick or injured.
4. Setting reasonable goals and keeping fit enough to meet them.

Equally important to conditioning is your pre-race attitude. I know of too many runners who run faster workouts than races because they lose their confidence as soon as they pin on a number. Mental toughness is important. You are what you think you are. And I think racing is 75 percent training, 5 percent luck, and 20 percent mental attitude.

Perhaps the toughest runner mentally was the late Olympian, Steve Prefontaine. He once got so psyched up for a treadmill stress test at Dr. Ken Cooper's Aerobic Center that they had to drag him off the machine; he wanted to beat the apparatus that bad! Before I race, I do two things. If I'm not serious about the run, I'll chat with anyone right up to the starting time, and then run for fun. But if I'm in it for blood, for an hour before the gun I concentrate. I think of my strategy: the expected time splits, the course, who I'll go out with, who I want to beat. I hide somewhere. Before the 1975 New York City Marathon I locked myself in a room off the locker area and then walked straight to the starting line. I was ready mentally, and knocked 10 minutes off my best previous time. The mental discipline of training daily in heat, rain, snow, etc. must be transferred to the race experience, and this must be finely honed in the pre-race concentration.

Concentration during the race is another factor. You must be prepared for the unforeseen—a sudden storm, a stitch, or an unpleasant course. An old-fashioned approach enters here, namely "guts." You can talk all day about "euphoria," and LSD running, but to be successful at serious competition you've got to take the best punches thrown by Mother Nature, your competitors and your own aching body. I think it's important, therefore, to prepare for tough races with "gut" workouts. Sometimes I'll run repeated intervals uphill until I feel "the bear on my back." Then I'll curse him, and run a few more. This is, of course, not for beginner competitors—not yet. But if you want to be better, you'll get to know "the bear."

## STRATEGY AND TACTICS

Racing strategy includes training for your event both physically and mentally. You will find that pre-race strategy may have to be changed suddenly during the race. You must be able to out-maneuver a rival in several ways.

Tactics are most important when you battle huge fields of runners, or on a track when the battleground is compact and the atmosphere tense. There are four basic styles of running a race: leading from the start, bursting open a lead in the middle, kicking at the end, or pacing evenly throughout.

Front running can be very dangerous. You don't know where the competition is, and you may go too fast and burn out. You can also get lost running unfamiliar courses. There are, naturally, exceptions. On an indoor track it is an advantage to lead because it's difficult to pass in a crowded field. Filbert Bayi, the Tanzanian 1500-meter world-record holder, normally bursts to the lead right away to avoid traffic jams. On narrow, rugged cross-country trails it's also sometimes better to lead so that you can have a clear view of upcoming obstacles and turns.

Bursting open a lead in the middle may work. But for some runners, sudden changes in speed will wipe out their stamina and pace. In long races, it may be a wise tactic to get rid of much of the competition (whatever your personal goals for that race) as you near the three-quarter marker and before the run to the finish. This will give you a clear view of the field ahead, and allow you to maintain your pace during the last, often grueling miles.

Kickers who burst at the end of the run love slow, tactical races. But relying too heavily on a kick can get you in trouble. First, it may not be there when you need it. More often, you can get caught in traffic, make your move too late (or too early), or, heaven forbid!, get outkicked from behind by another sprinter. Watch out: Speed is beginning to dominate even the long races now.

"Following" is a tactic that can work to your advantage. On windy days you can duck behind other runners and let them shelter you. You may also employ this method: Before a marathon a few people asked me what pace I would be running and the word spread. Five miles into the race I realized that a full dozen people were following me, and it was a strain. If you want to run in a group, fine; but share the lead. I picked up the pace and got rid of some, then slowed it down and got rid of the rest. I still like to follow someone whose time is good, and have them pace me to a good run.

### Pacing

Most races are won by pacers not racers. Steady pacing is the best bet, unless an elite runner is going for time. The average racer should be a pacer. After all, his goal is to improve his or her time, not beat others.

Pacing requires patience. If, for example, you're running a 6-mile race and your goal is to break the 8-minute-per-mile barrier, you should run close to that pace all the way. You shouldn't run faster than 5 to 15 seconds per mile below your goal so that you can spread out your energy over the race rather than wipe it out at the start. You must actually force yourself to go slow at the start, realizing you'll be stronger at the end. (See charts in Appendix for perfect pacing guidelines, pp. 406–407.)

You'll face three obstacles in running a well-paced race from start to finish. First, you're so full of adrenalin you just want to fly out of the starting line. Second, the mob always starts too fast; you must fight the tendency to go with them. Third, spectators and friends will unknowingly urge you to run faster. Remember: the tortoise always beats the hare.

How do you know your pace? Most races give "time splits" every few miles. Race officials are stationed at mile markers along the course. As runners pass they call out the time that has elapsed since the start of the race. From this time split runners can determine their pace. For example, if at the 2-mile marker, you are told that 17 minutes has elapsed, your pace is 8½ minutes per mile. The best way to keep track is to figure out in advance what your time should be at the mile markers and adjust your pace accordingly. If you hit a reference point too fast, you may be able to save yourself by slowing down a bit. Sometimes the splits that are given are inaccurate, so be careful. You may want to wear a watch and check the time yourself at each mile marker (most courses have them). Before deciding on your pace, try it out on a local track.

A marathoner must be wary: The pace at first is so leisurely and the distance so long that he or she may be tempted to blast out the first few miles. Reaching the halfway point oftentimes brings a new temptation, the urge to quit. In a typical marathon, 25 to 50 percent of the runners never finish. They burn out too early.

If you can, make sure you know the course well. This will help you anticipate obstacles and prepare your mind and body for them. When I reach a tough spot, I try to break the running into pieces: I pick a spot where I'll run hard, where I'll coast, and where I'll start my final push. It makes the race more exciting and less formidable.

Passing runners is an art form. On a track or in a cross-country race, you should pass decisively and get other runners out of your way—also psyching them out because you appear very strong. On a track, pass coming out of a turn, thus using the momentum. On the road you have more time. I often pick out a runner in the distance and gradually catch him or her. I may run alongside the runner for a while, then pull away if I feel him or her slowing the pace. On the other hand, if a runner passes me and looks strong, I'll often tag along letting him or her drag me into a brisk pace. I seldom pass on hills, except at the very top, when I churn by them with what strength remains, knowing that gravity will let me fly down the other side.

One final strategy that may help all of us. Before the race pick out some runners you know who have been running slightly faster than you. Try to stay close to them. If you do, and they are friends, you'll have a lot of fun over the postrace beers. If they are not, and you beat them, you'll have a private victory. Whatever, you'll run a faster race—and perhaps surprise yourself.

## RACING TIPS

There are several things to remember. Racing diminishes the fitness we build up, and we must have time (and patience) to rebuild. Lydiard recommends a simple solution to this: Race no more than 10 percent of your total mileage. Dr. van Aaken is even more conservative and recommends only 5 percent.

Going stale is another problem. Staleness often results from a program in which you set unreasonable goals. What reinforces your desire to race? If you try to work too hard, conquer too much too soon, you may get frustrated, stale or injured. Take a few days off. Swim, bicycle, walk, map out a new running route. Varying your racing pattern is also helpful. If you're tired of road races, try cross-country. If marathon training has you down, train for a mile on the track.

The racing schedule in New York City, for example, is broken into seasons. Runners are offered an automatic variety of challenges. The summer months feature track races and 3-mile "speed runs" in the city parks. Fall brings both cross-country in the hills of Van Cortlandt Park, and the city's marathon. The "winter series" offers weekend road races of 4 to 20 miles in Central Park. Spring, of course, brings the Mini-Marathon in Central Park, and a wide variety of other runs in other parks.

"Peaking"—simultaneously reaching the physical and emotional high point—is the trick. The average runner should try to "peak" only once or twice a year, for special races. For example, I plan for a gradual three-month buildup—running longer distances and incorporating speed work into my program—prior to the New York City Marathon in October and then return to a base-level program until I build again for Boston in April. Run a few races as "tune-ups" before your event. I'll run a half-marathon in late August and a 30-kilometer race in early March to test myself physically and mentally for the upcoming marathons.

Lasse Viren is a master at building to a peak that lasts for three weeks. Before the Olympics in 1972 and 1976, he carefully sharpened his fitness level for the big races. He won the 5000- and 10,000-meter races in both Olympics, but both before and after the Games he was soundly beaten. By contrast, Frank Shorter runs races all year round and believes in keeping racing-fit at all times.

However you train, remember the words of Dr. Sheehan: "My friend finished far back in the race. No matter. The race allows for this. The struggle that the Greeks called *agon* (from which comes our 'agony') is there for winner and loser alike—as are those briefly splendid moments that accompany it when we realize our finest potential.

"Only the race allows for this. The runs may be meditation and all that implies. But the race is experience—the transformation of you or me meditating to you or me as we are, to knowing who we actually are and what we actually can do."

## HOW TO START A RUNNING CLUB

Now that you have reached competition level, you may want to join, or start, a running club. There may already be local or national organizations like the Road Runners or the National Jogging Association in your town. These are administrative, not competitive, clubs. They promote running. (A list of officers and addresses is in the Appendix, p. 396.)

Clubs, formal or informal, give you the chance to run in a group. By working out together, runners often go farther and longer than they would alone. There is also the companionship of the group, the conversation, and even the protection against dogs in the country and muggers in the city.

A successful group needs a leader, a schedule of runs and a regular place to meet. The leader, not necessarily the best runner, makes sure the pace is not too fast, introduces new runners, organizes informal workouts, and so on. He or she must be sensitive to the group's and individuals' needs. He or she should set a pace comfortable for the slowest runner, or subdivide the club into smaller groups.

The Road Runners group I lead in New York City is typical. We meet at 6:45 on Wednesday, a time convenient for people who must arrive from work, change, relax and stretch. It is also convenient for their running schedules, and allows some runners to increase their pace or distance. We gather for announcements about upcoming races, parties and so on, and I ask how far each person is going to run and divide them into subgroups. We're very flexible. First, we run a loop in Central Park of a mile-and-three-fourths at a leisurely pace. Slower runners at the rear are accompanied for at least one loop. On the second loop we usually break into subgroups according to pace. Some runners quit after one loop, or two, or run loops up to 7 miles, or continue on with us to the George Washington Bridge, a distance of 17 miles. Those who wish can turn around halfway for a 10-mile run. Thus runners may select runs of almost 2, 3.5, 5.25, 7, 10 or 17 miles. The hard core group then runs to the nearest saloon to complete the workout.

Starting a club is easy. First, decide on the size of the group and the running schedule. A daily group generally runs either before work, at noon, or after work. The purpose is an obligation to a schedule: If you don't show, you catch hell. A weekly group meets for that one long run, and during the week members run alone or in twos or threes.

Contact as many runners as you can by advertisements in a runner's newsletter, on a community bulletin board, by word of mouth, or corporation house organ. Next, meet, and select temporary leaders. I've found by experience that these clubs often work best by "benevolent dictatorship." An active leader is important, and should be a person who motivates individuals and binds the group together. Plan to hold regular workouts—the best is twice a week for a long-and-short or interval workout—and regular meetings, perhaps disguised as parties.

Later, plan a monthly club newsletter that includes running tips, upcoming events, club business, race results for every club member, team "gossip" and lots of enthusiasm. Print as many club members' names as possible.

Also, develop a club bulletin board if you can. A local YMCA, a corporate board, or even a friendly pub may lend you space. Post records for club members in all age divisions: race results, profiles of top runners, race brochures, and so on.

Team identity is also essential. T-shirts are a basic must; warm-up suits and complete racing outfits with matching tank-tops and shorts (for men and women) can be ordered. Team spirit will soar when club members see each other during a workout or a race. When you do race, be sure that someone gets the race results for the entire team. Sometimes individual runners must leave before results are posted.

Also, for team spirit, parties are important—planned or un-planned. The social atmosphere of the club will affect athletic performance. I've been a member of a group that ran in the early morning, and then met for breakfast at a different member's house every other day. I've also been part of running clubs that met regularly in saloons. I'm still not sure which one I liked better, but both worked well.

Finances: Club dues and donations are essential unless you get a sponsor. Also, it is important for morale that your club go out and get runners at all levels. Actively recruit—with enthusiasm not aggressiveness. The best clubs have room for the jogger and the Olympian, and treat them equally, men and women, young and old. Our club's age range is ten to seventy-six, men and women in equal numbers. Times for the mile vary from 4:14 to 15 minutes, and for the marathon, from 2:27 to 7:24. The excitement of such a club comes from watching runners progress, the advanced runners helping the newer (although not necessarily younger) ones.

For more information on clubs order *The Road Runners Club Handbook: A Guide to Club Administration,* edited by past National Road Runners Club president Gar Williams. It can be ordered through the RRCA president (see Appendix).

# 4 THE ULTIMATE FITNESS CHALLENGE: THE MARATHON

"Marathon Mania" has swept our land. Nearly 50,000 men and women from ages four to eighty-four are running this classic event of 26 miles, 385 yards each year. Mention marathon, and most runners respond "Boston." The first Boston Marathon was run in 1897; 15 men competed. Until 1965, Boston usually had 250 to 400 starters, but by 1969 there were 1152, and in 1970 the field had to be limited by a qualifying time (now three hours for men under forty, 3:30 for men over forty and women). In 1964 there were six marathons in the United States. By 1977, there were 166. Not only are more of us running "the classic distance," more of us are running it well. In 1970, 812 men completed a U.S. marathon in under three hours. In 1976, 3600 men and women completed the distance in that time, or better.

A marathon, says the dictionary, is any test of endurance. But almost every marathon runner knows the legend of a fierce battle on the plains near the small Greek town of Marathon in 490 B.C. The invading Persian army was caught by surprise by the outmanned Athenians, who charged into their ranks and saved the Greek empire. Pheidippides, a Greek soldier, was ordered to run to Athens with the news of victory. His run of about 22 miles from the battlefield is considered the first "marathon," but poor Pheidippides wasn't as fit as the modern marathoner. He entered Athens, exclaimed "Rejoice, we conquer!" and collapsed and died.

The marathon was added to the first modern Olympic Games held in Athens in 1896, and was won by a Greek, Spiridon Loues. Spiridon Clubs (Road Runner Clubs) have been established throughout Europe (with the help of Dr. Norb Sander), and annual marathon runs are held over Pheidippides' route. In the United States, the first marathon was run in New York City (actually 35 miles from Stamford, Connecticut, to Columbus Circle). But the event was discontinued until 1970. Boston, with a marathon every year since 1896, remains the oldest, continuous marathon in the world.

The distance of the marathon has varied until recent history. Pheidippides ran 38 kilometers as compared to the present standardized 42.195 kilometers (think metric!). From 1896 to 1908, the Olympic marathon distance was unset, but in 1908 the Olympics was held in London, and the races began at Windsor Castle and ended at the new White City Stadium. An English princess, so the story goes, wanted to watch the start of the race from her castle window and then view the finish from her seat at the stadium. The distance, set to please her highness, was 26 miles, 385 yards. That was about 2 miles longer than previous marathons, but it became the standardized distance. As you puff along those last few miles, all obscenities should be uttered to "Her Royal Highness" whose vanity created the distance.

The Munich Olympics of 1972 saw Frank Shorter, Kenny Moore and Jack Bachelor finish 1-4-9 in the greatest performance in American marathon history. Millions of excited Americans watched on television. This American triumph in an event previously dominated by other countries signalled the start of the marathon boom in this country. Within an hour of Shorter's greatest moment, I was on the roads training seriously for the first time in eight years.

Why would anyone want to run a marathon? The glamour and tradition of "the classic distance" captures the imagination. It's also "there," like the highest mountain or the tallest building. As the longest, most grueling and most unpredictable running event, it is a symbol of superiority in physical and mental performance.

Most beginner marathon runners enter the first race to prove that their minds and bodies can meet the challenge, and their only goal is to finish. Then, they may set time goals of breaking three or three-and-a-half hours, and training becomes more specific. We search to find our limits and then reach beyond them. We also begin comparing ourselves to other runners; my original goal, for example, was to finish in the top 50 percent of the field, and now it has become the top 10 percent.

As a veteran of more than twenty-five marathons, I've learned many "secrets" of survival, although I never guarantee that any one of us will ever experience that beautiful, pain-free, fast marathon of runners' dreams. The marathon event is a true test of the runner. Proper training, diet, race experience, pacing and so forth are important, but among the elusive elements that make the marathon special are the combination of Mother Nature and Lady Luck, and your mental ability to overcome physical torture for 26 miles, 385 yards. The marathoner learns to discover the peace inside of pain.

Sometimes you first discover that strength from the words of others. When Carl Eilenberg was halfway up Heartbreak Hill during the 1975 Boston Marathon, he was about to stop. But Tom Coulter, a former Syracuse University All-America cross-country runner, came by and told Carl, in words that should be chiseled on those terrible hills, "Once you cross the finish line at Boston, there isn't anything you can't do." Eilenberg finished.

## GENERAL GUIDELINES

Here are some tips for all marathoners:

1. Work *from* a consistent base of endurance training. As you get stronger, you should increase your weekly mileage gradually at a rate of not more than 10 percent. Speed work and racing shouldn't even be considered until you've built a proper foundation of stamina. *Marathoning is a race where you avoid slowing down*, rather than try to gain speed. Consistency in training—"putting miles in the bank"—is the key.

2. The concept of "train, don't strain" that applies to the beginner runner also applies to all levels of marathon running. I feel that *all* workouts should be at a conversational pace for marathon training until the runner has built up a sufficient level of endurance to allow him or her to complete the race comfortably at a pace equivalent to or better than his or her normal workout pace for 5 to 10 miles. Then, to improve performance, he or she can practice going faster in intervals in order to develop the ability to push a marathon pace that is faster than the training pace. But beware of long, fast runs! Save them for the races.

A common-sense marathon schedule includes alternating hard or long training with easy or short days. The rest days are necessary so that the body can recover and strengthen itself for more progressive work. Tom Osler's plan for balancing long runs, average runs and recovery runs is listed in *The Conditioning of Long Distance Runners*, and includes:

|               |                                                                        | *40-mile week*                                  | *60-mile week* |
|---------------|------------------------------------------------------------------------|-------------------------------------------------|----------------|
| *Day One*     | 5% of week's total                                                     | 2 miles                                         | 3 miles        |
| *Day Two*     | 15% of week's total                                                    | 6 miles                                         | 9 miles        |
| *Day Three*   | 30% of week's total                                                    | 12 miles (add a few runs of 15–20 miles)       | 18 miles       |
| *Day Four*    | 5% of week's total                                                     | 2 miles                                         | 3 miles        |
| *Day Five*    | 15% of week's total                                                    | 6 miles                                         | 9 miles        |
| *Days Six and Seven* | Remaining 30% of week's total (use for race or just having fun) | 12 miles                                    | 18 miles       |

**3.** The "long run" is the key ingredient if balanced by a consistent base of endurance training. This run simulates the physical and mental stress you must endure in a marathon, and allows your mind to accept the fact that you can run long distances with some reasonable effort. Additionally, the body learns to adjust to different energy sources utilized in the late stages of a marathon.

The long run should be part of all marathon runners' weekly schedules and should cover a distance of 15 to 20 miles or extend for two to three hours of running. Anything longer than that is unnecessary. Several top marathon runners like to put in regular runs of 30 to 40 miles to build up confidence and strength for the late stages of a race. But for the average runner, this is not necessary, and runs beyond 20 miles could result in fatigue or injury.

Our club's marathon-running success comes from our regular Wednesday night "George Washington Bridge" runs of 17 miles. Not a single runner who was able to complete this run at least twice before the 1976 and 1977 New York City Marathon failed in the race. Mike Cleary, a sub–2:30 runner, Lauri Pedrinan and Jane Killion, both sub–3 hour runners—all marathon runners for less than three years—are products of this workout. The confidence gained from these long group runs at a conversational pace (you can hear us coming three blocks away) is invaluable.

**4.** Listen to your body and avoid injuries. If you become injured or overly fatigued, your training will be set back. (See chapter 11.)

**5.** Don't forget a proper warm-up and cool-down. I find a warm bath before and after long runs very soothing.

**6.** Run a few races before your marathon. A scattering of short races will toughen your mind for competition and provide you with good speed workouts. A strong, but not all-out, race of 10 to 20 miles four to six weeks before the marathon should be run at race pace or faster to establish confidence. Don't attempt a marathon until you've raced at least a half-marathon.

**7.** Don't peak too soon. Plan your workouts to build to a peak work load about two weeks before the marathon, and then taper off. Don't attempt to put in lots of last-minute mileage. You could "burn out," and besides, it takes several weeks for the training effects to take place.

**8.** Don't set unrealistic goals. If you do, you may become a race casualty. Establish an attainable race goal, and pace yourself. Set your goal a year away; it will be more likely within your reach after the training.

**9.** Respect the changes in your life, such as family or work problems, diet changes, a new baby, falling in love, or out of love. All may affect your training. Be flexible! A training schedule must not be a way of life. Stick to it as closely as possible, but be alert to the stress and strain of everyday life that may affect your training, too. You may have to take it easy for a while to get over, or around, bumps in your life.

10. Respect the "collapse point" theory. Ken Young's theory states that training mileage over the previous six to eight weeks sets the limit on how far you can hold a fast pace. The limit is about three times your daily average. If a runner averages 6 miles a day, he or she can expect to "collapse" or "hit the wall" at about 18 miles. Sub–three-hour marathoners who run 9 miles a day won't fit this point, but the undertrained runners will slow considerably in the late stages and should be mentally prepared. Twenty miles is the halfway point, psychologically, in the marathon.

A few years ago, researcher Paul Slovic compared finishing marathon times with weekly mileage, and came up with the following averages:

     1. Sub–3:00 runners      9 miles a day
     2. 3:01 to 3:30 runners    6 miles a day
     3. 3:31 to 4:00 runners    5 miles a day
     4. 4:01 and up runners    4 miles a day

11. Don't be stubborn! If you force yourself to train or race while injured, you may set yourself back for months, or longer. Adjust to the demands of Mother Nature, especially heat and humidity.

12. Be stubborn! Be consistent in your training. Force yourself out the door when you feel lazy. Enter the race well prepared and confident that you will meet your goals, but don't think it will be easy; I've run too many to take any one of them for granted. The marathon monster is always prepared to gobble us up; the unprepared is his favorite target. E. C. Frederick, author of *The Running Body*, wrote, "It's a rare person who has the fortitude and mind control to force himself to finish a

marathon when not properly trained for it. Even highly trained persons undergo much soul-searching and must dig deeply into their bag of tricks to endure those last 6 miles. Because they are prepared, most trained marathoners finish. Rarely does an unprepared person make it past 20 miles."

Most marathon runners, including me, want to quit at several points during the race. I push through these desires by thinking about all the hard work I've put in training for that one race. Only injury or illness that could cause further damage should be accepted as an excuse to drop out. The pain is part of the challenge. Most marathon runners swear after a race that they will never do it again. A few days later they are planning to better their time.

In 1977, at Boston, I ran with star marathon runner, Lauri Pedrinan, in an effort to get her under the three-hour barrier. It was just too hot that day to hold the pace. With 3 miles to go she developed painful thigh cramps, and considered (as we all do) quitting. I reminded her that I never said it would be easy, and she bravely fought on, defeating two-thirds of the world class field of men and women in 3:04. That's my basic point: "Don't think it's easy—it ain't!"

According to the Greater New York AA's Richard Traum, "Anyone who honestly takes the time to train can finish a marathon." On October 24, 1976, Dick finished the New York Marathon, despite an artificial right leg.

I first met Dick when he started in my beginner's fitness class. I asked him if he would think about the challenge of a 5-mile race. He completed a 5-miler in May, 1976, and then we set the goal to be a half-marathon—what I considered to be a full marathon for a one-legged man. He then decided to train for the New York City Marathon, and completed a 30-kilometer race as a test. He trains three times a week with two two-hour runs (9 miles each) and one five-hour run (18 miles) per week. He needs the days off so that the welts on his stump will heal. All of his training is done on a 23-laps-per-mile indoor track. We feel that he runs the equivalent of 60–80 miles per week for the average runner.

At New York, when the winner Bill Rodgers passed Dick Traum (Dick started at six a.m.—the Verrazano Narrows Bridge was closed just for him) they had run 16 miles. Bill turned and said, "Atta boy, Dick!" At the awards ceremony, Dick was given a roaring, standing ovation. When asked if he would have run the marathon if he had two legs, he replied, "Yes, the challenge is certainly there." His next goal: a 50-miler. How's that for inspiration!

I have also been inspired by other unique marathoners. California's Peter Strudwick runs marathons despite his club feet. I've run with blind marathoners Tom Sullivan, a California pop singer, and Joe Pardo, who often wins Master's awards in New York area races. In the 1974 Boston Marathon, I was in agony and considered quitting when Californian Harry Cordellos passed me. On the back of his T-shirt were the words: "Caution, Blind Runner." I was so inspired I had to try and keep up. He pulled me through the race—and beat me. But I finished. In the 1976 Boston Marathon, I ran a see-saw battle with Bob Hall of the Greater Boston Track Club. I'd pass him on the uphills and he'd destroy me on the downside. He finally rolled ahead of me. In 1977, at Boston, Bob won the National Wheelchair Marathon Championship over eleven other entries in 2:40!

Anyone can run a marathon, and finish, if trained properly for it. Teammate Hans Hartmann began running at age forty, and eighteen months later ran a 2:43 marathon in 77° F. heat in the 1977 race to Boston. He seldom runs more than 40 miles a week! But he's certainly an exception.

## TYPES OF MARATHONERS

I find that marathon runners fit into four general categories and training schedules: the survivor, the average marathoner, the above-average and the elite racer. You'll probably find yourself somewhere in these categories.

### The Survivor

Before running a marathon, you should first build up to 20 to 30 miles per week, or about 30 to 45 minutes of running a day. This may take six months to two years. The next goal is to work up gradually to 40 miles or more per week, depending on your age, weight, and previous experience. You should maintain this mileage for at least four months prior to the marathon, and include several long runs in your overall schedule. A well-planned three-month build-up schedule might look like this:

|  | Mon. | Tues. | Wed. | Thurs. | Fri. | Sat. | Sun. |
|---|---|---|---|---|---|---|---|
| First month (*40 miles*) | Off | 7 | 10 | 7 | 4 | 7 | 5 |
| Second month (*40–45 miles*) | Off | 5 | 15–20 | 5 | 5 | 10 | 5 |
| Third month (first two weeks follow same schedule as second month) | | | | | | | |
| Taper-off week one (*35 miles*) | Off | 4 | 10 | 4 | 4 | 8 | 5 |
| Taper-off week two (*16 miles and race*) | Off | 4 | 6 | 4 | 2 | Off | Race |

Slowly increase the mileage to 40 or 45 miles a week. The important workout is the long run, which gradually increases from 10 to 15, to 20 miles. Keep in mind that the duration of the run is more important than the speed. Your training pace, however, should be approximately the pace at which you want to run the marathon. Include hills in your training, and run several 10–15 mile races at slightly faster than your expected marathon pace during the three months before your marathon.

Your goal, again depending on such factors as age, sex, previous athletic background, and ability, should be in the three-and-a-half to five-hour range. But this goal is secondary to the first priority, which is to finish. Start the race slowly and run at your own pace. Don't get caught up in the excitement and start too fast. Take plenty of liquids throughout the race. (See chapter 14.) Dress properly for the weather conditions (chapter 9).

You do not have to run all the way. If you tire, try walking briskly, but don't stop. Late in the race you may be able to walk up hills faster than you can run them because you're using different muscles. The same run-walk theory used by beginner runners can be applied to the marathon. With 40–45 miles of training per week, you'll probably "hit the wall" between 15 and 20 miles. The last few miles may not be very pleasant, but you can make it if you let the spirit of the other runners and spectators help you along. Use common sense and be patient; the finish line will still be there when you arrive. Don't forget to smile when you finish, and shout "Rejoice, we conquer!"

After finishing, force yourself to stretch as soon as possible, and over the next few days take plenty of long walks, warm baths and stretching sessions. Run as soon as you can, preferably the next day; it will help pump blood to your leg muscles and the stiffness will go away sooner.

Two additional tips for the beginner marathoner need to be emphasized. Do not follow the depletion cycle of the carbohydrate loading program—your body is experiencing enough new strain already. Do not wear racing shoes—your trusty training shoes offer you comfort and reliability in your effort to complete the race.

### The Average Marathoner

The average marathon runner varies according to age and sex. This marathoner can be a man under forty aiming for a time of 3 to 3:30 hours, or a man over forty or a woman of any age aiming for a time of 3:15 to 3:45. The average marathoner has completed at least one marathon and should average 50 to 60 miles a week over a period of two months before the marathon race.

His or her schedule is similar to the Survivor's, except for three advantages. He or she has already been through the learning experience of a marathon, has more "miles in the bank" over a period of time, and has averaged more miles per week. Also, the "collapse point" is nearer the end of the marathon.

Set yourself a reasonable time goal and pace yourself toward it. For example, you might want to run an 8-minute mile for a sub 3½-hour marathon. But if you wish to break 3½ hours, you should run no faster than 15 seconds per mile faster than that pace for the first half of the race (starting a little faster allows for time lost late in the race when you begin to tire).

In the three months before the marathon, you should also run one or two races of 10 to 20 miles at a slightly faster pace than your anticipated marathon pace.

A typical schedule for the average marathon runner might follow Bill Horowitz' schedule. He's my dentist and teammate who at age forty-five ran a 3:24 Earth Day Marathon. Bill cut a half hour from his initial marathon time with this weekly schedule:

| Mon | Tues | Wed | Thur | Fri | Sat | Sun | Total |
|-----|------|-----|------|-----|-----|-----|-------|
| Off | 10 | 12 | 8 | 10 | 6 | 18 | 64 |

Remember, this was purely long, slow distance work. His only speed work was in races of 4 to 12 miles, which he often ran every other week during the six months between marathons.

### The Above–Average Marathoner

This is generally the below-forty male who aims for a 2:30 to 2:59 marathon, or the Master's or female runner in the 2:50 to 3:15 range.

This runner puts in 60 to 80 miles a week, and some reach 100. The runner also puts in speed work because he or she is racing at a faster pace than their training pace. The once-a-week long run is usually supplemented by two or three days of interval, fartlek or hill training. A sample schedule used by our club's sub–three-hour national class runners, Lauri Pedrinan and Jane Killion, follows:

*Sunday:* An "active rest day"; 5 to 10 miles easy.

*Monday:* Short interval day; jog three miles; four to eight 440-yard runs at 75 percent effort, equal distance recovery; two to four 220-yard runs at 90 percent effort, equal distance recovery; jog 3 miles. Alternate schedule: fartlek runs with 440-yard bursts and 220-yard bursts.

*Tuesday:* Active rest day; 5 to 10 miles easy.

*Wednesday:* Long run, 17 to 30 miles; first few miles slow, last few miles strong.

*Thursday and Friday:* Active rest days; 5 to 10 miles easy.

*Saturday:* Choose between hill day; jog 3 warm-up miles;

four times run a 1½-mile hill loop—up a steep ½-mile hill at 75 percent effort, an easy ½-mile recovery at the top, and downhill at good pace. *Or,* eight times up ¼-mile steep hill at 75 percent effort, jogging back down. *Or,* 5 to 10 miles hilly cross-country. But, whatever the program, jog 3 miles at end. Or, long interval day; jog 3 miles; run 4 1-mile runs at 75 percent effort, ½-mile-run recovery; jog 3 miles.

This schedule offers a flexible range of 60 to 80 miles per week. As the race draws near, the endurance base is sharpened by increasing the intensity and decreasing the recovery times of the interval runs. One month before the 1977 Boston Marathon, Lauri averaged 6:40 per mile while placing second by 10 seconds in the National 30-kilometer Bankathon in Albany. On the same day, Jane won the Earth Day Marathon in 2:59 (short course—projected time 3:05). Thus they both entered Boston full of confidence and placed thirteenth and fourteenth in a field of 144 national class women runners on a very hot, tough day. The following October they led the team to its second straight New York City Marathon Championship: Lauri, 252:32; Jane, 2:56:22. On the same day in Minneapolis, Nina Kuscsik ran a 2:50:22 marathon—giving our Greater New York AA team three of the top thirty times in the world.

A similar schedule can be expanded to 100 miles per week by increasing the distance of the long runs and adding additional daily workouts of 5 easy miles. This is my basic schedule during the weeks. I'm not either injured, traveling, or lazy.

### The Elite Racer
These are the fast national and world class runners. I once trained for a couple of days with Bill Rodgers, the American

record holder at 2:09:55 (a sub–five-minute mile pace!) and quickly found out that his six-minute training pace is faster than my race pace. He regularly runs twice a day for six days, with one long-run day, covering between 140 and 150 miles a week. Jacki Hansen, former American record holder for women at 2:38:19 (slightly more than six minutes per mile) averages 100 miles per week, including two workouts per day most days. Three times a week she is pushed through tough interval workouts by her coach. For these runners, there is nothing more central to their lives than the marathon.

## THE RACE

What's it like to run a marathon? I remember best the 1976 New York City Marathon, probably because it was New York's first marathon through all five boroughs and because so many runners entered and more than half a million people watched and cheered.

The bus ride to the Verrazano-Narrows Bridge was quiet and filled with a sweet mix of apprehension and excitement. As we approached the bridge, the unique love-hate relationship all marathon runners feel took over: We love to race and look forward to it, except for these last few hours before the gun when we all hate it.

The check-in was a madhouse of frantic runners. Officials shouted directions that no one could hear in the din. The smell of liniment and nervous sweat filled the air. Outside, runners forced themselves through a vast assortment of pre-race rituals. As the excitement rose, runners made countless trips to the water fountain and the woods.

Then, together, thousands of bouncing bodies, we made a wide, colorful, undulating train from Ft. Wadsworth toward the starting line, where the tension was almost tangible. Helicopters chattered above us, and television newsreel camera crews were filming the runners closest to the front. Thousands began shouting "Let's go! Let's go!" When Manhattan Borough President Percy Sutton, the official starter, finally fired the pistol, men and women screamed with excitement, and punched the air with their fists. More than 4000 feet pounded the asphalt approach to the world's largest suspension bridge. "Oh my God, it's so beautiful!" We were caught in a vacuum and swept up the incline as if it didn't exist—up, over, and across into Brooklyn, the first of five boroughs.

Brooklynites are great: Choir boys sang outside a church, signs flashed to local runners, Finnish and English flags flapped in the wind. Old and young cheered and cheered as we passed. They offered water and oranges, kids held out their hands for a touch, and handslap.

We passed through Queens, and into the Bronx. Glances exchanged at the Willis Avenue Bridge at the 15-mile mark reveal two types of runners at this point in the race: those who are feeling good, and those who are suffering. I was awakened from my painful, hypnotic state only by the sound of an incredible mass of cheering spectators along Central Park West in Manhattan. Stunned, tired, hurt, I pulled myself together; the cheering had picked me up. I ran across the finish line—and kept going until someone finally made me stop after an unforgettable journey of agony and ecstasy.

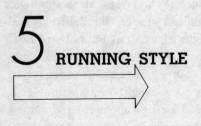

# 5 RUNNING STYLE

Every runner has his or her own form. I can spot a running friend at a distance. Some have faults in form such as a pronounced forward lean, high arm carry, bouncing motion, body sway or flailing elbows. Others stand out because of structural faults such as bowlegs, or feet that point outward, or inward. Others run with good form but are quickly recognized by such quirks of habit as a rolling head, or long-legged or short, choppy strides.

Running should come naturally. Many of our faults of style come from the way we grew up and what impressed us. When I worked at the Y in Rome, New York, I coached a youth track team. One regular event for our kids was a mile run. It was the first exposure to distance running for most of them. Rather than teach them how to run, I decided just to let them run naturally and then work on apparent faults in form. The top runners of the future aren't necessarily the fastest, but those with an economical stride, patience and will power. Form counts more than time when you're young.

I was amazed by the difference between the boys and girls. The majority of the girls ran very smoothly and gracefully with near perfect form. In fact, many of them ran faster over the mile than the boys. The boys, however, tended to run like football or basketball players. Physical education in the "ball sports" emphasizes this style which promotes power and speed. Therefore, many boys learn to run high on their toes and have a pronounced upper-body movement. Competitiveness, learned from a very early age and reinforced with Little League Baseball and Pop Warner Football, is reflected in their tense bodies. The girls, however, aren't exposed as much to highly competitive "ball sport" activities, and instead participate in sports that emphasize form, agility and patience, like gymnastics and dance. A ten-year-old girl is probably the most natural runner in our running world.

Unfortunately, young girls often develop a less efficient running motion as they become teen-agers. A girl at that age is sometimes told to run in a "lady-like" manner. She bounces on her toes, with her arms carried too high in front of her, elbows swinging in the air. The adult woman who begins to jog usually possesses these traits; she not only runs inefficiently but also bounces along with extra weight. She is susceptible to injury. Many women joggers complain of soreness in their upper back. This is usually because they carry their arms too high and force their shoulders back. Adult women also tend to lean forward too far, and have a lower knee-lift than men. The foot is often brought forward by swinging it out to the side rather than by raising the knee. All of this is correctable; women haven't had the "ball-sport" training, and learn new running methods quickly.

The teen-age boy often likes the power and speed of competitive sports. His coaches tell him to run on his toes with fists clenched and arms pumping. Later, men may be trained to concentrate on power and speed rather than relaxation and efficiency of motion. Sitting before the television set, watching football and basketball heroes, reinforces the running form of power-speed athletics.

We face a relearning process when we wish to "run for fitness." How can you teach running form? It can be detailed on paper, but must be practiced and refined in motion with a natural style that can be modified by a trained instructor. I don't tell my beginner runners how to run. I just allow them to start running naturally. Or, I'll observe them individually on the track. Either way, I can pick up obvious faults in their form, and correct them. I highly recommend that beginner runners start by running naturally, but under the watchful eye of someone who can correct obvious faults in running style before they become bad, hard-to-break habits.

Running, when done properly, is a complete, flowing action that takes place unconsciously. The following sections analyze the parts of this fluid movement, and will help you check your own style, or that of a friend. Keep the following guidelines in mind while analyzing your running form:

- Relaxed, efficient running form is essential to using your muscle energy well.
- An erect body carriage results in maximum movement and efficiency, and wastes less energy needed to move forward.
- Use your arms for balancing and power, don't just carry them along for the run.
- Footstrike and stride are aids to running speed, and must be adjusted to meet the demand.
- Improper footstrike and running form may lead to injury, fatigue and decreased efficiency.
- Your form should be the natural result of the best use of your body frame, and not someone else's style.

## FOOTSTRIKE AND STRIDE

Running is similar to walking. The heel of your foot makes the initial contact with the ground, followed by the mid-stance or support phase, the toe-off or propulsive phase and finally the leg swing.

In walking, one foot is always on the ground; in running, there is a "floating" phase between toe-off and foot contact when neither foot is in contact with the ground. Dr. Steven Subotnik explains in *Podiatric Sports Medicine* that running is divided into a support phase and a recovery phase. The support phase consists of footstrike, mid-support and takeoff. The recovery phase consists of follow-through, forward swing and foot descent.

Dr. Subotnik describes the biomechanics of running: "At the implant of footstrike, the foot makes contact with the ground initially in a supinated position and as weight is accepted proceeds into a pronation until the forefoot is securely fixed to the running surface. The hip is internally rotating and extending during this period. From this period of initial contact until toe-off, the limb then externally rotates. At toe-off, the lower extremity then begins to rotate internally. We can see an analogous situation between running and walking wherein pronation occurs at heel strike and supination occurs throughout the remainder of the period of time that the foot is on the ground, allowing it to convert from a mobile adaptor to a rigid level in order to accept stress and allow for a powerful thrust at toe-off."

When the foot has structural weaknesses—and more than 90 percent of our population have such weaknesses—then normal pushoff is impaired. The result is an abnormal turning at the hip, knees, ankle joints and within the foot, which can

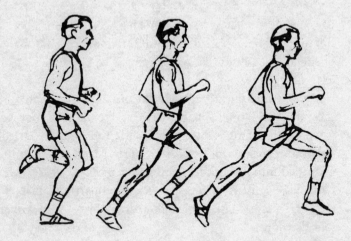

result in injury. These abnormalities may be controlled with shoe inserts or arch supports (see chapter 10).

All runners land first on the outside edge of the foot, and roll inward as the rolling action cushions the blow. Sprinters contact the ground high on the ball of the foot. Middle-distance runners hit on the metatarsal arch. Long-distance runners and joggers strike heel first. Some distance runners hit somewhere between heel first and ball first, landing on the outer edge of the whole foot. Some coaches, including Pete Schuder, Columbia University track coach, teach this method of foot-strike.

Running on the toes produces more speed and power for short distances, but in longer runs, it results in leg fatigue, calf tightness, shin splints and Achilles' tendonitis, among other maladies. Many joggers run with a slow "flat-foot" technique:

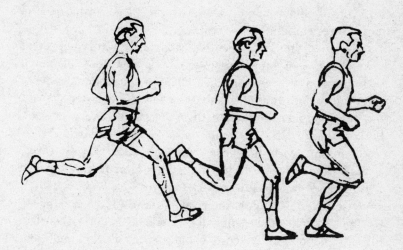

The entire foot strikes the ground at the same time. The wide surface area cushions this footstrike, and it's easy on the rest of the body. It is difficult, however, to run very fast or for long periods of time with this style. Some runners run flat-footed but with a "slap-foot" contact that can have a jarring effect on the body. Other runners land too far back on the heel, and hit the ground with a rigid rather than relaxed footstrike.

Proper footstrike for the long-distance runner and jogger is important. The foot contact should be as light and silent as possible. The foot should strike the ground on the outside, between the heel and the metatarsal arch, and, on contact, gently roll forward and inward to the ball of the foot, and then gently upward and outward to toe-off. A slight "rocking motion" between the heel contact and pushoff insures proper cushioning and effective forward propulsion. This "rocking action" results in a hitting and springing motion that is less jarring and increases acceleration.

The toes should be pointed straight forward, but don't force this if it is uncomfortable. Check your foot alignment by running in wet sand or mud. The individual components of stride are length, knee-lift and back-kick. The faster you go, the more you increase the length of your stride and your knee-lift and back-kick. The point of foot contact should be directly in line with the knee, with the knee slightly flexed. Actually, the foot should hit the ground after it has stretched forward and has already started to swing back. If you overstride so that the leg hits the ground ahead of the knee flex—the leg is straight—the result will be a braking action rather than forward propulsion. A short, choppy stride is also inefficient because more energy is used traveling a shorter distance. The short stride is often the product of inflexibility. If the runner is unable to extend his leg fully, then he is losing several inches of forward movement with each stride. The runner with a relaxed stride and flexible leg muscles will not have to work as hard as the runner with a short, choppy stride. Runners with pronounced knee-lift or back-kick (other than in short sprints) are merely wasting energy.

## RUNNING POSTURE

Bill Bowerman, former track coach at the University of Oregon, feels that an erect posture is most essential for a smooth running style. "Run tall," he preaches to his disciples. Running tall means running with your back as straight as naturally comfortable, the head up, and eyes straight ahead. The buttocks should be "tucked in" so that an imaginary line drawn from the top of the head through the shoulders and hips to the ground would be perpendicular.

A forward lean places an extra burden on the leg muscles and often contributes to back pain and shin splints. It should only be used when sprinting or going uphill. Leaning backwards has a braking effect; it places a severe burden on the legs and back.

The shoulders should "hang" in a relaxed manner, level to the ground. If you stick out your chest and throw back your shoulders you'll develop tightness in the upper back or even the lower back. Concentrate on not allowing the shoulder blades to pinch together. Tension first collects in the head and shoulders. Be aware of tension beginning at the base of the neck, in the jaw muscles, around the eyes, in the muscles of the forehead and in the shoulders. Occasionally, let the head roll from side to side, shrug the shoulders and let them drop, or drop your arms loosely at your side to promote relaxation. Allow the chin to drop and flap, as if talking. This keeps the jaw and neck muscles relaxed. The arms should swing from relaxed shoulders; the eyes should look straight ahead.

## ARM CARRY

The movement of your arms provides the rhythm that pulls you along. The faster your arm movement, the faster you will be able to move your legs. "Pumping" the arms in powerful strokes is as important to the sprinter as high knee-lift. But the jogger and long-distance runner don't worry about arm pumping unless competing in a race or running up a hill. These runners are interested in two important factors relating to arm carry: balance and energy conservation.

The arms balance the runner. The left arm should swing forward, balancing right leg action; the right arm should swing forward, balancing left leg action. If the arms are carried too high, the result is a shortened stride, shoulder twisting, muscle fatigue and tension in the shoulders and upper back. Arms carried too low often contribute to a forward lean, and to a side-to-side and bouncing motion. Arms moving across the body result in side-to-side motion and a shortened stride. Too little forward or backward motion results in lack of proper drive and balance. Flopping of the arms or rigidly held arms also contribute to inefficiency of motion, and thus waste your energy.

How should the arms be carried? The general guidelines are as follows:

- The arms should be carried low, between the waistline and the chest.
- At the midpoint of your stride, the forearms, wrists and hands should be parallel to the ground, as are the shoulders.
- In the forward swing, the forearm moves slightly up and inward; on the back swing, it moves slightly down and outward.
- The thumbs should rest on your index fingers, with your fingers lightly clenched, palm turned slightly up, wrist firm but not tight, hand in line with forearms. Some runners prefer to put their thumbs in their middle fingers, forming a meditative circle.
- The elbows should be relaxed, not locked, and should not dramatically point away from the body, but should be loose at your sides. They should bend and straighten a little with each arm swing.
- The shoulders should remain level and should not move appreciably, although there is a rise and fall as the arms swing forward and backwards.

It is important to concentrate on relaxing the shoulders, elbows, wrists and fists. Body tension is often the result of improper arm carry. Occasionally let your arms drop straight down at your side and loosely "shake them out"; this reduces the tightness that results from holding them up for a long time. According to the famous coach Percy Cerutty, "All running starts with the thumbs." Tension begins in the hands and improper hand carry can set off a chain reaction of form problems.

## BREATHING

Many runners ask, "How should I breathe while running?" or "Should I breathe with my mouth open?" There is a theory that runners should breathe in through the nose and out through the mouth. Supposedly this promotes relaxation and filters the air. But running calls for lots of air to satisfy the body's need for oxygen. You won't last long breathing in through the nose, and out the mouth. Open up your mouth and suck in all the air you need.

Some runners enjoy breathing in tune to their footstrike. They may inhale, for example, on every other left step, and exhale on every other right. Such breathing techniques may be relaxing during yoga exercises, but they would drive me nuts during a run, and I'm sure I'd get confused. If I had to blow my nose during the run, would it count as exhaling? What if I sneezed when I was due to inhale? Life is too short, and running too beautiful, to spoil with rigid rules. My advice is to breathe when you feel like breathing. On the other hand, Jack Shepherd—who will try anything once—has done special breathing exercises while running. He loves them, and we describe some in chapter 15. You decide what's best for you.

However, there are two basic rules. Breathing should be relaxed, and should follow "belly breathing" principles. Most of us breathe backwards. We tend to suck the stomach in, and breathe from the chest. With proper abdominal breathing the belly expands as you breathe in, and flattens as you breathe out. The expansion of the abdomen indicates that the diaphragm is fully lowered, inflating the lungs to their fullest and allowing a more efficient intake of oxygen. Improper breathing can also cause the dreaded side stitch (see page 266).

To understand how to belly breathe, lie on your back and place a light book on your stomach. (Try this one.) Take a deep breath. If you are "belly breathing" properly, the book will rise as you breathe in, and fall as you breathe out.

## THE THREE "R's" OF RUNNING STYLE

1. Run tall   2. Run relaxed   3. Run naturally

No one can teach you how to develop your running style. For the most part, you are born with a certain style that changes as you do. The best we can hope to do is clean up bad habits. The "natural" runners possess a beauty most of us who run can recognize, and partially imitate. They run, as Tom Sturak writes of the great Filbert Bayi in *The African Running Revolution*, "like water flows or the wind blows."

Some days I feel as though my whole body is in complete synchronization and towing my mind along for the ride. I cleanse myself in the pleasant breeze I create with my free-flowing body. On these days I don't need to emulate anyone's style; I've created my own.

Study the mechanics of a proper running style, but always be yourself.

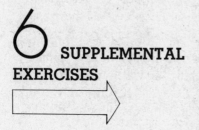

# 6 SUPPLEMENTAL EXERCISES

Training should be an enjoyable habit. And to make that habit more enjoyable, I suggest alternating your regular exercises, outlined in chapter 1, with the exercises below. Some of these are valuable for cross-country skiing, swimming, biking and other vigorous sports. Some of them also are for advanced fitness only, but all will benefit runners.

## WEIGHT TRAINING

In every sport, weight training exercises benefit the serious competitor, and running is no exception. A supplemental weight training program will not only improve your strength, but also your running time. Runners who compete in distance races need upper body strength and endurance; just holding the arms up during a long race, or finding extra leg power through those last few miles requires added muscular strength. Track coaches are now recommending weight programs for their men and women runners.

Several books give detailed programs and theories of weight training (see Appendix), but there are a few simple rules that I would like to mention here. There is one basic law in weight training: Heavy weights with few repetitions build strength and a bulky body; light weights and many repetitions build stamina and a lean, firm body. The rule that applies to developing a runner's body is the same for men and women: light weights, many repetitions. The goal is to firm the body, not to build bulky muscles.

You should exercise with weights two to five times per week. Fit them into your program after you have properly warmed up—either after stretching and before running, or after running and the cool-down exercises. If you plan to work out with weights at a time separate from your running, do some stretching exercises before and after lifting.

A Universal Gym is easiest because the weights can be changed quickly. A basic set of barbells, however, is also good. You also may wish to modify the program by sticking to one weight for each set of exercises, and doing 20 to 30 repetitions rather than changing the weights frequently.

Here's what I recommend. First, find a starting point for each exercise. This is whatever weight you can lift 10 times— the last few times being a strain. In each exercise, lift 10 times as briskly as you can. Then change the weight, reducing it 10 to 20 pounds, and repeat for a total of 3 to 4 sets. At first, 3 repetitions may be all you can do. As you get stronger, you may increase your starting weight, but never emphasize lifting an impressive amount of steel. Leave "pumping iron" to the gym-bound narcissists.

A good 15- to 20-minute program would include the military press; the quadricep exercises (sitting, weighting the ankle and straightening the knee; 10 times each ankle), curls, a few bent-knee sit-ups, and the bench press. (These are standard exercises found in any weight training book.) The quad exercises are important, for these are the muscles that lift your legs, the muscles that often tire in long races.

Remember to breathe out as you work against the resistance of the weights, and to maintain proper form through the workout. Don't arch your back, or get carried away and try to do too much in one session. Improper lifting can result in injury.

After a few weeks, you will notice results. Weight training over several months added strength to my own running as I prepared for marathons. My leg lift improved dramatically, and my upper body and quadriceps have held up better during those final brutal miles of a marathon. Both the men and women runners I train have noticed similar improvement, and I recommend weight training to all of them.

## EXERCISES

Too often I hear runners complaining because they can't keep up with their jogging programs; they've been injured, or are in pain. When I hear this I ask them: How long have you been jogging? How far do you run? Are you doing your warm-up and cool-down exercises? Too often, the slowed-down jogger is beyond the beginner stage, and has increased his or her mileage, while at the same time giving up the warm-up and cool-down "because it's boring." I offer these exercises as substitutes for those given earlier, with the encouragement that they may make the very essential warm-up and cool-down more interesting. Variety, as we all know, is the spice of life.

### Leg and Groin Exercises

1. *Hamstring Stretch, Standing*  Stand, feet slightly apart, hands clasped behind your back. Slowly bend forward from the hips. Keep legs and back straight, head raised. Bend down as far as you can comfortably, and slowly return. Repeat two or three times.

2. *Hamstring Stretcher*   Stand; cross one leg in front of the other. Toes of front leg, but not entire foot, should touch ground parallel to rear foot. Slowly bend forward from waist, hang, breathe deeply, touch toes. Keep rear leg straight, heel to floor. Hold for 20 seconds. Repeat each leg twice.

3. *Sprinter's Position*   On all fours, one leg forward and bent, rear leg extended. For thigh: on balls of feet, slowly lower hips as in push-up. For shin: Rear foot extended, with toes extended out. Slowly lower. Repeat and alternate. For calf: Cup heel of rear leg, and lower. Repeat and alternate.

4. *Thigh Shift*   Stand with feet far apart and somewhat turned out. Keep both heels flat on floor. Bend the right knee. Return to erect position. Alternate and repeat.

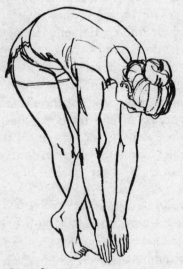

**Hamstring Stretcher**

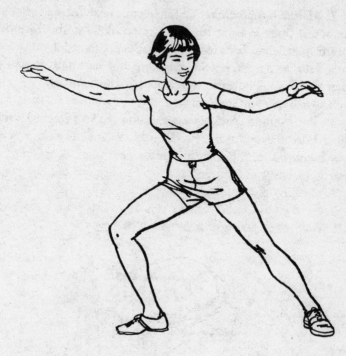

**Thigh Shift**

**5. *Calf Stretch*** Stand. Place one foot ahead of the other with weight on the ball of the back foot. Slowly lower the heel of the rear foot to the floor, and hold. Alternate.

**6. *Hamstring Stretch*** Stand, with knees flexed. Let fingers touch the floor close to toes. Slowly straighten knees while keeping fingers on the floor. Repeat.

7. **Medial Thigh Stretch**   Sit; bend knees so that soles of feet touch. Rest arms on thighs. Grasp ankles and force knees toward floor while bending forward as far as possible.

8. **Hurdler's Stretch**   Sit, extending one leg and tucking the other under your bottom. Reach with both hands toward toe, and hold. Repeat and alternate.

9. **Toe Pointer**   Sit on feet, toes and ankles stretched backward. Raise knees from floor slightly, balancing weight with both hands on floor just behind hips.

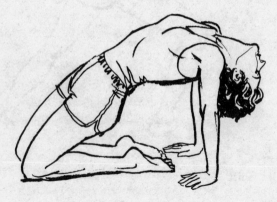

**Toe Pointer**

10. **Knee Hugs**   Stand or sit. Grasp right ankle or shin, and hug knee to chest. Alternate and repeat.

11. **Ankle Rolls**   Sit cross-legged. Grasp right foot with both hands and rotate ankle. Reverse direction. Repeat with left ankle.

**12.** *Extended Ankle Roll* Lie on back, left knee flexed, right leg raised 10 inches. Rotate ankle and reverse. Alternate.

**13.** *Ankle Stretch* Sit with your legs extended. Raise legs off floor, pointing your toes forward, and making circles with your ankles to the right and then to the left. Relax, and repeat.

### Groin Exercises

**1.** Sit, legs outstretched. Slowly spread legs, and hold.

**2.** Lie on back, curl legs overhead into bicycle position. Straighten legs, spread them and hold.

**3.** Lie on back, knees bent, feet on floor. Slowly open knees, and let fall toward floor.

**4.** Sit and place soles of feet together. With hands, easily push down on knees. Repeat.

**5.** Sit with one leg out straight. Bring the other leg in so that the sole of the foot is against your thigh. With hands, push down on the bent knee. Repeat and alternate.

**6.** On hands and knees, slide one leg out to the side with foot extended. Alternate and repeat.

### Hamstring and Groin Exercise

Stand with left foot pointing slightly outward, right foot straight ahead, hands behind back. Slowly lower forehead towards the left knee, and hold. Alternate.

### Arm and Torso Exercises

**1.** *Double Arm Circles* Stand, and extend arms forward. Do arm circles upward and overhead. Repeat to side and behind back.

**2.** *Shoulder Grapevine* Stand erect. Put left hand behind back, reaching up toward shoulder blades; move right hand behind head, reaching down to meet the fingers of your left hand (between shoulders). Repeat stretch in opposite direction.

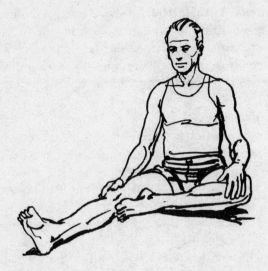

Groin Exercise #5

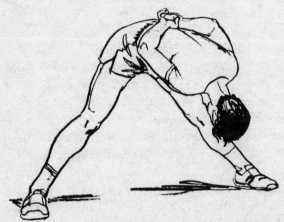

Hamstring and Groin Exercise

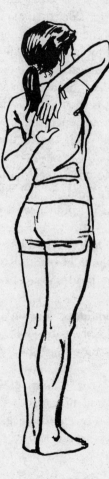

**Shoulder Grapevine**

3. *Static Trunk Stretch*  Stand an arm's length from a wall, left side facing wall, heels together, and left arm at side. Extend your right arm to your side, then slowly swing it backward and around to touch the wall. Your head follows your right arm. Force the stretch by inching down the wall with the fingers of your right hand. Repeat and alternate.

4. *Dynamic Trunk Stretch*  Stand with your back 6 to 12 inches from a wall, feet at shoulder width. Keeping knees straight, slowly reach down and touch the floor, then straighten up and slowly swing back and touch the wall. Alternate directions.

5. *Shoulder Stretch*  Lie on stomach, arms extended overhead, forehead on floor. Lift hands as high as possible, keeping elbows locked and forehead in contact with floor. Lower, rest. Repeat.

6. *Arm Down Under*  On hands and knees, bring right arm under left arm and touch shoulder blade. Reach up, extending arm straight up and twisting head upward towards outstretched hand. Repeat and alternate.

7. *Hip Raiser from Shoulders*  Lie on back, arms folded across chest, knees flexed. Raise and arch body on shoulders and feet by thrusting hips upward. Hold for a count of two or three. Repeat.

8. *Hip Raiser and Knee Hug*  Alternate the above hip raiser by drawing knees to chest and hugging them.

9. *Lower Back Stretch I*  Lie on back, legs extended. Lift and bend right knee and hip, grasping leg below the knee. Keep left leg on floor, and pull right knee to chest. Repeat and alternate.

10. *Lower Back Stretch II*  Kneeling, slowly lean back until your bottom touches your heels. Arch back, and return to starting position. Repeat.

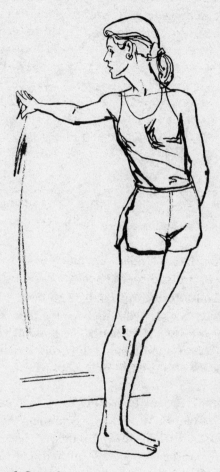

**Static Trunk Stretch**

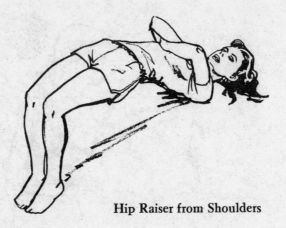

**Hip Raiser from Shoulders**

11. *Lower Back Stretch III*   Kneel with toes pointed toward each other. Slowly lean back and either let weight fall on hands placed beyond your toes, or grab ankles.

12. *Cobra*   Lie on stomach. Arms at side. Arch your back and look towards ceiling. Hold, and repeat.

### Multiple Benefit Exercises

1. *The Crawl*   Stand. In a swimming motion make a crawl stroke forward while slowly bending at knees toward almost a squatting position. Down and up, and repeat.

2. *The Swim*   Stand with feet well apart for balance. Keep legs straight, and bend forward from the hips. Using crawl strokes, bend left, center and right, and repeat. Reach out as far as possible. Keep knees straight.

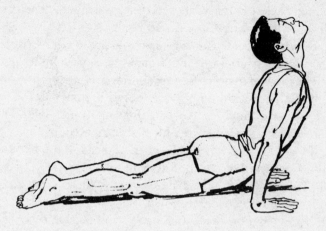

**Cobra**

**3.** *Arm Circles* Stand with clasped hands together, feet apart. Keep arms straight, and make circles with hands, slowly raising arms up, overhead and back, and then slowly all the way down between your legs, and up. Also repeat to each side.

**4.** *Standing Alternate Toe Touch* Both hands together, feet apart. Belly breathe up, and stretch arms overhead, rising on toes. Flatfooted, both hands together, exhale, slowly reach down toward left toe, and hold. Repeat and alternate.

**5.** *Hamstring and Back Stretch* Sit with legs straight and together. Reach forward with both hands on legs, and lower head toward your knees. Go as close as you can comfortably, and hold. Repeat.

**6.** *Bend and Reach* Stand, heels apart, hands overhead. Slowly bend forward, reaching toward the floor; continue stretching back toward your heel line. Slowly unbend to a standing position, breathing in and stretching. Repeat.

7. *Rotator*  Stand with legs apart, hands on hips. Rotate body by bending at waist and forming a circle: front, right, back, left, forward and up. Repeat and reverse.

8. *Twist I*  Stand, extend arms outward from sides. Twist body to left and hold, center, and then right and hold. Turn head in opposite direction to add to stretch. Repeat.

9. *Twist II*  Stand with hands behind head. Raise left knee and touch right elbow to it. Alternate and repeat.

10. *Twist III*  Sit; knees flexed, hands behind neck. Alternate touching of elbow to knee.

11. *Knee to Forehead*  On hands and knees, tuck head toward stomach and bring right knee toward forehead. Then slowly raise head, looking up, and stretch right leg fully to rear and up. Alternate and repeat.

12. *Leg Swings*  Lie on left side. Slowly swing right leg forward and twist your head back to the right while swinging right arm back and to the right. Repeat by swinging right leg backwards while swinging head and right arm forward. Repeat. Roll over and do other side.

13. *Arch and Stretch*  Lie on back. Thrust hips into air, raise up on hands and heels—bending knees if necessary—and arch back. Hold. Repeat.

14. *Triangle Pose Forward*  Stand with feet wide apart, right foot at a right angle, and body twisted to right. Bend right knee so that your right thigh is parallel to floor, left leg straight. Place right hand outside right heel; left arm stretches forward, pulling away from body. Tuck head below arm, with face turned up. Weight is forward on right foot. Hold and alternate.

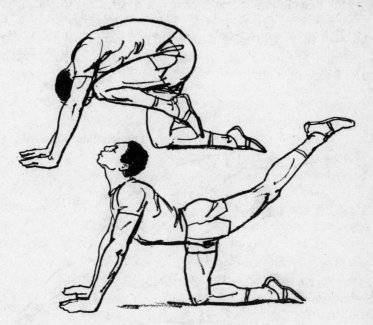

**Knee to Forehead**

**15.** *Fencer's Pose*  Stand, feet wide apart, right foot at right angle and body twisted to right. Bend right knee so thigh is parallel to floor, left leg straight. Extend both arms and stretch out and up with spine. Rotate head to right, stretching back muscles. Pretend someone is pulling both arms. Hold. Alternate.

**16.** *Praying Pose*  Stand, feet wide apart, right foot at right angle and body twisted to right. Left leg is straight. Bend right knee so thigh is parallel to floor. Clasp hands overhead and pull straight up, looking up with head. Weight shifts forward. Hold and alternate.

**Triangle Pose Forward**

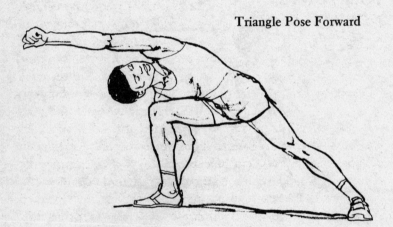

# 7 NEVER TOO YOUNG, NEVER TOO OLD

If you're young enough to walk, you're young enough to run. And if you're old enough to walk, you're old enough to run. Children run as a form of play, while adults run for more complex reasons. But there are millions of Americans between the ages of two and one hundred and six who get both pleasure and comfort from running. Two-year-old Scott Adam of Albany, New York, ran in a special 550-yard race during the 1976 Road Runner's Club National Age-Group Championship. Larry Lewis ran every day up until his death at one hundred and six, ending a string of ninety-seven years of running life.

## YOUNG RUNNERS

Running is growing fast as a sport for kids. In some areas of the country it already rivals swimming and Little League baseball. Kids should be encouraged to run year round for fitness and fun. Running in longer races with adults, however, should be a low-key effort. The Road Runner's Club of America has more than 25,000 kids in its age-group program; most of them are competing on organized teams. The most successful single program is the annual National Road Runner's Club Age-Group Cross-Country Championship held each fall in New York's Van Cortlandt Park. The 1976 races, under the direction of the NRRC's Age-Group Chairman, Barry Geisler, were a joy to watch but a headache to administer—3429 kids participated. Even Kurt Niemand, the six-year-old son of Arno Niemand, who sponsored the Championships, made a successful debut—he finished. Most important, all 3429 kids were winners—each got a trophy.

Geisler runs twenty-eight weekend age-group meets a year in the New York area. The meets are informal and low pressure, but they encourage kids to start running. Geisler, an ex-football player, took up running to keep in shape. He encouraged his two sons to run, and found that there were no programs for kids. Also, the AAU forbade children under the age of eleven to run longer than 220 yards in any meet. Geisler sponsored legislation through the Road Runner's Club to change this ruling, and began the age-group program.

The RRC developmental races are set up in groups of four race series. Each child who runs in all four races gets an award, such as a patch. The RRC program starts with the six- and seven-year-olds competing at distances of 1½ miles. As the youth ages, he or she moves up from one group to another, spending two years in each competitive level. "They normally experience one bad year and one good year," says Geisler. "It's good for them to face varying levels of competition and success as they mature."

I started working with kids and running in 1971, and now encourage pre-schoolers to run a little. I've coached championship teams in baseball and basketball, but for a coach, nothing compares with the excitement of track. And no one sits on the bench.

I feel very strongly that any youth running program must be low-keyed and begun with the objective of teaching kids long-distance running for fun. Here are some suggested guidelines:

- Sportsmanship and the Olympic ideals should always be emphasized.
- The teaching of skills should be stressed. This includes proper form and technique in all aspects of track and field. Kids should participate in several track and field events to learn as much as they can, and to avoid specialization.
- Each runner should be praised and given attention, regardless of ability. Records should be kept to give incentive for both team and personal improvement. This has proven to be a major motivating factor.
- The season should be just eight weeks, and practices scheduled only three times a week. The program should begin with two weeks of conditioning and skill development, and then intra-squad races for interest.
- All practices should be fun, and divided into four skill areas and four age groups and rotated every half hour. We never do interval work, long-distance running, or weight lifting.

Low-key. That's important. Noncompetitive. But why bother? One day, after handling a group of a hundred screaming and yelling nine- to twelve-year-olds on a hot summer afternoon, I also wondered why. As I packed away our equipment, a shy eight-year-old came up, eyes sparkling with excitement and pride, and asked, "Coach, could I please run another mile?" My outer smile didn't match the one inside.

Running is a natural extension of play. Dr. Ernst van Aaken, who has spent much of his life in sports medicine and working with children, spoke in 1976 at a RRC clinic in New York City. He said that "a child is born a long-distance runner, his play is running, and innumerable X-ray exams have demonstrated that the heart of a child has a more favorable volume relative to body weight than adults." Studies show that the typical nine-year-old has the biggest heart volume for his weight that he will ever have, unless he trains hard to be a world class endurance athlete.

Dr. van Aaken added that the play of children is really a long-distance run interrupted by several breaks. He once measured the total distance covered by a seven-year-old boy at play. The lad covered 5 miles in 90 minutes, taking 400 breaks. A healthy child, according to Dr. van Aaken, can run and play all day long and thus should be encouraged to participate in endurance sports rather than "ball sports" that only promote speed and power.

Other recent medical research shows that even "untrained" children have high rates of oxygen intake, which is considered a good measure of endurance fitness. In fact, many nine- and ten-year-old children score higher than all the highly trained distance runners. Most interesting is the fact that the untrained children scored as high as the trained children, which may indicate that endurance is something we are blessed with as children, but squander as we age.

I like to see children introduced to running at an early age, but not pushed into it. Running should be self-motivated. Bennett Gershman is a New York attorney and a top marathon runner, representing the Central Park Track Club. In the 1976 WBAI Six-Mile Race, I was surprised to see Bennett far back in the field. Then I noticed that he was running with a big smile on his face, accompanied by a similar one on the face of his eight-year-old son Seth, who was running his first race. Was the father pushing the son into his sport? Bennett said absolutely not. "During the summer I often run along the beach at Fire Island. Seth would see me run and occasionally, as a five-year-old would, ask if he could come along. It was his idea from the beginning. We now run together early in the morning a couple of times a week. We go an easy 2 or 3 miles in Central Park. It gives us a chance to be alone together and creates a stronger father-son bond. Seth used to watch me at races; he asked if he could run one, so we did. He was really excited about the whole thing, especially when he received a trophy for being the youngest finisher, as well as lots of applause from a big crowd. We ran another race and he didn't get a trophy. He was disappointed, but I think he understood. I definitely believe that my son enjoys his running, and I don't want to see his fun ruined due to either one of us taking it too seriously."

He was right; I think there are specific guidelines for working with kids interested in running:

- Don't let the sport shift from being playful to being too goal-oriented. An adolescent especially can be helped or crushed by running competition. As a shy, skinny teenager, I felt that no one recognized me until I was a track star. Suddenly my confidence rose and I became more outgoing. The discipline of running can also give a kid a steadying influence—as it can an adult—at a time when life may seem to be "a real bummer." One of the teenage girls on our team recently asked me to write a letter of reference for her college résumé. I did, emphasizing the fact that anyone who could make the sacrifices to train for and successfully complete long-distance races— in her case a marathon—would indeed have the self-discipline to make a good college student.

- Beware of the pressures involved with the sport. Dr. George Sheehan warns that "Competition and parental ego are the main stumbling blocks to young runners." I've seen parents scream and yell at children after races because they didn't perform as well as the adult thought they should. Parents and coaches should step back from the kids and leave them alone. Adult training methods are for adults, not kids. (Incredible as it may seem, I once discovered that a parent was introducing a young runner to carbohydrate loading before a marathon, a process that includes the possibly dangerous depletion cycle.)

- Let kids learn to lose. You can only appreciate winning by losing a few. I also think we are too award conscious. The New York RRC used to give out awards to the youngest finishers at races. It was a cute idea—until the parents began arguing over the trophies and withdrawing kids from races.
- Praise the child, win or lose.
- Practices should be fun. There's enough competition in the races. Parents should encourage their children to run with them, but only at the child's suggestion and his or her pace.
- Remember, children, like adults, have their ups and downs. Geisler emphasizes that "The body has just so much energy. When more is needed during growth stages, less will be available for running, and performance is affected. Coaches need to be aware of this concept."
- If the child wants to join a team, be sure that the coach is responsible and that he puts the emotional and physical health of team members before winning.
- The ultimate goal should be long-range: It should be the fun of running and the need for fitness, not the compulsion to win. There's a whole, big overcompetitive

world waiting for the child when he becomes an adult. A balance should be maintained between preparing the child for competition and depriving him of his right to grow up at his or her own speed through play and sports.

How far should kids run? As far as they want to, and as far as they can without hurting themselves. Most races for young-sters are between ½ and 2 miles. Several teen-agers I know run 4 to 10 miles regularly. Beyond that distance there is a problem. Marathons are increasingly becoming testing grounds for children. A child may negotiate a marathon comfortably, provided he or she takes rest breaks, if necessary. If the child feels forced to finish despite injury, illness, boredom, bad weather or whatever, then he or she could be emotionally or physically harmed. I also feel that children running long distances should be accompanied by an adult in case of diffi-culty. (The child may take care of the adult!)

Barry Geisler is quick to point out that he made mistakes with his own kids. But age-group running is so new that we sometimes learn through errors. At age eleven, his son Barry, Jr. ran a string of ten marathons, one every other week. His best time of 3:17 was of national caliber. Both his sons ran 50 to 80 miles per week, and even some 50-milers. But they developed Osgood-Schlatter disease as a result of all the pounding on their young, growing bones. The growing end of the bones knobbed out, resulting in pain and a knock-kneed running style that caused further injury. The only solution was rest.

Children shouldn't be encouraged to race more than 6 to 10 miles, even if they can handle more. High mileage places a stress on growing bones. Barry says, "Also, if the kids only run long and slow as they are growing up, they develop a shuffle style of running. I'd rather see them run all out more often, which is a natural thing for kids. Most of our teams have two long, slow workouts per week and one session of speed work. On the other hand, the CYO team of Washington, D.C., which completely dominated the RRC Nationals, won't allow kids to make the trips to meets if they don't put in at least 60 miles of distance work in addition to speed work the week of the race."

What is best? We can take the East German approach and train kids seriously at a young age for possible future stardom (which our age-group swimmers and gymnasts are now doing), or we can take the run-for-fun approach. Perhaps the Road Runner's Club method of something in between is best.

The greatest dream of the addicted adult runner may be for a young son or daughter, who wakes them up on a Sunday afternoon snooze with the plea: "Daddy, would you like to go for a run with me?"

## SENIOR RUNNERS

When President Jimmy Carter stepped out of his limousine, and walked back to the White House after his Inauguration in 1977, people were shocked and surprised. What they missed might have surprised them even more. On the President's-Council-on-Physical-Fitness-and-Sports float in the parade not far behind the president was Paul Fairbank, on an exercise treadmill, jogging in place for the two-hour march. Still not surprised? Fairbank is seventy years old, and a marathon runner. He started running when he was sixty-two, and completed his first marathon in 1976, in 3:58. Moreover, after "jogging" the Inaugural route, Fairbank rested two days and then ran a 20-mile race sponsored by the D.C. Road Runners.

Yet Paul Fairbank is not unusual. More middle-aged and older Americans are running now, and even entering competition. The masters group is getting larger, and in some major races more than half the field consists of men and women over forty years old, although all age breakdowns vary around the country. In 1975, Toronto hosted the first World Master's Track and Field Championship and several hundred runners participated.

In most parts of the country, men and women in the Masters category (over forty) race against each other and are scored separately in ten-year age breakdowns. The Road Runner's Club of New York, for example, categorizes runners this way: Sub-masters (ages thirty to thirty-nine), Veterans (forty to forty-nine), Masters (fifty to fifty-nine), and Seniors (sixty and older). Some races now even have a seventy-plus division.

The result of this breakdown by age is that the older runner gets a "new life." How many sports allow a fifty-year-old to compete against his or her peers for a trophy? Runners secretly watch the calendar as they await their chance to move into a new age group, and be called "the new blood" or "kids." Team competition further reinforces the athlete's acceptance and pride in being fit. The spirit of the Masters runner is very high. Dr. George Sheehan, himself a fifty-eight-year-old Masters champion, notes in *Dr. Sheehan on Running,* "We are continually capable of doing everything we did in our prime—a little slower, perhaps, somewhat weaker, surely, but if they wait around long enough we'll finish." One of the Masters groups that has a lot of fun is the Scarsdale Antiques. This club was formed in 1971 by men and women in their fifties, sixties and even seventies to promote running for young and old alike. The Antiques often place several members in races around the metropolitan New York area, and entered 20 runners in the

1977 Marathon, inspired by Stanley Newhouse, a sixty-seven-year-old insurance executive.

As we age, our bodies betray us; we recover more slowly from hard runs, and we are much more brittle and inflexible. At a recent RRC sports medicine clinic, a middle-aged runner complained of a series of chronic injuries. Dr. Richard Schuster summed up his problem by saying, "Look at the calendar, my friend."

Studies made by Dr. L. E. Bottinger, a professor of medicine at the Korolinska Hospital in Stockholm, showed that distance runners peak in performance between the ages of twenty-six and thirty. His study indicates that racing times become slower from that point almost linearly with age, while decreases in performance drop about 6 to 7 percent with every decade. Maximum oxygen consumption and response of blood flow to the stimulus of exercise decrease with age. Maximum heart rate is the key to performance because it controls the oxygen needed during exercise. The faster you run, the more you need. But the older you are, the less you get.

Muscular strength also peaks between twenty-six and thirty, and decreases very slowly during maturity. By our fifties strength decreases at a greater rate, but even at age sixty the loss does not exceed 10 to 20 percent of maximum.

Still, physical exercise, and especially running, does make us feel better. It may not prevent heart disease or promote longevity, but it does increase the size of our coronary arteries, and turn our hearts into better pumping machines. It is believed to have a positive effect upon the condition of the bones in old age and the functioning of the joints. Exercise, then, plays a key role in relief of two of the nemeses of old age: osteoporosis and osteoarthritis.

According to Dr. Hans Kraus, a skier and rock climber at

the age of seventy-two, "Unfit persons age more quickly. They suffer from a deficiency of sufficient exercise and all the benefits exercise means to the body." When I return home and see the deteriorated condition of some of my classmates, I'm convinced that too many of us get old before our time. It may be that the elderly do not exercise because society doesn't expect it of them. An old man jogging along the road is still considered a nut. But fitness programming for the middle-aged and elderly is now becoming more popular as a greater percentage of our population consists of men and women over sixty. Dr. Kraus believes that we need to do more than mere "reclamation jobs" with the elderly. Since many of the disabilities we associate with old age result from years of inactivity, he recommends regular exercise (preferably begun in childhood) followed by a program of flexibility exercises, walking or swimming to prevent aging.

Women runners in the Masters category seem to get better with age. Miki Gorman of California's San Fernando Valley Track Club began running at age thirty-three. Five years later, in 1973, she held the world's record for the women's marathon —2:46:36. In 1976, at age forty-one, she ran 2:39:11 at the New York City Marathon, the third fastest women's marathon in American history.

Toshiko d'Elia, who teaches the deaf, was a mother in her late thirties when she started jogging. Her first race was a 2-mile cross-country run which her twenty-year-old daughter Erica suggested she run so that none of the high school girls would come in last. But Tosh finished third and won a trophy, and has been hooked on running ever since. Toshika is now a member of the Greater New York AA.

Within two years, she was a nationally known runner. In 1975, at the age of forty-seven, she competed in the United

States Masters National Track Championship and ran third in the 5000 meters. She then went on to Toronto for the First World Masters Track Championship and won second place in the same event with a time of 19:26.5—only a tenth of a second off a world record! In 1977, she finished second in the forty-five to forty-nine age group at the World Masters Marathon Championship in Sweden. Her time was 3:05:20.

Her first marathon was the Jersey Shore Marathon, run in 1976 in icy, snowy conditions with a windchill factor of —19°. She intended to run only halfway, but the friends who had arranged to pick her up in a car never appeared and she was forced to finish—running a 3:25 marathon that qualified her for Boston. She finished in 3:04 in the 1977 Boston Marathon, copping a twelfth place.

The Pike's Peak Marathon climbs from 6500 feet to 14,110, and Marcie Trent of the Pulsators Track Club of Anchorage, Alaska, ran up and down the 28-miler in 5:23:10 in 1974, which at the time was a course record. She was fifty-six years old! Brenda Ueland ran and hiked halfway up the mountain in 1975 when she was eighty-three. She's vowed she'll return.

Ruth Baker, a fifty-four-year-old soap opera actress, enrolled in our beginner's fitness program, lost twelve pounds and found running "a natural high." Says Ruth, "I find that the more I run, the more confidence I get. It's really increased my belief in myself. Now I have proof that I don't have to be limited because of my age." Ruth ran in the 1976 Mini-Marathon, and finished with a huge smile. Later that evening on her way to dinner with her husband, she was wearing her medal proudly around her neck for all to see. With a bit of encouragement, more older women could know the joys of running. It's too easy to say, "Hey, I'm too old to do it." That's just not true. Nobody should give up because of her age.

Joe Marinucci of New Windsor, New York, is the oldest competitor on our club and is a real ball of fire. He ran the 1976 New York City Marathon, his first, at the age of sixty-eight, and finished in 4:16:05, ending in an all-out sprint for the last 100 yards "to give the people a thrill." Joe asks, "Why do I do it? Well, to demonstrate physical fitness to kids and their parents, mostly. I hope that people will notice and ask themselves how come a sixty-eight-year-old gets younger every day. Maybe it will lead some kids to cut out the cigarettes and beer blasts, and discover that working out is a better thing to do."

Joe's main goal in life is to catch Johnny Kelley, currently the top marathoner in the sixty-five to seventy age group. Joe states, "I want to be the national champ at age seventy." Catching Kelley may be tough. The amazing Kelley has run forty-six Boston Marathons, winning in 1935 and 1945. The former Olympian is honored at Boston each year by wearing the number one, and his fans cheer him every step of the route. At the age of sixty-eight, he ran the 1976 Boston Marathon in 3:20 despite 100° heat.

However, there are other young upstarts moving in. One of our club members, Don Dixon, threatens the records of such greats as Clarence De Mar and Johnny Kelley. Dixon, fifty years of age, ran the 1977 New York City Marathon in 2:39:57. Don started running at age forty just to get in shape, and became a typical YMCA 2-mile-a-day runner. At the age of forty-four, he entered his first race, the Yonkers Marathon, and ran 3:35. He later found he could maintain a fast pace throughout a race, and he discovered something about himself: "I think the secret of my success is consistency. I run year around and thus have accumulated lots of miles in the bank." Don feels it takes longer now for him to recover, but he picks his races and runs with the best. He adds, "I plan my running schedule better now. Also, when I lose the desire to run and my body tells me I need rest, I don't hesitate to take a day off. I feel it's important for older runners to ease off in training at least twice a year and come back strong, keying for a big race. As we get older, we need more rest. Many of the Masters runners run too much, or run too little and then try to race too hard." Don trains 40 to 60 miles a week, and leaves many younger competitors far behind. Most important, he says, "I feel as good as I ever have in my life. The more I run, the younger I feel."

Another older marathoner, Flory Rodd, says he runs 120 miles per week because he needs the stamina work. The fifty-three-year-old Californian noted, with a twinkle in his eye, "I couldn't even finish a marathon on less than 60 miles per week." To each his own.

Ted Corbitt is so famous as a runner that a book was written about him (*Corbitt* by John Chodes). He ran his first marathon at age thirty-one and at age fifty-eight is still running them. In 1968, at forty-eight, Ted won the National 50-Mile Championship in 5:39:45, and became the oldest runner ever to win the national distance racing title. The next year, he ran 100 miles on a track in 13:33:06, and cut three-and-a-half hours off the American record. At the age of fifty-three, in 1973, he ran twenty-four hours on a track and completed 136.4 miles. Corbitt, who was the first New York RRC president in 1958, says that as runners age they must learn to adapt to the changing condition of their bodies. "Fitness can't be stored," he says. "It must be earned over and over, indefinitely. If a man runs for twenty years and stops completely, it is just a matter of time until he is in the same condition as the fellow who has never done any running."

The oldest noncompeting member of our running club is

Sam McConnell, who at age seventy-seven runs 6-mile workouts four times a week at the local Y. He also often ice skates twice a week. Sam began running in 1921 in high school, and later at the University of Pennsylvania. He never stopped, and during business trips ran in cities around the U.S. and overseas. "I attribute my success as a person, and certainly my longevity, to running. I recently went to a college reunion. It was pathetic! All of my classmates had either passed away or were dead on their feet. I feel great, running keeps me young!"

The oldest member of the National Jogging Association is 107-year-old Zachariah Blackistone of Washington, D.C. In the March 1977 *Jogger*, Blackistone commented upon his great physical condition and mental awareness (he's an active millionaire), "I owe it all to exercise, especially jogging. When I wake up I think I'm dead. Jogging brings my blood pressure up and I feel like a man. I'm ready for the whole day."

Larry Lewis may be the most celebrated runner in history. He was 106 years old when he died, in 1974, of cancer. Up until his death, he ran 6.7 miles every morning at 4:30 a.m. around San Francisco's Golden Gate Park; he then reported to work as a full-time waiter at the St. Francis Hotel. Sometimes he walked the 5 miles to work as well. In the March 1974 issue of *Runner's World*, Larry Lewis said it all, "Never say a person is so many years *old*. Old means something dilapidated and something you eventually get rid of, like an old automobile or a refrigerator. I'm not in that category. You may become mellow, but never old."

# 8 WOMEN ON THE RUN

There have been several obstacles placed before women who want to run. One is mental, another physical, and a third is the reaction of men. Even so, women runners are more and more evident. They are running in races with men, and even in special long-distance races for women competitors, who are no longer uncommon.

The mental barrier to running may be the toughest. Some women still believe that it is unfeminine to put on shorts, a T-shirt and running shoes, and get out and jog and sweat. Some wouldn't think of running when pregnant. Yet many are overcoming these inhibitions and today even pregnant women runners are becoming almost commonplace. Take the case of Mary Jones, thirty-two, of Dallas, Texas, who in her eighth month of pregnancy, ran a 2:05 half-marathon at the White Rock Marathon in December 1976. Her preparation was jogging 40 miles a week. "My doctor told me to listen to my body and as long as I felt good about running, continue to do it," she said. "My idea of a beautiful delivery would be to run 13 miles in the morning and have the baby later that day."

Physical characteristics make women runners different from men. Researchers Dr. Ernst van Aaken and Herbert A. de Vries (author of *Physiology of Exercise*) point out that women have only 85 to 90 percent of heart size of men, and they also have smaller lungs. They have more body fat, but smaller bones and less muscle. Women generally weigh less than men of the same height, and have less power to propel the mass. They are slower over short distances.

But women have more endurance, and they may suffer pain better. Dr. van Aaken believes that "Women are born with greater natural stamina. Men, on the other hand, will always throw farther, jump higher, run faster for shorter stretches. Forty percent of man's body weight is muscle; in women, muscle amounts to only twenty-three percent. Instead of this, women have more hypodermal fatty tissue—and that is the source of energy for hours' long exertion." Women runners, Dr. van Aaken suggests, may become very competitive with men at long distances.

So, in the long run, these differences may not be obstacles at all. Still, the woman who runs must be concerned with her menstrual cycles, and possibly birth control devices, pregnancy and motherhood. All may be shared with the man in her life, but only two can be exchanged: You can let *him* watch the kids while you run, and you can let him practice birth control.

The biggest obstacle women runners have faced has been men, especially some officials and organizers. For too long, women have had to run behind men—separate and unequal. Most major track events, even the Olympics, limit a woman's participation. Only recently have women been welcomed into such prestigious contests as the Boston Marathon.

In the early 1900s, women were allowed (by men) to whack a tennis ball in ladylike fashion, or swim—if well covered up. British women who dared to race were called "brazen doxies." Not until 1928 could women run in the

Olympics, and when several untrained ladies collapsed at the finish of the 800-meter race, the race was labeled "frightful." The event wasn't held again until 1960. Even today, the longest running event for women in the Olympics is the 1500 meters —less than a mile.

Luckily, the feminist awakening of the 1960s gave women tools to fight for their rights, and one is the right to run as far and as fast as they are able. One myth women faced was that long-distance running would make them muscle-bound. Chris McKenzie, a former world record holder at 800 meters while living in Britain, decided to convince American male officials they were wrong. She arrived at a monthly meeting wearing only a bikini and a coat. When the subject of muscles came up, Ms. McKenzie peeled off her coat and asked if she was too muscular. Only then was she given permission to run longer distances.

Still, men were slow to learn. In 1966, Roberta Gibb Bingay ran the Boston Marathon—unofficially because her entry was refused. The next year, Kathrine Switzer got an official entry number when she sent in her application as "K. Switzer." Race officials, thinking she was a he, let her run; she was several miles into the marathon before being discovered. When Jock Semple, the race director, caught up to her, he tried to rip her number off. Kathy Switzer's boyfriend deposited Jock on the curb, and because the action took place before the press bus, the media couldn't miss the message. Kathy's plight and photos were in newspapers coast-to-coast.

A few days afterward, she was thrown out of the AAU. They gave her four reasons: She had fraudulently entered the race; she had run with men; she had run longer than the allowable distance; and she had run without a chaperone.

Yet, she had completed the race in 4:20. In 1973, in her

home town of Syracuse, she paced me to my first sub-3:30 marathon, which qualified *me* for the Boston run. In 1975, she was the first American woman across the Boston finish line, running a 2:51:37 marathon. The boys behind her ate their hearts out.

As barriers fall, it is difficult to remember how ridiculous they were. Before the 1972 New York City Marathon, for example, the AAU suddenly decided that women would not be allowed to run with men. The women would run separately, beginning their race 10 minutes ahead of the men. (Ladies first!) But when the starting gun fired, the women, in protest, sat down behind the starting line and waited for the men's race to begin 10 minutes later. When the men started, off went the women, too—all of whom voluntarily had 10 minutes added to their running times. This discrimination prompted a civil rights lawsuit against the AAU, which finally gave in and ruled that men and women may start "from a common line at a common gunshot," but must be scored separately and compete for separate prizes.

This took place a year after an important New York Marathon—as important to women's running as Englishman Roger Bannister's classic race in May 1954 in which he broke the four-minute mile barrier was to running in general. The goal was for a woman to break the 3-hour mark. On a hilly Central Park course, Beth Bonner made history by holding off the challenge of Nina Kuscsik, 2:55:22 to 2:56:04. The current women's record, set in 1977, is 2:34:47, held by West Germany's Christa Vahlensieck.

In 1976, Nina Kuscsik, American record holder for 50 miles, spoke at a Marathon Conference held by the New York Academy of Sciences. "Girls and women, ages ten to seventy, have become marathon runners," she told the conference. "It is an exciting time to be a female long-distance runner. National and international competition exists for us.

"Since the marathon is an event that comes to the people, we and the public share a unique spontaneity; that of our reactions toward one another. And in only a few years the reaction has changed considerably. Spectators appreciate our athletic abilities more and have become less concerned that we are women.

"Like our male counterparts, we sometimes wonder what cravings keep us on the road. Pre-race nerves and the fatigue that inevitably envelopes us en route have no sexual preference. Women, too, feel a tiredness that affects our whole psyche. . . . Indeed, we love to run and we welcome the intensities of a life-time that can be captured in the span of our races. There we find an admirable interdependence of our mental, emotional, and physical energies. We've concluded that marathon running is a truly human and healthy endeavor. This, however, is a very contemporary conclusion."

Nina is right. Only recently have we become accustomed to seeing women run with men in Boston or New York or other marathons. One of the best races for women, in my opinion, is the Mini-Marathon, organized by the New York Road Runner's Club. The Mini was the first race in the world for women only. In 1972, 72 women showed up in Central Park to run it. The sponsor was getting sued, and the race was unknown. In 1973 and 1974, the RRC itself sponsored the race, and in 1975 and 1976, my friend Arno Niemand provided sponsorship. By 1976, the Mini had grown to 429 women runners.

Just one year later, the 1977 Mini was a spectacular event. More than 2064 starters began the race, including several pregnant women and thirty-six mother-daughter teams. One pair was sixty-five and forty-one years old. The field also included some top competitors, some beginners, and a lot in between. They ranged in age from five years old to sixty-eight! The sponsor was Bonne Bell Cosmetics. Its chairman Jess Bell is an enthusiastic runner and his wife Julie participated in the race. The Mini in 1977 was a Maxi: the largest "women only" running event in the world.

What a celebration of feet! Before the start, these more than 2000 women held hands and sang "America the Beautiful," and a national championship all-girls band led the runners to the starting line. Balloons filled the air, and more than 500,000 people lined much of the route around the park— attracted by the race and the annual "Taste of the Big Apple" festival. Mayor Abraham Beame counted down from ten, and fired the starter's gun.

The race covers 6.2 miles, a little more than a complete loop in Central Park. The run offers any woman the chance to race. Kathy Switzer, writing in the RRC *Newsletter*, caught the true magic of the Mini, "Here was a race with publicity, planning, a strong competitive field and one other ingredient for spice. When you add that elusive element—the individual, noncompetitive, otherwise ordinary woman—the race fairly bulges with hundreds of hearts all pumping wildly with determination to succeed personally, to accomplish, and to mix dreams and fantasy with sweat, sisterhood and liniment. It seems only for that one day, but indeed!—the Mini is that one moment in time that pulls hundreds of women through the months of slogging rainy-day workouts, carping secretarial pools and screaming kids, and it is the one moment that they can savor and use for fuel the rest of the year."

In 1977—the race is usually held in late May or early June —Peg Neppel of Iowa State ran the Mini in 34:15, a new record by 50 seconds. Chantal Langlacé of France, former holder of the world marathon record at 2:35, was third. Miki Gorman, the little super runner from California, had a choice of taking the First Place National AAU Masters Trophy (she's forty-four) or the eighth-place AAU Nationals Open. She took the open as a symbol of her youth and to pass the Masters Trophy on to encourage more older women to run. Toshika d'Elia of the Greater New York AA, then forty-seven, won that trophy, and said, "Never mind your age, just keep running."

It was Laura Craven from Cleveland, a twelve-year-old who finished seventh at a sub-6 minute pace, who summed it up, "What a great day for us *women* runners!"

The old myths are dying—slowly. I am certain that we will see women long-distance runners breaking men's records. Remember those physical differences? According to Dr. van Aaken, "Psychologically, men are more explosive, inconsistent, not enduring, and in pain and exertion—especially among high-performance athletes—somewhat sniveling. A woman is the opposite: tough, constant, enduring, level and calm under the pain to which her body exposes her (during childbirth). On the average, she is more patient than a man. Armed with these advantages, women are in a position to do endurance feats previously considered by men to be impossible."

Physically, and psychologically, women may be prepared for great runs. But will men allow that to happen? I think so, but with time. While male runners are usually supportive, there are still some men who grumble about women in *their* race, and others who insist upon following the fastest woman during a race, and gleefully sprinting by her to avoid losing to the opposite sex. When I once wrote that men whose pre-race strategy was not to let a woman beat them are male chauvinists, an apparently guilty man threatened me physically and announced that he could beat any woman any time. He also called me a communist.

Further, too many women I have helped train get onto the jogging paths full of enthusiasm and spirit, and run smack up against the worst kind of male chauvinism from nonrunners. They become targets of verbal and sometimes physical abuse. They become afraid of running alone. I tell them just to keep running; with their improved fitness they can usually outdistance the old-fashioned male jogger. Male runners, however, are usually supportive—at least until the race begins.

Still, I'm afraid there are some safety guidelines that men and women runners together outline for women:

- Try to run with a friend. Run alone only in daylight in safe areas populated with other runners and strollers.
- If you run alone, wear a loose shirt, ugly gray sweat pants, and a plain old hat. Look as though you mean business, and are headed somewhere (even if you're lost).
- If you hear someone coming up behind you, pick up your pace slightly, and look back.
- Avoid obvious places of ambush: alleys, bad neighborhoods, thick bushes, and so on. Run along streets on the road, away from buildings.
- Carry a hat pin or dog spray.
- Be in shape. I know of several women who have broken away from attackers and outrun them.
- Don't be careless: A lonely country road, no matter how lovely, can be as unsafe as a city park.

One solution to this problem is for all of us—men and women—to educate men. Let them know clearly that women runners are out there for the same reasons they are: to get into shape, to compete, to feel healthy, to meet friends and enjoy companionship.

Dr. Kenneth Foreman wrote about men for the United States Women's Track Coaches Association newsletter: "The reasons for our attitudes toward women who participate and excel in sport are complicated at best. I submit, however, that for most men the problem is this thing called ego. In western society, sport constitutes one of the last frontiers wherein the male can assert his superior strength. For females to engage in sport, or show superiority in the male domain, is an open threat to the male of the species. Perhaps it is understandable that a threatened male would be critical of a female who makes him feel ill at ease with himself. What is not understandable, however, and can no longer be tolerated is the insistence that the female athlete be accepted only on the male's terms—that is, poorly coached, inadequately supported, and publicly recognized only if she passes the 'pretty' test."

Despite the obstacles—and not one is insurmountable—women should run. They need the exercise as much as men. Like men, they suffer from sedentary jobs that add fat, not tone, to their bodies. And, as women become more liberated, they, too, are suffering from diseases of high-pressure occupations: high blood pressure, stress, heart attacks—in fact, the rate of heart disease among younger women is increasing dramatically.

I am amazed at the scarcity of information available to women who *want* to run. Women are easy to coach, especially beginner runners wanting to move up into competitive running. However, I strongly suggest that women who are just beginning avoid being coached by a husband or boyfriend. Either one may be condescending as you make him run slower than usual at first. Then, he may get hostile when you run faster than he does. Don't run at all with your husbands or boyfriends in the beginning unless they really enjoy and encourage your running. Runners may make better lovers, but sometimes lousy spouses. The New York City Marathon has been named in at least one divorce proceeding for causing "incompatibility" between husband and wife runners. Another caution: I know three world class women runners who married their coaches.

One woman runner, a good friend of mine, is Kathryn Lance, author of *Running for Health and Beauty: A Complete Guide for Women*. Kitty started as a beginner runner at age thirty, and now is one of our club's noncompetitive runners. I helped her with her book, and she helped me with this chapter. She also gives a woman good reasons to run. "You have been cheated," Kitty writes in her book. "Throughout your entire life, your family, your schools, society itself—all have systematically cheated you of one of your most fundamental rights: the right to a healthy, active body.

"Studies show that girls tend to reach their peak of physical fitness at about age thirteen or fourteen—and from there on it's straight downhill. This is because from the time we are very young our culture simply doesn't encourage females to take care of their bodies. Worse, in subtle and not-so-subtle ways, we are actually discouraged from using our bodies in a truly athletic way. . . .

"Today, almost everyone agrees that women have a right to earn as much money as men for equal work. But where you stand on the question of woman's place in society is irrevelant. . . ."

Women runners have helped prepare this chapter, and

here are several topics they feel important to women who want to run. They are listed somewhat in the order that they occur during life.

## MENSTRUATION

Most women occasionally experience bothersome symptoms related to their menstrual cycle. These symptoms may include cramps, depression, irritability, backache, nausea, weakness, a feeling of "heavy legs" or of being bloated due to water retention.

Medical opinion suggests that women not exercise strenuously during the first two days of their menstrual period. A heavy flow may make exercise impractical, or severe cramping may make it uncomfortable.

Most doctors agree, however, that reasonable exercise during menstruation is not only acceptable, but also helpful. Exercise that improves blood circulation and muscular strength and flexibility in your abdominal area is desirable. Further, it frequently relieves the discomforts of cramps and backache. Exercise may also relieve irritability and other emotional symptoms. A conditioned body is simply better prepared to handle this monthly stress.

Women report that their menstrual periods do not affect their performance in races. One study of Olympic athletes found that they won gold medals during all phases of their monthly cycle. In fact, training may be more troublesome than racing. The reason is logical: The runner will overcome discomfort in the excitement of a race, but not in the drudgery of practice.

Most women runners we talked with find that running doesn't make menstrual cramps worse, but running may be slower during this time. Many find that cramping actually diminishes or disappears while running. Some women runners report that running regulates their periods, but others, who are training with high mileage, report that amenorrhea, or total cessation of their periods, sometimes occurs for a few months during this training. This condition certainly worries them, but it is not considered harmful and generally returns to normal either by your body adjusting to the demands of training, or by cutting your mileage.

Running may help eliminate some physical problems by increasing blood flow and reducing body water retention through sweating. Moreover, as a runner experiences various pains associated with running, she may more easily adjust psychologically to the pains involved with her period.

Painful menstrual cramps may be caused by the swelling of pelvic blood vessels that supply the uterus, ovaries, Fallopian tubes, and upper vagina prior to menstruation. Doctors and women alike realize that there are also complicated psychological reasons that may create painful cramps, many of them created by the attitudes of the woman's mother or peers toward menstruation.

Kathryn Lance has some good insights into the psychological factors of women and menstruation. "Many of us have been taught that we are in a weakened condition at this time, and so we are used to doing as little as possible while we are menstruating, if not actually taking to bed. Because of these years of conditioning, the thought of any really strenuous activity seems foreign and a little dangerous to most of us— almost against the laws of nature.

"Unfortunately, what most of us *didn't* know all these years was that doing something strenuous might have been just what we needed to help avoid menstrual problems in the first place. Running not only seems to relieve cramps in many women, but also helps to *prevent* them in some cases."

## ANEMIA

Blood loss from menstruation results in a depletion of iron, which may lead to anemia. Mild anemia may not affect the average woman, but it will affect the performance of the average jogger because anemia limits the oxygen-carrying capacity of the blood. Hemoglobin, the substance that carries oxygen, is composed mostly of iron. Jogging with little evidence of improvement, or dramatic decreases in performance for trained athletes may be caused by anemia.

One solution is taking more iron. The average American diet for women is deficient in iron, and women runners may want to supplement their diets with iron capsules of at least 30 milligrams daily or more iron-rich foods such as liver, leafy green vegetables, wheat germ, soyflour, edible seeds and blackstrap molasses. Your doctor should be consulted first, of course; he or she may want to give you a blood test.

## CONTRACEPTION

Women who are taking birth control pills probably don't have any problems with their running. However, Nina Kuscsik, a registered nurse, believes that as women become more attuned to their bodies through running, they may not want to use a drug like the Pill. It does make some women runners feel bloated and unenergetic at times.

The Intra-Uterine Device (IUD), however, has caused pain and discomfort in some women, which worsens when they run. Others have complained that the IUD makes them bleed so heavily during their periods that they can't run long distances. In that case, if you are wearing an IUD, you might want to have it removed for long-distance running, and switch to some other form of birth control. Or, have your husband or lover practice birth control so you can run free.

Running can work in other ways, too. We know of women with sterility problems who became pregnant after starting a regular exercise program. Of course, their inability to become pregnant may have been due to psychological reasons, but running does put women (and men) more in touch and tune with their bodies; it makes us aware of how we are caring for ourselves.

## PREGNANCY

Should you jog during pregnancy?

Deborah De Witt began exercising regularly when she reached thirty. Her husband, a member of the New York Road Runner's Club, convinced her that running was fun and healthy. Little did she know just how healthy. "I would typically jog three times a week for a mile or a mile and a half. I am not a gung-ho runner by any stretch of the imagination, but I was getting to the point that I could run two miles with not much effort and some enjoyment. Then, we decided to have a baby. I had read Cooper's aerobics book, and I consulted with my obstetrician, who assured me that I could continue jogging as long as 'everything was going well.' "

Everything went well, and Deborah kept running. Six months came and went. She reported to her doctor monthly and told him she was still jogging. He encouraged her. "Since I felt good, I decided to continue. Of course, my pace was slowing because I was carrying a lot of extra weight, twenty pounds in all. And by the end, I was having swelling in my legs which frequently caused cramps during running, but I tried to push through. Since I was jogging three times a week regularly, I never had any sensation of a large belly swaying back and forth. But I was a sight at the YMCA track in my green man's extra-large T-shirt and my maternity shorts."

Deborah ran a 10-minute mile during her exercise class on a Monday, and on Wednesday began labor. She was in labor eighteen hours with no medication. "Because I was in good shape from the jogging and exercise and had been through childbirth classes, I was able to rotate the baby's head—it came out face up instead of face down—and did not have to have a forceps delivery." She gave birth to a 7-pound, 13-ounce boy. "I came home from the hospital with a flat stomach (I did sit-ups until about two weeks before Andrew arrived), weighing what I did before the pregnancy.

"If this sounds like a testimonial to running, it is. But it is a testimonial from an average, run-of-the-mill jogger, not a super athlete." Deborah continued her jogging after her six weeks' postpartum checkup.

Even well-trained athletes are not stopped by pregnancy; some have won Olympic gold medals while pregnant. Dr. Gyula Erdelyi of Hungary studied 172 women athletes through their pregnancies and found that two-thirds of them were able to continue training through the fourth month. The quality of their performances did not decrease during the first three months.

Dr. Erdelyi found that pregnant runners had fewer complications during pregnancy, and 50 percent fewer cesareans. He also found that duration of labor was shorter for athletes than for nonathletes.

Unfortunately, little information and few exercise classes exist to prepare pregnant women physically for childbirth. Carol Dilfer of Palo Alto, California, jogged through her pregnancy and was so excited by the way she felt that she started a Prenatal/Postpartum Aerobics Fitness Program. She found that by exercising during pregnancy, women develop firm, elastic bodies that can handle delivery better than unconditioned bodies. Women who have developed a strong cardiovascular system also recover much faster from childbirth.

Dr. Evelyn Gendel, director of the Kansas Division of Maternal and Child Health, sees no reason for women not to continue running during pregnancy if that is what they were doing before they got pregnant. But run first, get pregnant later. It is not a good idea to start a vigorous exercise program after pregnancy occurs.

There are some other rules to follow. Dr. Joan Ullyot notes in her book *Women's Running*: "A general rule for any form of exercise during pregnancy is, 'Do what you're accustomed to, as long as it feels comfortable.' If you've been jogging five miles a day, keep it up. If you find yourself getting tired more easily, cut down the mileage. If your uterus contracts wildly whenever you jog late in pregnancy, walk or swim instead, so there's less jostling.

"Using the 'talk test' while running, you'll be assured that both you and the baby are getting plenty of oxygen. The increased circulation will be as beneficial as the continued muscular toning during exercise."

Of course, before you run off, consult your obstetrician. Pregnancy is a much different physiological state than normal, and you may have complications that would make jogging inadvisable. Sadly, there are still many physicians who are anti-exercise. If your physician tells you not to jog, you should ask the reason. If the answer is satisfying, respect the opinion. But if it isn't, seek other medical advice. Find a physician who will support your desire to maintain a healthy body.

When Pamela Mendelsohn Burgess became pregnant, she continued running with her child's father, Peter. "We had always enjoyed running together," she wrote in the March 1977, issue of *Jogger*, "and I had wondered whether we would have to start going separately because of my slowness due to the added weight. Peter began to carry rocks of increasing size to slow him down. His last rock weighed in at twenty-eight pounds!

". . . The day before Rebekah was born, we went for a long run on the beach in the fog. I felt like a huge friendly cloud about to burst as I lumbered along. Peter was doing circles around me, disappearing into the fog only to reappear seconds later. He said I looked like a voluminous pillow floating through space. We found a perfect sand dollar that day, jumped into the icy ocean, had dinner out, and went to bed early. The next morning labor began, and we were off and running."

Pamela's labor lasted twelve hours. "Running had helped to prepare me, having taught me endurance, pacing, acceptance of a little fatigue, and the discipline to push on to that marvelous second wind."

The next joy is getting back into shape. One day at one of our fitness classes I noticed a woman who had been away for a few weeks. She was back, jogging along with her friends—pushing a baby carriage. She was delighted to be back, and so was baby!

## MOTHERHOOD

Dr. van Aaken believes that motherhood may improve running performance. A German study of fifteen champion women athletes who bore children during their careers found that five gave up sports after childbirth, but that two of the remaining ten maintained their performances, and the other eight improved measurably. All of the women runners agreed that after childbirth they were "tougher" and had more strength and endurance.

Many women, including nationally ranked American runners, have started jogging for the first time after they had children. Nina Kuscsik didn't start running competitively until her thirties, when she had already given birth to three children. Since then, she has run six sub–3-hour marathons, and won the women's division of the 1972 Boston Marathon. Miki Gorman was forty when she came in second in the 1975 New York City Marathon, only eight months after giving birth to her first baby.

As Kathryn Lance writes, "In short, there is no more reason (other than lack of time) for a woman not to run after becoming a mother than for a man to stop running after becoming a father." Both need to run, and perhaps the only obstacle is to convince Dad to watch the kids while Mom works out.

## MENOPAUSE

Regular exercise is even more important after menopause. With a diminished supply of the estrogen hormone—the hormone believed to make arteries more supple—women quickly become as susceptible to heart disease as men.

Further, menopause sometimes causes depression in women, for a variety of reasons. Running can provide a challenge and create goals at a time when a woman may feel her skills and value—especially as a mother with grown children—have diminished.

As we age, moreover, we become more susceptible to illness and disease. By being physically fit, we can overcome illness more quickly, and recover from surgery and other traumatic medical events more rapidly.

But, whatever your age, or physical condition, don't be cheated any longer. Our bodies are made for lifelong physical activity, and we should use them. Most women—afraid to sweat, convinced that their physical differences from men mean that they can't perform well athletically, or intimidated by husbands, boyfriends or sour lovers—have stopped regular physical activity. If you are one of them, don't be cheated any more. Start running.

# 9 RUNNING WITH MOTHER NATURE AND HER CHILDREN

Mother Nature provides us with seasons for running—from the brisk snappy weather of autumn to winter's sometimes windless mornings with light, fresh snow, or summer and spring's flowers, green hills, fresh gardens and new breath of life. She is a runner's greatest friend—and teacher.

Runners go out in every season, in every environment, in clothing invented and selected to protect us, and to please our demanding Mother. As we expose ourselves more and more to running, we also expose ourselves to the vagaries of the environment. We need to know the challenges, and to prepare for them.

## CLOTHING

Clothes provide comfort and warmth, protect against the weather, and satisfy moral custom. Unless you're running with the Suncoast Nudist Camp Joggers, you'll fulfill all these requirements.

Running clothes should be your own creation. Wear what feels best and protects you most. Forget style. Last year's fashionable jogging suit is next year's dust cloth.

### Socks

Socks are meant to protect your feet from rubbing against the shoe, which can cause blistering; to absorb sweat, which can harm your feet and cause your shoes to deteriorate quickly; and to provide cushion. Most runners wear socks all the time, while some never wear them in the summer or in races (to reduce weight) and others never wear them at all.

There are three types of athletic socks: tube, anklet and cushioned. Tube socks are long, without a shaping at the ankle or toe, and generally stay up well when you run. The elastic top does tend to loosen with laundering, and the socks will slide down the leg during long runs. The anklet covers only your foot, just up to the rim of the shoe. They are light, but offer little cushioning. They sometimes come with a little tassle in the back that keeps the sock from slipping down into the shoe, although some runners cut this off, thereby losing much of the sock's benefit. The cushioned, formed socks are shaped at the heel and toe, and are lined in the foot with terry cloth. These are comfortable and offer a cushioned pad.

Socks may bunch and fold causing blisters during hard runs or when they get wet. For this reason, I prefer the low-cut anklet (with tassle) in races and during rain storms. Switching from regular socks or tubes to anklets does reduce weight, and psychologically you feel lighter in the feet, and thus more competitive. Beware of deformities in the socks, or rough spots that can cause trouble. Also, always wear clean socks. Dirty socks can cause blisters, and they wear out sooner. At the very least, socks should be rinsed and dried prior to a second wearing.

Cotton socks are generally best. They absorb sweat and last longer. Wool socks are warmer in winter, but much hotter in summer. Wool retains warmth even when wet, and is a good choice on cold, rainy or snowy days. This type of sock wears out fast, however, and soon develops the bad habit of "drooping," often slipping into the shoe. Nylon socks are great in the rain and dry off quickly, but are hot. If you're wearing nylon shoes and socks and are passing a lake, stream or open hydrant, just soak the sock and cool off. You'll have dry feet in no time.

### Underwear

Most men run in some sort of undergarment. The preferred one is a cotton athletic supporter, or "jock," but some men prefer jockey shorts or even nylon bikini briefs to reduce chafing. "Speedo's" or other similar racing swim briefs are also used as undergarments, and new European racing shorts come with built-in supporters.

Women runners—most of them—wear underpants. Cotton absorbs sweat, but nylon, which is not particularly absorbant, doesn't get heavy or droopy with moisture. Tightly elasticized bikini panties can become uncomfortable during a run. Some women like nylon brief swimming trunks, worn without underpants.

Some doctors, mostly male, say that women should always wear a bra when they run, or risk damaging the tissues of the breast with bouncing, and develop "sagging breasts." Dr. Joan Ullyot notes in her book *Women's Running* that sagging breasts are not the result of bouncing while running, and the only reason for wearing a bra is comfort. Many small-breasted women run happily without the need of this added piece of equipment. And most large-bosomed women wear bras for comfort and discretion.

The preferred choice of bra is a stretchy nylon, one-size-fits-all type without hooks and metal strap joints, if possible. Sometimes it is necessary to wear protective tape on the skin or over these metal annoyances to prevent blisters. Large-bosomed women may need to wear a full-support bra to reduce bouncing.

### Shorts

Comfort is the key. The waist should be loose and the shorts not tight in the leg or crotch. Pants with zippers and belts are uncomfortable.

Most runners wear cheap, loose-fitting cotton shorts. Cotton, however, can cause chafing along the insides of the legs. (Vaseline applied to the inner thighs reduces this chafing.) Nylon racing shorts are lighter and preferred for competition, and are good for running in the rain because they don't absorb water and sag like the cotton models.

Some people like to run in swim trunks or cut-offs. My favorite shorts are the double-knit, stretch type. They are tight-fitting, but give with the motion of running. Women's briefs are also available in this material, and seem to be the choice of most serious female runners.

### Shirts

Cotton T-shirts are worn by almost all runners because they are comfortable, absorbent and a high-fashion item. Get your running T-shirt a size larger than your tight walk-around T-shirt to ensure freedom of movement.

Nylon mesh tank tops were supposedly invented to let air flow around the body and keep you cool. But our running club voted unanimously to do away with them because they clung and nearly suffocated the body in hot, humid weather. Of course, nylon is good in rain because it dries fast. Cotton tank tops are comfortable and popular in the summer.

But when that ole summer sun rolls around, I usually run

without a shirt. I may start out with a T-shirt, but soon remove it, tuck it into my shorts, and carry on. Why spend hours lying in the sun to catch the rays when you can run and sun at the same time?

### Rubberized Clothing

Plastic or rubberized clothing *is not* recommended and can be dangerous. People wear these outfits because they think that if they sweat more, they'll lose weight. But the weight loss following a run in a rubber suit is only temporary; as soon as you eat or drink, your weight will return to normal. Permanent weight loss comes only from burning calories, which comes from exercise. (See chapter 13.)

Plastic or rubberized clothing prevents evaporation of perspiration, which is nature's way of cooling your body. Running in rubber suits builds body heat to dangerous levels, and promotes dehydration, which can lead to muscle cramps, fatigue and perhaps heat exhaustion.

As far as I'm concerned, there is only one valid use for a rubber suit: to acclimatize the well-conditioned runner in a cool climate for a race in a hot one.

### Outer Wear

Cotton sweat pants, usually gray or blue, combined with a matching pullover cotton sweat shirt are probably the most preferred cool-weather outer wear. The sweat pants are inexpensive and have elastic at the ankles and a drawstring at the waist. They are absorbent, nonbinding and, because of their looseness, comfortable in warmer weather. But they are ugly, shapeless, don't have pockets, and shed cotton fuzz when new. They may shrink when washed, and the drawstrings—unless tied together—often disappear inside the pants during laundering. The elastic ankle bands can also cut off circulation and cause foot or leg injuries. If it's raining, cotton sweat pants get waterlogged and may droop and chafe. A pair of loose-fitting bluejeans can be an acceptable alternative if they are not too tight at the crotch or in the legs.

A common top is the cotton sweatshirt jacket with hood and zipper. You can unzip it in hot weather, or pull up the hood when it rains or snows, and the pockets, an important feature, can carry gloves, hats, keys, money and a wad of toilet paper. A pullover version, minus zipper, has a pouch.

Nylon windbreakers, sometimes coordinated with matching bottoms, protect against biting wind and repel rain. They are brutally hot, however, and can be as dangerous as rubber suits.

Warm-ups—brightly colored, striped, color-coordinated—are increasingly popular and increasingly expensive. Don't buy a "cheap" outfit here. The cheaper suits lose their form and stretch out of shape, or shrink. Make sure your warm-ups have two important items: pockets, and a zipper up the ankles to facilitate removing the pants over your running shoes. The cotton outfits are preferred in colder weather, the lighter double-knit suits in warmer weather.

### Head Gear

Short hair is cooler (in temperature) and less of a hassle. Men and women with long hair will tie it back in a pony tail, braid it, or pin it up. Hair flopping in your face can be annoying, and long hair will make you feel sweatier around the neck and head. Sweatbands keep sweat from dripping down your face or neck. Most sporting goods stores sell headbands, or you can fashion your own from colorful bandanas. Steve Stack, my friend in Rome, New York, wears the elastic band off discarded underpants as a cheap headband. Cotton hats with small visors, made for bicyclists, also make excellent hats for running in the sun. There is usually room to tuck an ice cube inside during a summer race for extra cooling.

Shepherd protects his balding head from the sun with an old African game warden's hat, similar to the soft fatigue hats worn in Vietnam. In winter, we both wear knit watch caps; they itch a little when you sweat, but they do keep you warm. Protect your head from the sun and the cold; after all, you can always take the cap off (and doing so will let heat escape from the top of your head, cooling you).

### Other Items

Some runners carry accessories to help with their runs. You may want to wear a watch to know how long you've been gone. Make sure that the band isn't too tight, and wear a cloth wristband under the watch to protect it from absorbing sweating and causing discomfort. Some women wear jewelry (and perfume) on a run; if it feels good, why not. Be comfortable. Other runners wear pedometers to measure distances. Shepherd uses one in Vermont when he plots new routes, but he also finds them inaccurate, and has to drive the route anyway to check the pedometer against the car's odometer! Other runners like lap counters to click off the mileage indoors. All of these are okay if they don't interfere with your run.

Some items are essential. I always tuck a wad of toilet paper into my shorts for emergency use. It's also wise to bring your own paper to a race; chances are they'll run out in the overworked johns. I thread my apartment keys with my shoe laces, and tie them in a double knot. Also, carry money for an emergency. You may have to take a taxi home, or make a phone call if you get hurt or lost. Paper bills can be pinned to your clothing; spare change can be wrapped in a plastic bag and pinned on. Change should be carried with bills; you may want a soda from a machine. In New York City, I pin a subway token (they have a hollow center design) to my shorts. Safety pins come in handy for pinning your keys to your shorts too. Once, while running along Riverside Drive, I felt my jockstrap snap. Luckily, my running partner, dentist Bill Horowitz, always carries an extra safety pin, and I was soon pinned together and happily on my way. Sometimes, men (or women without bras) need to put Band-Aids or Vaseline over their nipples before a long run to protect from chafing. I frequently bled from the irritation before learning this trick. Finally, I've seen a lot of runners with small radios, or even radio headphones. They look a little weird, but they really rock 'n' roll down the highway.

## WEATHER

### Heat and Humidity

Heat threatens everyone who exercises no matter how well-conditioned. A stroll on a hot day doubles the body's heat production, and a day that feels cool when you walk may be disastrous for the unprepared runner.

There are three types of heat disorders:

- Heat cramps are painful, sudden involuntary contractions of specific muscles or muscle groups.
- Heat exhaustion occurs when the cardiovascular system is overworked. Symptoms include an increased heart rate, palpitations, nausea, vomiting and, finally, fainting. The skin remains moist and cold as the runner continues to sweat.
- Heat stroke occurs when the heat regulatory system suppresses sweating. The skin will be hot and dry, and the runner may develop convulsions, collapse or go into

a coma. Heat stroke is an extreme emergency and can be fatal. It can hit without warning, but most often the symptoms are evident. Warning signs include
—not sweating although very hot
—flushed red skin
—a burning feeling in the legs
—difficulty breathing
—burning in the chest
—headaches
—feeling dizzy and delirious
—inability to think straight or run a straight line
—a chilling sensation
—suddenly finding yourself on the ground.

Treatments are different for heat exhaustion and heat stroke. With heat exhaustion (pale, clammy skin), the immediate treatment is fluid replacements and rest. After heat exhaustion, the next critical condition is heat stroke (skin dry, red and hot). A common—and wrong—first-aid treatment is to cover the victim with a blanket: This drives up the temperature even higher, and could be a fatal move. Body heat must be reduced immediately. Dr. Gabe Mirkin says: "Forget about giving the victim fluids by mouth. It is worthless. You are interested in cooling him off immediately. His temperature may be 110°. Place the victim in the shock position: legs up, head down. Evaporation is the key. Pour anything you can on the victim immediately (water, milk, Coke, Gatorade, etc.). Rub his skin vigorously to open up the surface blood vessels. Hose water on him. The best thing to do is rub ice cubes all over his body. Get him out of the sun. Above all, keep pouring something wet on him. If the patient is not lucid and able to communicate with you intelligently, get him to a hospital immediately."

Heat exhaustion can occur as a delayed reaction. I was one of the speakers at the National YMCA's Cardiovascular Health Conference in 1976. Early in the morning, I ran 20 miles in warm, humid weather, then took a quick shower and went off to the lecture without eating or replacing fluids. The room was warm and stuffy and held more than 400 people, mostly doctors, who listened intently as I delivered my slide presentation. Suddenly, I was having trouble remembering my carefully written speech; I began asking the slide projectionist to please focus the slides. The next thing I knew, I was on the floor. I was okay, and finished my lecture with an important added message: Always eat and drink plenty of fluids after a long run.

Dr. David Costill, an exercise physiologist, says a runner faces four physical limitations to performing well in a race on a hot day. First, he or she must understand that a runner can only partially adjust to heat. You cannot run faster in heat, so the next choice is to prepare yourself to be more competitive in the heat than the other runners. Second, when running, your muscles produce eleven times as much internal heat as they do at rest, and thus require more blood. But on a hot day more blood is also demanded by the skin. The result is that the runner involuntarily decreases his or her pace because of reduced circulation to the working muscles. If you ignore these restrictions and continue to push the pace, you face a third limitation: Under any heat stress the skin can only eliminate body heat at a limited rate. If heat is produced by the muscles faster than the heat is removed from the skin, an unfavorable balance results between internal heat gain and heat loss. The fourth physical limitation is the runner's heat tolerance. If the runner forces himself or herself to perform despite a critical imbalance between heat gain and heat loss, his or her body temperature may exceed 105° F., and heat exhaustion may be closely followed by heat stroke.

Air temperature is one factor to consider when running. Humidity is another. The key to body heat removal is sweat evaporation, which accounts for as much as 90 percent of heat removal. Under very humid conditions little sweat can vaporize; it is difficult for the body to lose heat. An air temperature of 60° F. with 95 percent humidity could be more dangerous than a 90° F. temperature in a dry climate.

A head wind facilitates evaporation, but a tail wind eliminates most of the air flow over the skin and therefore reduces sweat evaporation and heat loss. The position of sun and clouds is also a factor. Direct sunlight at high noon results in a rapid rise of body heat; cloud cover, of course, shields the runner. Running on an indoor track with little ventilation could be a concern on hot days, or even on cool ones if the gym is overheated.

The following guidelines to running in the heat apply to all runners, regardless of level of ability:

1. Avoid the heat. If you don't plan to race in it, don't train in it. Run during the cool of the early morning or late evening. Look for running paths that are shaded, and run on the shady side of the road.

2. Be in shape. An unconditioned runner places an extra burden on his body by running in heat.

3. Acclimate yourself to the heat. Allow 10 to 14 days of slowly progressive training to get used to new heat conditions. Your body needs time to improve the efficiency of its sweating mechanism, and its ability to reduce salt and mineral loss.

If you live in a cool area, you can "heat train" by running

three or four times a week for several weeks in double sweats to create an artificial heat stress. Buddy Edelen trained in double sweat suits in cool England and won the 1964 Olympic Trials Marathon at Yonkers, New York by more than 9 minutes. It was 90° F.

Ron Daws, an Olympic marathoner, suggests leaving on your winter wraps when spring arrives. Training in rubber suits and jogging in steam rooms are also effective. But these methods should only be used by highly conditioned athletes and plenty of liquids should be consumed before, during and after these "heat training" workouts. A slightly more human method is to train for summertime races by running during the hottest part of the day.

4. Run on cool surfaces. I once ran a 15-kilometer race on an airport runway at Griffis Air Force Base (Rome, N.Y.); the surface temperature of the asphalt was 115° F.! Hot pavement burns your feet, and the heat from the road pushes your temperature up. Try running on the dirt shoulders. Search for dirt or grass surfaces, or even a wet beachfront, on hot days. Pavement sprinkled with water is cooler. Also, the white lines on the road reflect heat, so run on them (if you can run a straight line).

5. Adjust your pace. Start out slowly and run a steady pace in both workouts and races. During workouts, take periodic rest breaks.

6. Keep your body wet. During races, pour water over your head, and allow helpers to spray water on you. Accept sponges offered to you, and douse your body with water. Be warned: I once unexpectedly doused myself with ice water and discovered agony and ecstacy. During workouts, dunk your shirt in water where you find it, and drape it over your head and shoulders. Ice is great on hot days. Put it under your hat, and

just let it melt. Or, rub it across the base of your neck and under the arms. Chew it. Carry it in your hands.

7. Drink plenty of liquids before, during and after your workouts. (See chapter 14.)

8. Dress carefully. In direct sunlight, provide the body with shade. Wear white or other bright colors that reflect the sun. A hat should protect your head and shoulders. It should be white, lightweight and well ventilated.

During the 1976 Boston Marathon, with temperatures approaching 100° F., I wore a white painters' cap with a white handkerchief attached, white shorts, white T-shirt and carried a small towel to wet myself with along the course. Golf hats, bicycling hats, terry cloth tennis hats (great for dousing in water, because they remain damp and cool), and handkerchiefs knotted at the corners are all good in hot weather. Often handkerchiefs are pinned at the back of the hat to protect the back of the neck, one of the key areas of heat absorption.

Wear a full T-shirt on sunny, hot days, not a tank top, to protect your shoulders. Cotton is preferred to nylon because it absorbs water and "breathes" more readily. On the other hand, nylon shorts may be preferred to cotton ones which tend to droop when doused with water. The best shirt may be an old cotton T-shirt with holes cut into it. It should fit loosely and not be tucked in. Some runners cut off the lower half of the shirt to aid air circulation. You may want to eliminate socks and insoles on hot days if you expect to get doused with water; they'll get wet and bunch up on you. Also "Spenco" insoles may make your feet become very hot.

Dehydration may cause a 6 to 10 percent loss of body weight, which can be very dangerous. Respect the elements on hot muggy days, but remember, you can also suffer from heat disorders in cool days, too, if you overdress.

## WINDCHILL FACTOR CHART

| Estimated wind speed (in mph) | Actual Thermometer Reading (°F.) | | | | | | | | | | | |
|---|---|---|---|---|---|---|---|---|---|---|---|---|
| | 50 | 40 | 30 | 20 | 10 | 0 | -10 | -20 | -30 | -40 | -50 | -60 |
| | EQUIVALENT TEMPERATURE (°F.) | | | | | | | | | | | |
| calm | 50 | 40 | 30 | 20 | 10 | 0 | -10 | -20 | -30 | -40 | -50 | -60 |
| 5 | 48 | 37 | 27 | 16 | 6 | -5 | -15 | -26 | -36 | -47 | -57 | -68 |
| 10 | 40 | 28 | 16 | 4 | -9 | -24 | -33 | -46 | -58 | -70 | -83 | -95 |
| 15 | 36 | 22 | 9 | -5 | -18 | -32 | -45 | -58 | -72 | -85 | -99 | -112 |
| 20 | 32 | 18 | 4 | -10 | -25 | -39 | -53 | -67 | -82 | -96 | -110 | -124 |
| 25 | 30 | 16 | 0 | -15 | -29 | -44 | -59 | -74 | -88 | -104 | -118 | -133 |
| 30 | 28 | 13 | -2 | -18 | -33 | -48 | -63 | -79 | -94 | -109 | -125 | -140 |
| 35 | 27 | 11 | -4 | -20 | -35 | -51 | -67 | -82 | -98 | -113 | -129 | -145 |
| 40 | 26 | 10 | -6 | -21 | -37 | -53 | -69 | -85 | -100 | -116 | -132 | -148 |
| | Green | | | Yellow | | | | | Red | | | |

(Wind speeds greater than 40 mph have little additional effect.)

| LITTLE DANGER (for properly clothed person). Maximum danger of false sense of security. | INCREASING DANGER Danger from freezing of exposed flesh. | GREAT DANGER |
|---|---|---|

## Cold

Too many runners stop running when the weather turns cold. The greatest obstacle to winter running is really just getting out the door. Those who fear the cold, however, cite two reasons: "freezing of the lungs," and frostbite. Freezing of the lungs is a myth. The air we breathe is warmed by the upper air passages, thus cold air never reaches the lungs. Frostbite, however, is a very real danger; it can result in the loss of fingers or toes, and has even caused death. To prevent frostbite, keep covered, keep dry, keep moving and avoid strong head winds, especially when wet. Frostbitten skin is cold, pale and firm-to-hard to touch. The first step in treatment is to warm rapidly without excessive heat. Use water about body temperature. Do not massage or, in the case of toes, walk on the injured area. Do not rub with snow. Take the frostbitten runner immediately to where he or she can get medical aid.

Then get yourself properly bundled, back on the run. You shouldn't miss the fun and excitement of running in cold weather. Dressing properly is the key. The danger of cold includes the wind, which when combined with air temperature produces something called a windchill factor. The attached chart from the *Encyclopedia of Sports Medicine* will help you find the true temperature before setting out. Running into the wind creates a lower windchill factor, while running with the wind may speed you along enough to produce a sweat.

Plan your workouts in the cold carefully. Warm up properly indoors (good advice even if you're going to shovel snow), and prepare the body for the sudden change in temperature. When running an out-and-back course, always begin running into the wind. Otherwise, you'll build up a good sweat with the wind at your back, and then turn into the biting wind for the return, which may cause frostbite or at least extreme discomfort. Be sure to remove wet clothing immediately after running to avoid getting chilled. Winter runs, also, should be shorter and slower. But they are very important in building up an endurance base for warmer weather racing, or just maintaining a fit body.

Use your own body heat to protect you from the cold. Even a slow run on a cold day produces enough internal body heat to warm up comfortably. The key is to trap this heat with insulative clothing, yet allow enough of it to escape before overheating.

Runners can overdress, especially on cold but windless days. Several layers of lightweight clothing, rather than one bulky winter coat, are best. The layers of clothing trap warm air between them. Also, as you heat up, you can unzip or remove (be careful about this) layers, replacing them as you cool off. Shepherd, running in cold Vermont winters, wears (from the skin out): athletic supporter, T-shirt, long underwear—both shirt and pants in temperatures below zero—bulky turtle-neck sweater, warm wool socks, sweat pants and shirt (with turtle neck pulled high), insulated U.S. Army gloves, knitted watch cap, running shoes and a down vest. His arms are free, and the vest can be unzipped.

If you get too hot, first remove your gloves (fold them together and carry them in one hand, or tuck them into your pocket). Next, loosen your collar, and if you're still hot, pull back your hood. A zippered top is preferred because you can unzip and zip it as you wish, to allow heat loss. Your hat or cap comes off as a last step; this results in a major loss of body heat. Reverse these steps to re-warm yourself as the temperature drops. Be careful not to discard any clothing early in a winter workout, or wait too long to get warm again. Better to be slightly too warm than slightly too cold.

Your feet are sure to be safe and warm as long as you keep running. But if you stop to rest, walk, or chat, be alert. Nylon running shoes will cool off quickly. Wool socks are warmer than cotton; one pair will usually suffice. You may wish to wear a pair of cotton socks under the wool, but be sure both pairs of socks are pulled tight and smooth to avoid blisters. A plastic bag may be tied around each foot to keep it warm and dry.

The legs usually stay warm with one layer of clothing. If two layers are needed, try tights, long underwear or old pajamas under sweat pants. Tights or long underwear are preferred by many runners to sweat pants as a single outer layer because they are less bulky. They are covered with shorts, which will help keep your privates toasty.

Cover the upper body with as many as four layers. The first should be an absorbent and nonirritating T-shirt or other undershirt. The second layer should be a good insulator, like a long-sleeved turtleneck that protects both the arms and neck. Soft, double knit ski turtlenecks are terrific. The third layer could be a wool, hooded sweat shirt, wool sweater, or the tops of your longjohns. I combine the second and third layer by wearing a hooded thermal sweat shirt with built-in layers. In extremely cold weather, when it's windy, a windbreaker of nylon is effective as is Shepherd's down vest. Nylon won't let sweat evaporate, so be careful you don't overheat.

Mittens are warmer than gloves, although I still prefer gloves for an unknown reason. Wool gloves are preferred, but if you have a habit of wiping your nose with them as I do, they can be abrasive. Thus my cotton gloves serve double duty as a handkerchief, and no one ever borrows them, either. When buying gloves, be sure that they cover your wrists. When it's really cold, I wear my G.I. woolen inserts covered with leather gloves (as does Shepherd). They have a pull-cord over the back of the wrist that traps warm air. Extreme cold also brings out my ski gloves, or even a plastic bag wrapped around my gloves. Some runners prefer to wear old socks as gloves. They can be tossed away at no great loss if they become a problem.

The most important area to keep protected is your head, from which a great amount of heat can escape. A wool ski cap that pulls over the ears does the job in most weather. A single wool band across the ears can replace a hat, or be worn with a hat for double protection of the ears.

To protect your face against stinging cold a pullover ski mask is good. I prefer models with single eye slits that cover the bridge of the nose; I also like a mouth opening because I spit a lot while I run. Still, ski masks without a mouth opening protect the lips and help to warm the inhaled air. Some runners tie a woolen scarf over their mouths for the same reason. Ski goggles will protect the eyes, which sometimes get so cold you can barely see out of them.

When racing into cold winds, I smear Vaseline all over my face to cut down on wind burns. In very cold weather be careful about touching your face with water, or even with your snow-covered gloves. The result could be frostbite. Ice forms on beards and moustaches, and according to my bearded teammate Jerry Mahrer, the ice formations on his beard serve as air cushions and actually warm the face. However, ice can be troublesome. Frequently when running in snow-bound upstate New York I had to take a warm shower with my hat on until the ice melted so I could remove it.

A good cold-war story comes from Dr. Melvin Herskowitz of Jersey City, New Jersey, who wrote the following tongue-in-cheek account, warning about the danger of frostbite for the inadequately dressed male runner. It appeared in *The New England Journal of Medicine* (January 20, 1977):

To the Editor; A fifty-three-year-old circumcised physician, non smoker, light drinker (one highball before dinner), 1.78 meters tall, weighing 70 kg with no illnesses, performing strenuous physical exercise for many years, began a customary 30-minute jog in a local park at 7 p.m. on December 3, 1976. He wore flare-bottom double-knit polyester trousers, Dacron-cotton boxer-style undershorts, a cotton T-shirt and cotton dress shirt, a light wool sweater, an outer nylon shell jacket over the sweater, gloves, and low-cut Pro Ked sneakers. The nylon shell jacket extended slightly below the belt line.

Local radio weather reports gave the outside air temperature as −8°C, with a severe wind-chill factor.

From 7:00 to 7:25 p.m. the jog was routine. At 7:25 p.m. jogger noted an unpleasant painful burning sensation at the penile tip. From 7:25 to 7:30 p.m. this discomfort became more intense, the pain increasing with each stride as the exercise neared its end. At 7:30 p.m. the jog ended, and the patient returned home.

Physical examination at 7:40 p.m. in his apartment at comfortable room temperature revealed early frostbite of the penis. The glans was frigid, red, tender upon manipulation and anesthetic to light touch. Immediate therapy was begun. The polyester double-knit trousers and the Dacron-cotton undershorts were removed. In a straddled standing position, the patient created a cradle for rapid rewarming by covering the penile tip with one cupped palm. Response was rapid and complete. Symptoms subsided 15 minutes after onset of treatment, and physical findings returned to normal.

Side effects: at 7:50 p.m. the patient's wife returned from a local shopping trip and observed him during the treatment procedure. She saw him standing, legs apart, in the bedroom, nude below the waist, holding the tip of his penis in his right hand, turning the pages of the *New England Journal of Medicine* with his left. Spouse's observation of therapy produced rapid onset of numerous, varied and severe side effects (personal communication).

Pathogenesis of the syndrome was assessed as tissue response to high air velocity at −8°C, penetrating the interstices of polyester double-knit trouser fabric and continuing through anterior opening of Dacron-cotton undershorts, impacting upon receptor site of target organ to produce the changes described.

The patient continues to jog, wearing an athletic supporter and old light cotton warm-up pants used in college cross-country races in 1939. No recurrences are expected.

Apocryphal? I'd hate to be the one to test it.

I know of runners who work out in a windchill temperature of −125° F. Now that's cold enough to frostbite any appendage! The coldest I've ever run in was −19° F. during the 1976 Jersey Shore Marathon. Three months later I was in Boston running when it was 119° F. Mother nature is an extremist.

### Snow, Slush and Ice

Snow affects your running while it falls and when it is on the ground. Running into a driving snow can be troublesome. Keep your head down, and look only a few feet ahead. Ski goggles may help protect your eyes. Sounds will be muffled, so be careful to run on the edge of the highways facing traffic. Listen for approaching cars.

Running in newly fallen snow, or during a light storm, can be a joy, with the silence, broken only by your breathing. However, running on hard-packed snow is dangerous. You must run defensively, avoiding both the highway and the ruts.

In a 1977 marathon at Newton, Massachusetts, Vin Fleming (fifth at Boston in 1977) held a sizeable lead at the halfway mark, but was knocked down (and out) by salt sprayed from a vehicle. Perhaps you should try running on paths away from roads; hard-packed snowmobile trails are excellent, but don't tell the snowmobilers I sent you.

Ripple or waffle soles seem to grip snow and ice best. Galoshes or plastic bags may be slipped over your running shoes to keep feet dry and provide better traction. Be sure to do stretching exercises. Snow running requires a higher knee-lift and pulls harder at the hamstring muscles. But do get out in it. Shepherd runs best when it snows in Vermont. Each step may be a treacherous one, and yet the concentration makes the miles pass. The woods are silent, the animals out, tracks criss-crossing in the powder.

Ice is another thing. Be careful turning corners. If you run smoothly, and hit flat-footed, you won't have a fall. I've never fallen while running on ice, but I have slipped many times walking across the parking lot after a workout.

### Rain, Sleet, Hail and Storm

I ran my first marathon during a tornado warning in Kansas. First it rained, then sleet followed and then hail. Thunder and lightning capped the act. I was beginning to think Mother Nature didn't want me to run the race, but it was exhilarating and I felt like a kid running under the sprinkler.

If you run in the rain, wear a light nylon shell over a T-shirt, and nylon shoes, all of which will dry fast. Take off wet clothing as soon as possible after your run.

If lightning begins, bolt for the nearest shelter. Do not seek shelter under tall trees. Get away from them if that is your only choice, and lie flat on the ground. Don't stand upright in an open area, but lie flat on the ground.

### Wind

You can run for an hour into the wind, turn around, and run for an hour in the opposite direction only to find that it, too, is into the wind. I'll never forget the 1975 Skylon Marathon. We ran the first 6 miles full throttle into a strong head wind, expecting to turn around and fly along the Niagara River to the Canadian Horseshoe Falls in record time. When we turned, so did the wind, and we fought 30- to 40-mile-per-hour winds all the way to the finish. The 1975 Boston Marathon was a runner's dream, with 30- to 45-mile-per-hour tail winds that pushed runners to records they haven't come close to since.

A head wind of 10 miles per hour will slow your forward progress by five percent, while a 10-mile-per-hour tail wind will push you along at about three percent faster time. A head wind will cool you on a hot day or chill you on a cold one. (See page 185.) A tail wind can substantially increase your heat stress. Dr. Peter Cavanagh, associate professor of biomechanics at Penn State University, told a clinic before the 1976 White Rock Marathon in Dallas that as much as 8 percent of a runner's total expenditure of energy goes into overcoming wind, and that running twice as fast results in a wind resistance increase of four times. A 10-mile-per-hour wind requires an 8 percent energy increase, while a 25-mile-per-hour wind requires a 44 percent energy increase.

When running into a head wind, lean into it to decrease wind resistance. If possible duck in behind another runner or group of runners, and let them act as a wind break for you. If you're racing, take advantage of a tail wind, and really fly.

## OBSTACLES: MAN-MADE AND NATURAL

### Night

Running at night requires precautions. Try to work out on
well-lighted roads; a business district may be best. If you must
run on dimly lit streets or in the country, carry a flashlight,
and wear white, reflective clothing. Another trick is to tape
bicycle reflector tape to your clothes and shoes; wear one of the
small, white/red arm bicycle flashlights; wear a bright orange
reflector vest. Be defensive in the dark. You may also want to
purchase a pair of phosphorescent running shoes if you will be
doing a lot of night running.

### Air Pollution

A lot of runners want to know whether or not they should
run in polluted cities. The answer is mixed. Contaminants include sulfur dioxide, particulate matter (soot), various oxi-
dents which irritate the eyes and carbon monoxide. Studies
by architects in New York City, and by doctors in several
cities in California, show that the worst place to run is along
a highway or busy city street, but the good news is that pol-
lutants from cars dissipate quickly beyond fifty feet from
roadways. If you run along a roadway, keep your distance!

Large cities publish a daily "air pollution index." Too often
it reads "Air Quality: Unacceptable." Actually, city air is getting better on the average. Even so, runners with a medical
history of lung or heart problems should not run during air-
pollution warnings.

But what about the rest of us? Dr. George Sheehan, the
running cardiologist, states, "People who worry more about air
pollution than about attending to their physical condition

are deluding themselves. They would feel much better running in the city and becoming fit than they would sitting around doing nothing in the pure air of the country."

If you're a country dweller and are planning to race in a city, it is wise to spend several days acclimating yourself. Shepherd, the Vermont runner, finds it takes two workouts in New York City before he can run there without thinking his arms and legs have turned to concrete.

### Hills

Without hills, we wouldn't appreciate the flat stretches. Any workout, like almost any race, should include uphill and downhill runs. Only beginner runners, especially if overweight, should stay on level ground, because the extra work of carrying the body up a hill places severe stress on the cardiovascular system and the legs.

Many runners do hill training at a vigorous pace because it is really speed work in disguise, and it increases your anaerobic capacity and leg strength. Downhill work will improve your stride, although fast downhill running should be saved for races since it puts a severe burden on your legs and back.

Some people actually enjoy hill running. I often run from my parents' home in Dansville, New York, to my grandparents' home in South Dansville—an 8-mile run from a valley to a hilltop where the view is spectacular. After hills there is the challenge of running mountains. Along with several hundred others I ran the 1976 Mount Washington (New Hampshire) Race to the top of the East's highest peak, 6288 feet above sea level. The temperature was 90° F. at the bottom, and 52° F. at the top, with high winds above the tree line. It was torture all the way, and at times the grade was enough to make walking faster than running, but at the top we could extol the view and look down on the little red barn where we had started.

Exercise physiologists have proven on treadmills what hill runners have known all along. There is a large net energy loss when running hills compared to running flat or rolling countryside. There are ways to save some of that energy, to beat the hill before it beats you. I advise beginners on hills to run as far as they can comfortably and then alternate walking and running. But keep going. Pick a spot 50 yards ahead and run to it, then another goal and run to that. Shepherd runs the Vermont hills from farmhouse to farmhouse.

Also, follow this hill-running technique. As you approach the hill, shift into a lower gear and maintain a steady rate of effort and rhythm going up. Pick up the pace near the top, and maintain a steady rhythm going down. Use the hill to build momentum as you head into the flat beyond.

*Uphill:* Going up the hill, drop your arms low, pump them parallel to the plane of motion in an exaggerated fashion. Use them! Don't pump them across the body, but rather downward, like a cross-country skier. Your stride should be short, knees raised high. For short, steep hills you should get up on your toes, springing forward. You should lean slightly forward, back straight, hips in, chest forward. The head should be kept up. Avoid clenching the fists and tensing the upper body. Concentrate on pumping, running relaxed with a smooth, powerful and even rhythm.

*Downhill:* Again, the arms should be kept low. The upper body should be tilted forward so that it is perpendicular to the slope of the hill. Now gravity will assist you as you fall forward down the hillside. The hips are tilted back as the torso leans forward. Stretch out your stride, but don't overstride.

Keep the stride close to the ground. The arms should be held away from the body for balance on the downhill. Footstrike should be normal, but on steep downhills the heel should hit a little harder to provide slight braking.

The key to downhill running is control. If you go too fast, you'll burn excess energy and risk falling, or straining the body. If you go too slow, consciously leaning back and "braking" as many beginners do, you'll place a severe strain on the legs and lose time in races. Running up or downhill it's important to hold yourself together, to stay relaxed while maintaining control of your movement.

### Altitude

Beyond 3000 feet above sea level, you will notice altitude changes as you run. If you visit a high-altitude area (Denver, Colorado, for example) you should spend two to four weeks adjusting to the change. If you're visiting for a short while, and want to run, do so slowly and at a shorter distance. The casualties at the 1968 Olympics, held at high altitude in Mexico City, demonstrated the dangers of all-out exercise under these conditions without preparation. Many world-class runners purposely train at high altitudes, although they race at lower ones, to improve their ability to transport oxygen.

### Automobiles

Most of us have to run on roads, where we are second-class occupants. The auto owns the road—at least their drivers think so. I've had cars swerve at me, and drivers swing at me with their hands—and even with a car door. But I've also seen runners who thoughtlessly run in traffic lanes, or hit the road as though *they* own it. One of our runners, deep in meditation, ran smack into the side of a car—twice.

Here are some rules for road running:
- Always be defensive and expect the worst.
- Stay off high-speed roadways.
- Run on the shoulder of the road, or a sidewalk. Even then be on the alert. Three of our club's runners were knocked out of action one month prior to the 1977 New York Marathon when a drunk driver crashed into them as they were running on a sidewalk.
- On narrow, dirt country roads, run in the center of the road. It's softer; you can see cars easily, and they can see you. *Listen* for cars all the time. Move into the bushes quickly if you have to.
- Run facing traffic on paved roads.
- Be alert when approaching blind curves, and on hills.
- Run in an area you know, over a regular route. Eventually, you will develop a following of admirers, including dogs, who will watch for you, wave (or bark), and enjoy this craziness that brings you by their homes regularly in all kinds of weather.

### Hecklers

They will test your patience. "Hut, two, three, four" and "faster, faster" will compete with "Want a ride?" and "Look at those legs!" Women running alone will hear much worse—mostly from men being boys. Kitty Lance would hear things like "If I catch you, can I keep you?" from fellow runners. One reply: "Only after fifteen miles." The witty rebuttal is one good approach. For "Where did you leave your pants?" I've enjoyed replying, "With your girlfriend. She likes skinny lovers!" However, if your reply is nasty, be sure that you can up the juice a little to outdistance angered hecklers. Always remember that if your hecklers are in cars, you can reverse directions, go up a path, or down a one-way street. If it gets bad, head for a well-lighted home.

Sometimes kids run out and mimick my actions. I invite them to join me, and mention that I'm running 20 miles. Before long, they drop out. But one persistent runner was a drunk who started chasing a group of us from an outdoor party. His friends thought he was hilarious, and so did he. Amazingly, he jogged with us for 2 miles before he stopped to vomit.

### Dogs

I've stepped on snakes in Vietnam, tripped over rats along the Hudson River, been stung by bees, swallowed bugs, and was barely missed by a bear in Yosemite Park. But dogs can be the worst.

Some wary runners plan routes to avoid passing the houses of certain dogs, and others, in their anger at being chased and snapped at, have almost fulfilled that great journalistic reversal: man bites dog.

Not all dogs are interested in runners but any dog that comes out to check on you as you run is a potential danger. Never take your eyes off him, especially as you pass by. Dogs bite from behind. Shepherd was jogging in Riverside Park when he passed two well-dressed ladies talking and letting their little poodles sniff and scratch. Just as he got by, Shepherd heard the growl and snap. One poodle had lunged at him, and missed only because it was on a leash. The owner said, "My, my Tootsie, it's only a silly man."

Always talk to dogs in a soft, but firm voice. Say things like "good doggie" over and over (most owners address their dogs in this tone), and tell him to "stay home, stay, stay."

Try to anticipate a dog's intentions. If the tail is erect, ears straight up, lips curled open, hair raised on the back of its neck, he means business.

If you find yourself confronted with such a dog there are four techniques you can use to deal with it:

1. You can run. This works only if you are challenged by a Daschund, or a dog on a leash (do not rely on a rope). If you run, a dog will sense your fear, and chase you. Or, imitate the fleet Masai of East Africa, who know that if they encounter a lion they must face him and stand still. To run is to die.

2. You can stop, and try to make friends. This, too, contains risk. Some dogs are trained guard dogs. That hand offered for a sniff will appear to be a threat. If this tactic doesn't work, at least your arm gets the bite, not your legs, and you can still run.

3. You can threaten the dog. Shouting or growling—and some runners are excellent growlers—sometimes works. Often, dogs will retreat if you bend down and pick up a stone. (Be sure not to let the dog come too close before you bend down; in that position, you are vulnerable to a fatal bite.) If you grab a stone, and the dog halts, *slowly* raise your arm to throw it. He'll get the message, and retreat. But if he doesn't, begin to back off slowly, always facing the dog. Put some distance between you and the dog. To reinforce the threat of the stone, always throw it. Don't strike the dog, but the ground near him. He may even stop threatening you altogether.

4. Carry a stick or (better) a can of "Halt" with you. Some runners carry small water pistols with a half-and-half mixture of amonia and water. That's effective, although the water pistols sometimes leak. Also, one time I tried out my trusty dog spray, but blew it into a strong head wind. I cried all the way home; the dog ran off laughing.

As a last resort, you might try my father's trick. He was out for his nightly walk, when a dog that had been bothering him for weeks came up. My father knelt down quietly, and when the mutt came within range, he punched him in the nose. He hasn't been bothered since.

Be especially wary of any dog whose owner loudly proclaims, "Oh, he won't bite." He will, you can be sure. Also, if you are bitten, remember what the dog looked like, and preferably where it lived. This will save you from going through the extremely painful and prolonged rabies injections.

Owners of dogs can be nuts. When two large German shepherds attacked and bit me, the owner said I had provoked the attack by throwing rocks at his dogs as they slept innocently on the front porch. Jack Cohen, a New York Road Runner, ran a favorite course in upstate New York where he was continuously harassed by the same dog. He began calling the owner in advance so she could tie up the dog until he had passed. But when ole poochie howled, the lady got tired of tying him up. One day she suggested that Jack change his route, "After all," she told him, "the dog was here before you were."

# 10 ANALYZING RUNNING SHOES: IF THE SHOE FITS...

Each of your running shoes strikes the ground about 800 times per mile. If you run 10 miles a week, then each shoe strikes the ground more than 400,000 times a year. I run a lot, and each of my shoes pounds into pavement, grass and dirt almost 3,000,000 times a year. Obviously, we should be concerned about the quality of these running shoes.

Inside our shoes are two of the most abused parts of the human anatomy: our feet. They absorb the initial impact of running, and pass it upward to the ankles, legs, knees, hips, back, neck and head. Most people have weak feet, which when pounded on the earth thousands of times a week, cause a wide range of injuries.

Dr. George Sheehan states in his *Encyclopedia of Athletic Medicine*, "The worst thing that ever happened to feet was shoes. Or perhaps the second worst, after concrete. These two products of urban civilization have finally conquered the human foot which in its primitive state crossed continents, pursued wild game and danced for days on end."

It's not quite that bad, for with the running revolution has also come a running-shoe revolution. When I recall the flimsy items my cross-country coach in college told me were running shoes, I shudder—and my feet ache. Shepherd remembers playing 90 minutes of soccer in college in heavy leather shoes. When it rained, he felt like his feet were encased in cement blocks.

Luckily, there are many well-made, lightweight shoes on the market now—but perhaps too many. Runners need a manual to sort out the good from the bad. We won't analyze brands of shoes in this chapter because the styles (and prices) change too rapidly. Competition is intense between shoe companies, and quality is improving constantly.

*Runner's World* annually prints a special running-shoe issue that analyzes all the top running shoes in great detail. This issue is valuable to you as a runner: There are hundreds of quality running shoes available, and companies are making shoes to fit the specific needs of a variety of runners. As I said, you need a manual to tell them apart.

The leading companies have come into existence through family feuds, competition and rising demand. The Dassler brothers of West Germany were the first to take advantage of the tremendous market for good running shoes. But profit leads to greed, and the brothers fought. Brother Adi formed one company (Adidas) and brother Rudi another (Puma). For years they dominated the American market until the Japanese (Tiger) introduced nylon uppers. Another dispute followed, and the Tiger people in the United States split from the parent company and formed Nike, manufactured in the United States. Now, the big two became the big four: Adidas, Puma, Tiger and Nike. Along came Patrick from France, Pony from Canada, Reebok from England, Karhu from Finland and E.B. Sport International from West Germany. Today, other American companies are challenging the foreigners: New Balance, Brooks, Converse and Eaton. The competition is good.

For one thing, it keeps prices within reach, and the companies sponsor races. Unfortunately, competition also leads to world-class athletes being paid under-the-table to wear brand names for profit—but this happens only occasionally.

The following guidelines in buying running shoes come from personal experience with two dozen different models of shoes, and the advice of foot experts, including Dr. Richard Schuster, "the runner's podiatrist"; former Olympic marathon runner Ted Corbitt; world class ultra-marathoner and shoe salesman Gary Muhrcke of "Super Shoe on Tour"; and information from the *Runner's World* shoe supplements.

## WHAT TO LOOK FOR IN A RUNNING SHOE

A good running shoe protects the foot from the ground, supports the foot structure, and enables the body to move easily over the running surface, sometimes as fast as possible. Dr. Harry Hlavac, chief podiatrist at the Sports Clinic in San Francisco, says, "Shoes are for protection, support, traction, cushioning from the ground, balance of foot deformities and the accommodation of foot injuries. A proper shoe should provide support and cupping of the heel, firm arch support, protection of the ball of the foot, and flexibility of the front sole for easy push-off." Cushioning and stability, I feel, are the key factors.

The purchase of a good pair of running shoes is the one critical investment that a runner must make. Does it fit right? Can I afford it? Does it give adequate cushioning and support? How heavy should it be? Is it fashionable enough? Behind most veteran runners you will find a whole closetful of discarded running shoes. I recommend the following five guidelines for choosing your shoes:

**1.** Understand what is generally required in a running shoe, then decide which available shoes meet your requirements. (I'll help you do this in a minute.)

**2.** Inspect all the shoes you can, try them on. Make certain they fit properly. Try a short test; run in them if you can.

**3.** Beware of the advice of fast-talking salesmen, who don't answer your questions but downgrade the competition, and make excessive claims like "this is definitely the shoe for you." It probably isn't.

**4.** Give the shoe a break—but gradually. Too often runners discard shoes after one or two workouts because they "didn't feel right" or "caused a blister." It takes time to adjust to your new shoes, and eventually they'll adjust to you.

**5.** Don't be a faddist. If you are happy with one brand, stick with it.

One of the funniest conversations I ever heard involved a hyper runner who bought a pair of expensive widely advertised shoes from Gary Muhrcke, and wanted to return them. Gary asked him why, and the shoe buyer replied with anger, "They didn't work!" He had evidently wanted a pair of sub–3-hour-marathon shoes—guaranteed! The moral: Don't expect your shoes to do your work for you. You should do the work finding a good pair of shoes.

Not all models of a brand fit all feet. Take your time buying shoes, and wear socks that you will use with the new shoes. Obvious as it seems, try on the shoes in the store before you buy them. Shepherd was buying running shoes at a very busy athletic store in downtown New York City when a furious customer stomped into the showroom and demanded to return a pair of running shoes. "Why?" asked an innocent clerk. "Because they don't fit," replied the irate customer. "Did you try them on before you left here?" the clerk inquired. "Hell no," said the buyer, "I didn't have time." They didn't take back the shoes, either.

The shoe you buy—and try on—should fit your needs and requirements best.

## WHAT ARE YOUR NEEDS?

I believe all runners basically need the same quality in a shoe. Beginner runners and competitors must not settle for a "cheap" shoe for any reason. Your feet are important, whether you are just starting out or entering your first marathon. A competitor may want to buy a heavy training shoe and light shoes for racing, although many serious runners race and train in the same shoes.

If you are overweight, or built with a large frame, you will need lots of cushioning between you and the ground. This is also true if you suffer from arthritis, knee damage or other difficulties. Very lightweight runners, on the other hand, can often get away with a lighter, "faster" shoe.

Dr. Hlavac, in a 1977 *Runner's World*, said that people with normal feet and no injuries are able to wear almost any type of shoe with no pain or disability. But if a person has recurrent problems, then certain types of shoes may help and other types may aggravate them.

"For instance, relief from Achilles' tendonitis requires a flexible shoe with cushioning of the bottom of the heel and good elevation. Ankle sprains and instability need a shoe that will provide support and balance at heel contact. Arch problems and flexible feet require shoes that have a good shank area (under the arch) and a conforming arch support. Callouses on the bottom of the foot require a deep toe box and proper fit."

Additionally, shin splints require adequate cushioning under the ball of the foot. Heel problems may require cupping and elevation or more flexible cushioning. Many of these foot problems and solutions are discussed in chapter 11. But it is important to select a shoe that *feels* right and gives support and cushioning.

Anything of quality costs money, and lasts longer. You must plan an investment of twenty to forty dollars for a good pair of running shoes. It's your only major investment; cheaper shoes will cause aches and pains, and perhaps doctor's bills. Tennis shoes are out; they can lead to stress on your body, your pocketbook and mind.

Find a store that specializes in running shoes. Or, you can order shoes by mail, although I highly recommend that you personally inspect, try on and fit each shoe before you purchase it. A size 10 in one brand, for example, will vary slightly from another brand, or even from another pair of shoes of the same brand. When Shepherd bought his running shoes, he rejected the first pair because a "suction cup" on the sole rested exactly beneath the ball of his foot. He liked the design, weight, support and cushion of the brand, and asked the salesman to get the same brand and size, just another pair. The second pair fit perfectly.

If you must order by mail, I suggest the New Balance Company (38-42 Everett Street, Boston, Massachusetts 02135), which will take tracings of your foot that you mail to them, and assist you in selecting your proper shoe size. This was the first company to make shoes in a wide selection of widths and custom-make shoes for people with special needs. I emphasize

again, however, that there's nothing like going into the store
and trying on the shoes.

In my experience, runners make the best shoe salespeople.
Gary Tuttle, a two-time National AAU Marathon Champion,
"runs" his own store in Venture, California, and offers personal advice on shoes as well as training and racing. Well-
known runners like Frank Shorter, Bill Rodgers, and Marty
Liquori have opened up sports equipment businesses. In the
East, Gary Muhrcke works out of his home in Huntington,
Long Island, and "takes the shoe to the runner" in a van
converted into a shoe store on wheels. He travels around to
local schools and race sites selling shoes, talking and sometimes
getting out and running with his customers. He's a Millrose AA
runner and finished third in the 1976 London-to-Brighton 52.5-
mile race. That's my only complaint about Gary's shoe operation: By the time I finish a race he has not only finished
ahead of me, but had enough time to sell ten pairs of shoes
as well.

Selection, information from a good salesperson, price and
the condition of your feet are all considerations. When shopping, remember to bring your arch supports, insoles or anything
else you normally wear inside your running shoes. Carefully
lace up the shoe (with your running socks on), and bounce
around in several different pairs before selecting. Look for
minor defects such as improper tongue placement, rough
stitching on the inside of the shoe (which might cause
blisters), or crooked lasts. Place the shoe on a flat surface,
and make sure that the back goes straight up and down.

Even the best companies mass produce a few "lemons."
Take your time, and don't let the salesperson be your final
judge. Consider the requirements you want in a running shoe,
and make sure the pair you buy fits.

## SHOE REQUIREMENTS

### Size and Fit

Most shoes are available in men's sizes 3–13 in D width. Women with smaller and narrower feet are most often forced to buy men's shoes, although some companies, like Brooks, do make running shoes in women's sizes. Japanese-made shoes are frequently too narrow, especially in the toes, for most Americans. But if you need a narrower shoe than the average person, these may be good running shoes for you. New Balance and a few others produce shoes in variable men's widths (AAA–EEEE).

The shoe's toe box should allow free movement of the toes without pressure. Many of the shoes with pointed toes restrict movement. The forefoot area of the shoes should fit snugly. If it's too loose, the foot will slip as you run, causing

**Anatomy of a Shoe**

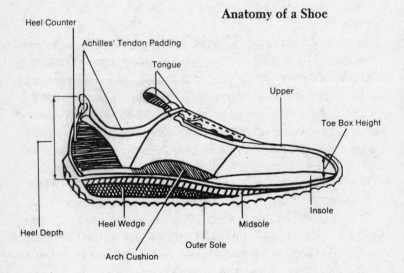

blisters. If it's too tight, it can cause cramping and nerve pressure. The cup around the heel should fit firmly, but not too tightly. If it's too loose or too tight, it could cause blisters or Achilles' tendonitis.

Ted Corbitt, and other experts, feel that the shoe should be large enough to allow half-an-inch between the big toe and the end of the shoe. This allows for foot expansion during running, and can compensate for narrow shoes. Some runners develop other problems (such as "curling of the toes," see p. 225) if the shoe doesn't fit fairly snug. You will need to find out what is best for you. Dr. Hlavac in *Runner's World* notes, "Given the choice between a slightly larger or slightly smaller shoe, select the larger size. If one foot is larger than the other, choose the larger size. Use the 'standing' rather than 'sitting' size of the foot." On the other hand, Gary Muhrcke suggests, "Fit the large foot snug or the small foot will fit too sloppy."

### Sole Makeup

A shoe should have a tough outer sole with a soft layer under it, and adequate cushioning from heel to toe. Look for a "2-ply" sole under the ball of the foot, and a "3-ply" sole under the heel, including a heel wedge. The "wedge" is usually a different color. The shoe should have a half-inch or more sole under the ball of the foot to insure adequate cushioning. The type of sole surface is important for traction, with the "ripple," "waffle" or "suction cup" soles preferred.

### Flexibility

The foot flexes about 30 to 35 degrees as you push off your toes. The shoe should flex, too. If the shoe isn't flexible under the ball of the foot, then the front and back of your leg take up extra stress which can cause injuries to the Achilles' tendon, calf muscle and shin. A balance must be achieved between cushioning and flexibility.

Check the ball—the widest part—of the shoe. Dr. Schuster says that if the shoe is difficult to bend at the ball of the foot with your hand, it is probably too stiff. If you can, take the shoe to a scale and apply pressure while flexing the toe. The pressure shouldn't exceed 10 pounds, but some top shoes take 20 to 30 pounds of force to bend. Dr. Schuster sometimes solves this problem by slicing across the widest point of the sole of the shoe under the ball with a hacksaw. Three cuts, spaced one inch apart and deep enough to cut through the first layer of rubber, may make the shoe more flexible. Or, you can choose a shoe that fits and is flexible in the first place.

### Shank Support

The sole of the shoe in the arch area should lie flush with the ground. In some shoes, the arch is "cutaway" in order to save weight or produce cheaper shoes. This bridge buckles under the severe stress of your footstrike causing potential heel and arch injuries. Avoid running shoes with such a design.

### Heel Lift

Runners need some elevation in the heels of their shoes to relieve the strain on the calf muscles and Achilles' tendon, which are accustomed to support in street shoes. Heel lift is measured by subtracting the thickness of the sole under the ball of the foot from the maximum thickness of the heel. The lift should be half-an-inch or more. Beware of a vast difference in heel lift between training shoes and racing flats.

### Inside Support

Most running shoes have built-in arches that range from a contoured leather interior to a removable sponge-rubber arch cushion. All of them are worthless. The supports are flimsy, and often runners need individually prescribed supports. I recommend Dr. Scholl's #610 arch support, or custom-made devices. Supportive stripes or other stitching on the exterior sides of the arch help keep the foot from sliding around in the shoe from side to side.

### Types of Uppers

Brittle leather causes blisters, and after getting wet stays soggy for days. However, leather gives good support and lasts longer. Suede shoes start off fitting very comfortably and feel already "broken in." But they also lack firm support. Nylon tends to be too warm, but will stay soft, dries very quickly, and is also very light. It can also be tossed in the washing machine (but not the dryer). Nylon uppers tend to wear out faster than leather, at about the same time the soles give out. Nylon shoes should have suede or leather strips of reinforcement along the heel and the sides and toe to give support. The nylon mesh upper is an improvement which allows the feet to breathe easier. After years of running in leather and suede, I definitely prefer nylon.

### Heel Counter

Thet heel counter is the firm wrapping around the back of the shoe; it stabilizes the heel. A rigid heel counter that covers the entire heel area is desirable.

### Shoe Weight

Most racing shoes weigh less than 10 ounces. All-purpose racing-training shoes may weigh between 10 and 12 ounces. Some heavy-duty shoes weigh more than 12 ounces. I prefer a 10-ounce shoe that can double as a racing and training shoe, but foot protection should be the deciding issue. I use Nike Elites for racing, but I use the heavier, well-cushioned New Balance 320s for long, slow workouts on hard pavement.

Beginner runners shouldn't be concerned with shoe weight, nor should beginner racers. Dr. Schuster notes that "more injuries occur during training than during racing. Thus it is most important to have good training shoes. During racing, shoe weight doesn't make all that much difference. I prefer to emphasize cushioning, support and comfort."

## CARE AND REPAIR OF YOUR RUNNING SHOES

Breaking in a pair of shoes is not much of a problem. New shoes are much softer today. Minor rough spots in the toe and tongue may need cutting away to avoid blistering. Vaseline inside leather shoes keeps them from developing "hot spots." Also, Neats Foot Oil, saddle soap and castor oil can soften and preserve leather. Stitching flaws or tears can be repaired with dental floss and a needle.

Carl Eilenberg, president of the Roman Runners in snow-bound Rome, New York, warns that shoes get stiff after sitting overnight following a run in rain or snow, and should be flexed before putting them on, to prevent injury. Shepherd, who runs in the snow and ice of Vermont, pulls open the tongue of his Adidas SL-76s and stuffs the shoes with newspaper balls to dry them out. He also carefully washes the rubber soles during winter to get salt from the roads off them.

A major cause of injuries is worn-down heels that allow the foot to hit the road at an unnatural level. Normally the rubber under the ball of the foot and at the outside edge of the heel will wear out first if you are using the proper foot-strike pattern. Some world class runners wear out the toes from their powerful drive at push-off.

Shoes that have a colored "heel wedge" have a built-in safety system to let you know that it's time either to get new shoes or fix the heels. When the blue coloring of my heel wedge begins to show through, I know it's not safe to continue using the shoes. The "uppers" often outlast the soles. If you wish to resole or reheel your shoes to save some money or maintain the "broken in" comfort of miles of running, you have several options.

1. Various substances like "Goo," "Sole Saver" and "Sole Patch" come in a tube and can be spread over the heel. They need to be applied frequently, and wear down quickly, but a thin, even layer of any of these materials is effective in preventing the wearing down of the heel of the shoe. They can be applied before the sole shows signs of wear.

2. "Glue guns" are available from Starting Line Sports (Box 8, Mountain View, California 94040). Sticks of glue are "hot melted" in the gun and then spread over the heel. Be sure that the repaired heel is level. If you put too much glue on the worn-down area, you may create a problem of imbalanced footstrike. In cold weather, this glue will get hard and brittle, and may crack and break off.

3. Ted Corbitt, a frugal man, repairs his shoes with old tire inner tubing or crepe and barge or contact cement. The inner tubing can be obtained from scrap heaps or a garage, and the cement from most shoemakers. You must be careful to cut the strips to the exact size of the area to be repaired, and shave it to match the taper of the wornout area.

4. A plastic tap, such as neolite, can be placed over the outside edge of the heel after the shoe has been worn down somewhat. Be sure to keep the heel even. The tap will keep the heel from rapidly wearing down.

**5.** Many shoe repair people will reheel your running shoes for a reasonable price. They just cut out the heel, and replace it. Be sure that the new heels aren't too hard or too soft. A friend once had a cobbler put an extra-hard rubber heel on his running shoes so that they would last longer. The result was a stress fracture because the shoe didn't absorb enough shock. Also, be sure that the repair person doesn't stick long nails into your running shoes which may stick into your foot.

**6.** Shoes can be rebuilt. Tred 2 (Dept. 125, 2510 Channing Avenue, San Jose, California 95131) and the New Balance Company will rebuild any make or model shoe for about half the cost of a new pair. They will put in a new sole, replace shoelaces, and repair various tears and stitching weaknesses. I've used the New Balance service with great results. I get about 1000 miles out of my running shoes, and with rebuilding I'll get close to 2000. It's great not breaking in new shoes. Some people even get as many as three or four "lives" out of their "uppers."

### Civilian Shoes

"Fashionable shoes" are almost worse than cigarettes, cars and concrete. Women and men who wear platform shoes, high heels or other faddish styles place great strain on their legs and shorten their Anchilles' tendons. I wear only soft suede shoes (they are not blue, but you better not step on them) with thick, well-cushioned, flat soles. This type of shoe helps my run-weary legs make it through the day at the office. Dr. Kraus even has running shoes painted black and wears them with comfort at work.

Various shoes, like the Earth Shoe, with the heel lower than the toe are advertised as helpful for runners because they correct defects that cause back pain, and stretch the backs of the legs. These shoes have indeed been helpful to some runners, and harmful to others.

The best shoe to wear when not running may, in fact, be no shoe at all. You should walk barefoot on grass or at the beach, and as much as possible elsewhere.

## "SHOE STUFFINGS"

The following are often inserted into running shoes:

### Heel Lifts

These may be used to soothe shin splints, Achilles' tendons and calf tightness. A lift of one-fourth to one-half inch allows the runner to hit farther back on the heel, thus decreasing the pull on the Achilles' tendon. Makeshift lifts may be constructed from surgical felt or similar material. Dr. Murray Weisenfeld suggests using powder puffs, which can be purchased at the cosmetic counter of any five-and-dime. You place first one, then up to three or four, under the heel to find the best level for you. Dr. Schuster says, "Ideally, the lift should extend to the middle of the arch so the foot doesn't sag in front of the lift. The lift should be tapered to the arch. Three insoles cut at different lengths can be used to obtain the desired results."

### Heel Cups

These are used to stabilize and cushion the heel and to prevent or contend with injuries such as heel spurs and bruises, callouses, shin splints and ankle sprains. Heel protectors can be ordered from M-F Athletic Company, Inc., P.O. Box 8188, Cranston, Rhode Island 02920.

### Arch Supports

The supports that come with running shoes are usually in-adequate. Many runners rip them out right away. Cheap supports can be purchased, but why treat your feet so poorly? The best mass-produced support is Dr. Scholl's #610 or Athletic A Arch Support. They are not always available in your local stores, but can be ordered from Dr. Scholl's Foot Comfort shops (see Appendix).

### Inserts

Most runners might find comfort in wearing a quality, mass-produced arch support. But many runners need orthotics, custom-made supports, designed by a podiatrist. Inserts are fashioned after a plaster mold of your foot, and are corrected to adjust to structural weaknesses in your foot. The most common insert is a flexible leather model with a corklike bottom that can easily be adjusted by sanding off or building up areas. Rigid supports made of hard plastic are favored by many podiatrists. When breaking in arch supports or insoles, you should first wear them while walking, and gradually increase your mileage while running. An insole can be worn over the arch support at first to prevent blisters. (See chapter 11.)

### Insoles

These cushion the feet and help prevent blisters. Foam rubber and other insoles don't hold up under the pounding and the exposure to sweat, rain and snow. The Spenco insole (Starting Line Sports) is the best in the market. It lasts a long time, and is made of neoprene sponge, which absorbs some of the shocks of running, and helps prevent blisters. If you ever run in them in the rain, however, you may have problems, because they soak up water and may bunch up in the toes or slide right out at the heel. It is better to remove insoles on rainy days rather than take a chance. Also, be sure that they are not too long because they will bunch up under your feet. After the insoles are worn for a while, they do become saturated with dirt and sweat and should be replaced. The Spenco can cause foot burning in the summer months.

One problem with "shoe stuffings" is that you can over-stuff your shoes. When you try on new running shoes, bring whatever you may put inside them. You might take a half size larger than usual. Be sure you don't raise your heel up so far that you lose support in the back of the shoe for your Achilles' tendon, or crowd the toes against the top of the shoe.

# 11 INJURIES: DISEASES OF INACTIVITY, DISEASES OF EXCELLENCE

In 1955, Dr. Hans Kraus presented a theory, based on his studies, to the annual meeting of the American Medical Association. It was a radical idea for the time, and one for which he was widely criticized. Dr. Kraus proposed that underexercise was the cause of a large number of illnesses. He reported that 57.9 percent of 5000 healthy American children between the ages of six and sixteen failed one or more of the Kraus-Weber Minimal Muscle Tests, while only 8.7 percent of 3000 children in Austria, Italy and Switzerland had failed the same tests. Dr. Kraus was accused of being unpatriotic!

When Dr. Kraus presented his report to President Eisenhower, however, it became the catalyst for the establishment of the President's Council for Physical Fitness. In 1960, President John F. Kennedy, a patient of Dr. Kraus, wrote in *Sports Illustrated*, "The harsh fact of the matter is that there is an increasingly large number of young Americans who are neglecting their bodies—whose physical fitness is not what it should be—who are getting soft."

Even today, the disease of inactivity is still with us. To the automobile, which Ulick O'Connor likens to a plague killing middle-aged men, we can add the elevator, golf cart, fast-food chain and other conveniences. All are mechanisms of twentieth-century life that either rob us of activity, or fatten us. The result is overwhelming "hypokinetic disease"—the disease of inactivity. The results of this habitual physical inactivity are heart disease, nervous disorders such as ulcers, headaches, insomnia; and musculoskeletal deficiences like lower back pain.

In 1955, the medical profession laughed at Dr. Kraus' suggestion that underexercise was a cause of disease. Heart patients and those with back pain were ordered to remain inactive. Twenty-one years later, however, the medical profession had changed. Several hundred doctors and scientists packed the 1976 New York Academy of Sciences conference to study the value of marathon running on human health. The American Medical Association, which was once unreceptive to the value of exercise, now has its own American Medical Jogger's Association, with hundreds of members running anywhere from a few miles to marathon events.

All runners overcome two physical obstacles: the diseases of inactivity, which are discovered when one is getting into shape; and then the diseases of excellence that sometimes come from running too well.

Injury is often part of an active life, but it can also be avoided, or minimized. The rush to get into shape, the tension of our society, the lack of information about relaxing, stretching and running all lead to a variety of frustrating injuries. A 1976 poll in *Runner's World* showed that 34 percent of the sub–25-miles-a-week runners suffered injuries, but among runners covering 50 miles or more a week 73 percent developed injuries. When runners strive for excellence at 100 miles or more a week, further injuries are possible.

What are the most common injuries? Dr. Richard Schuster selected 100 random cases from his files on runner-patients, and compared the types of complaints. Not surprising, since Dr. Schuster is a podiatrist, he found that "most of the complaints appear to be partially or completely related to structural shortcomings of the foot, the manner in which the foot functions, or in the environment in which the foot functions— foot gear and running surfaces." He found that knee and Achilles' tendon complaints headed the list.

*Runner's World* surveyed 1000 runners who had been hurt during the previous year. More than 60 percent of them had to interrupt their normal running schedule. They, too, complained of knee, shin and Achilles' tendon as the leading areas of injury.

## TEN REASONS WE GET HURT

In my work, I have found ten basic causes of injuries that occur to the runner moving from being underexercised to reaching a level of running excellence.

1. *Weak feet* Dr. George Sheehan reported in 1974 that a "revolutionary" concept had been developed by sports-oriented podiatrists. The concept was that the biomechanically weak foot held the key to the majority of foot, leg and knee injuries in runners. The reason is simple. A distance runner's foot strikes the ground 1000 times during every 7- to 10-minute mile. The force of impact of each foot is approximately three times the runner's weight. Surveys now indicate that 35 to 60 percent of all runners have weak feet. If the feet are weak, then the force exerted upon footstrike causes an abnormal strain on the supporting tendons and muscles of the foot and leg. The result is muscular or skeletal damage.

Further, the abnormal stress may cause a twisting of the foot on the ankle, or the leg or knee. The result may be stress fractures or "runner's knee." Arch supports, either commercially made or custom fitted, may help runners with weak feet.

2. *Unequal leg length* Perhaps 15 percent of all runners

have this problem. In many cases, unequal leg length causes no injury. But in other runners, the problem may force the shoulders and scapula to be out of alignment, the spine to curve causing nerve irritation, the pelvis, knees, ankle and foot to rotate abnormally. The result can be a whole variety of back, hip, foot and leg injuries. Dr. Schuster finds that most injuries first occur on the long side. Structural shortages may occur anywhere in the leg: the upper leg, the lower leg, and below the ankle. Heel lifts or inserts to balance the leg length difference may help, and should be placed inside the shoes, never exceeding half an inch. Exercises to stretch and strengthen the affected areas are also beneficial (see chapters 1 and 6). *Caution:* According to Dr. Schuster, "The general rule relating to the management of leg shortages in runners is to do nothing if the runner is pain free."

**3. *Poor flexibility*** Tight or shortened muscles can be more easily injured than stretched muscles and cause a variety of biomechanical problems. Stretching both before and after running is essential for the Achilles' tendon, calf and hamstring muscles and the back and hip. This is the only way to gain and retain adequate flexibility.

**4. *Weak anti-gravity muscles*** The back and leg muscles become overdeveloped and tight with running. Therefore, strengthening exercises for the opposite muscle groups are essential. These include exercises for the abdominal muscles (easing back pain), shin area muscles (shin splints) and quadriceps or thigh area (knee pain).

**5. *Stress and tension*** As mentioned in chapter 15, stress and tension may cause a variety of injuries, including lower back pain and injuries related to tense muscles forced into action. Relaxation exercises before and after workouts will help alleviate this problem.

**6. *Overuse syndrome*** Overtraining, or packing too many things into your life in addition to running, can make you susceptible to musculoskeletal injuries as well as illnesses. Early symptoms of overexertion such as fatigue, chills, frequent colds, insomnia and diarrhea should be recognized, and avoided. Listen to your body. Ease back in your running schedule, decrease your speed, time and/or distance. Run slow, run easy, but if symptoms continue, see a runner-doctor.

**7. *Improper training habits*** Sudden changes in intensity, duration, or frequency of your runs should be avoided. Work into changes slowly. Also, if you are running on dirt and switch to hard pavement, watch for signs of stress or injury. Run slower, or shorter distances at first. Proper running style should always be observed. Stay off your toes, and run tall by standing more erect.

**8. *Environmental factors*** Good running shoes are vital. Since running costs so little, treat yourself to a solid, comfortable, well-made pair of shoes. (See chapter 10.) Keep your shoes in good repair. If possible, avoid hard and uneven surfaces.

**9. *Injury rehabilitation*** Take your time! Allow any injury to heal before running hard, far and long again. Recover slowly from illnesses as well. Relapses are common if you don't take the time for recovery. Many serious injuries result from ignoring a minor injury.

**10. *Poor advice*** Sedentary doctors used to be blamed for many of our ills. They favored "staying off it" or "don't do anything strenuous" prescriptions. There are still too few sports-oriented, exercising doctors, and the medical profession has been slow to acknowledge the value of exercise as preventative medicine.

Be wary of nonathletic, out-of-shape doctors who prefer

inactivity and pills as cures. Also be very skeptical of poorly trained physical educators or boot camp drill instructors who believe in getting you into shape at any cost. The price may be your health. Unfortunately, the most dangerous "expert" of all is your fellow runner. Give some runners a few miles in their training diaries, a new warm-up suit—and suddenly they're experts.

Your best bet is to seek advice about running and injuries from running-oriented physicians, competent and cautious physical educators and physical therapists, and veteran, level-headed runners. Finally, remain skeptical.

Runners can run without injury. But like any one of us, runners tend to jump in and start out without a thought about *preventing* injury. The warm-up, flexibility and cool-down exercises are excellent ways to prevent injury on the run. If you are increasing your mileage beyond normal maintenance, for example, perhaps you should see a running-oriented podiatrist.

The next section, and the chapter that follows, may prevent unnecessary injuries. I learned the hard way; they happened to me. But I also know from runners I work with that most of us don't worry about preventing injury we haven't experienced. Thanks to the work of such people as Dr. Kraus, Dr. Sheehan, Dr. Schuster, Dr. Subotnick, Dr. Rob Roy McGregor and Ted Corbitt, we are learning more about ourselves as runners who battle first the "diseases of inactivity" and then the "diseases of excellence."


## "MY TEN MOST FAVORITE INJURIES FROM HEAD TO TOE"

Maybe I should call them "Infamous Injuries." I've had all of them, to my great displeasure. But I still want to emphasize:

You can prevent injury by observing the ten warnings above. While you shouldn't be afraid of getting injured, you should run as defensively as you should drive.

### The Black Toenail, and Other Toe Problems

Toenails may cause many problems. If the nails are too long, they can jam while you're running and cause a blood blister under the nail. After cutting the nails back, however, be careful to cover them or spread Vaseline over them before running; if not, the freshly exposed skin may blister. Or, tight shoes may cause your toes to jam and create blisters on the ends as well as under the nails. Shoes that are too big can cause slippage, resulting in blisters, too.

A blood blister under the toenail may cause several things to happen. The blister may go away by itself, and the toenail return to normal. A blister may force the nail away from its bed, leaving it slightly tender: the nail will grow back normally. Or, the blister will hurt so much that the pressure on the nail will have to be relieved. Hemorrhaging under the nail will cause it to turn black.

I used to develop painful blood blisters under my big toenail after long races. They were caused by my toenails rubbing against the top of my shoe. My foot rides high in the shoe because I wear inserts and insoles. In treating this injury, which once resulted in a 4 a.m. ambulance ride to a hospital, I learned that a blister may need to be popped to relieve the pressure. A doctor may sterilize a needle and gently probe beneath the nail. A common procedure for a podiatrist is to drill through the nerveless nail to the blister, which bursts; the relief is instant. Once, in desperation, I heated a paper clip red-hot, and melted a hole into the nail. It hurt like hell for a moment, but worked! I told a runner-doctor, and he assured me that the medical profession had known this intricate method for relieving pain for years, and some people even find that it doesn't hurt them. The next day I was able to run comfortably. This technique is difficult to face a second time, even after several shots of brandy. In defense, I've discovered preventative measures which have, so far, ended the problem.

Dr. Richard Schuster suggested that I cut a slit into the top of my shoe over the toe, and two smaller ones to either side, to allow the foot to expand during long runs and to eliminate friction above the toenail. After several months of questioning his sanity—What, cut up $30 shoes?—I finally gave in. It worked, and my shoes haven't fallen apart either. If you're hesitant, try cutting up an old pair first.

Another effective preventative method for me is to wrap the toe with gauze. Tape it securely, forming a cup of gauze to protect the nail. Foam rubber caps may work, and can be purchased commercially. They sometimes fall off while running, however, and may turn into sponges in wet weather. "Sanding" the toenail with an emory board also helps prevent blisters.

Another problem may be "tingling in the toes." This is frequently caused by nerve pressure in tight shoes. "Curling of the toes" is another ailment on my long list. My right foot is smaller than my left, so I face the decision of whether to have one shoe very tight or one a little loose. Looseness is less dangerous. Since I have lots of room in the right shoe, I often curl my toes under, sometimes causing tightness in my calf. An extra pair of socks on the one foot, or a shoe length appliance under the foot may help. I found that after slitting my shoes, my toes were more flexible and the problem went away.

Ingrown toenails can also be painful. Small cotton balls

can be placed under the corners of the nails to allow the nail to grow properly rather than cut into the skin. The cotton balls should be replaced daily, but used until the nail properly grows out.

### The Crusty Callus

Calluses develop from the constant rubbing of the foot in the shoe and the pounding of the foot onto the ground. They are usually found on the bottom and back of the heel, and under the ball of the foot. Calluses can be helpful in protecting the foot, but they can also cause painful problems. Thick callouses protect the outer skin layer, but also increase pressure on underlying tissues and bone.

Although calluses are surprisingly rare in runners compared to the general population, according to Dr. Schuster, they do cause us problems. Calluses form by a combination of friction and shearing action. I develop thick calluses on the ball of my foot. This is caused primarily by the rubbing of my foot in the shoe and the resulting friction developed between the metatarsal bones and the underlying skin and shoe. As the callus is allowed to grow, pressure is exerted on the subcutaneous tissue and eventually it results in an infected blister deep under the callus. The area has to be lanced by a physician, and the callus surgically removed.

To prevent this, calluses should be sanded down regularly with pumice stone, although some calluses should be encouraged, to protect the foot. Vaseline or some other type of skin softener may be regularly applied to keep the skin moist. Inserts or metatarsal pads are sometimes required to eliminate the pressure on the foot that can cause calluses. Spenco insoles or a similar friction-reducing device will also help prevent calluses from building up.

## The Bloody Blister

Blisters are caused by "hot spots" from shoes that are too loose or too tight, dirty socks, rough spots in the threading of your shoes, running in thin-soled shoes on hot pavement, holes or seams in socks, and many other things. The best way to prevent blisters is to prevent the friction that causes them.

High-quality, thick-soled shoes will help. Avoid those with improperly placed stitching and rough edges. If a rough area does develop in a good shoe, soften it with Vaseline. Never wear new shoes in a race or long workout. The shoes must be broken in gradually, and the feet must become accustomed to them.

Many so-called experts insist that socks prevent blisters, and argue that two socks should be worn to minimize friction. However, modern running shoes are thick, and don't need several layers of sock for added cushioning. With socks, the runner risks creating irritating skin folds, bunching, and slipping (especially if the socks get wet) which cause blisters. Socks should be clean, dry and snug-fitting.

Beginner runners tend to get blisters because their feet are tender and need to be toughened gradually. Avoid the commercial "skin tougheners"; they may be good for other sports, but not for the continuous motion of running. Foot powder or Vaseline generously applied to your feet before running usually prevents blisters. Special care should be taken prior to races, when your "blistering pace" may result in increased friction within the shoe.

I used to develop incredible blisters under the arch from the friction of my foot rubbing against my inserts—a common problem with insert wearers. Podiatrists can adjust inserts to minimize friction, and, frequently, they prescribe insoles that are specifically designed to reduce friction and can also be valuable in reducing foot shock. However, don't race with insoles in rainy weather because they'll absorb water like a sponge, slip around inside the shoe and cause blisters. Also, remember that insoles go *over* your inserts. I had been wearing my Spenco insoles underneath for extra cushioning until one day, slightly hungover, I reversed them, and my blisters went away.

If you do get blisters, be cautious. Stubbornly training on them may chew up your feet and knock you out for days. Stop and treat the problem, and you may return to your workouts immediately.

Small blisters should not be punctured immediately. Keep the area clean and protected; the skin may reheal itself. Taping, especially with Band-Aids, may only aggravate the blister further. Dr. George Sheehan paints the blister area with tincture of benzoin and then applies a tape, such as Zona, a standard product found in most pharmacies. The tape is left on for a few days, and reapplied if the blister is still present.

A blister that gets bigger and becomes painful to step on must be "popped" to relieve the pressure. Clean it with an antiseptic solution, and puncture it with a sterilized needle. Most of the fluid should be gently squeezed out with a sterile gauze. Do not remove the skin. An antiseptic, anti-fungal agent should be applied to the open area, and the blister should be covered with a sterile gauze pad or Band-Aid until it disappears. To prevent infection, be sure that all fluid is out of the blister, and no foreign matter remains.

Tinactin solution should be used for wounds on the bottom of your feet. Dr. Murray Weisenfeld, whose podiatry practice handles both runners and dancers, notes that a favorite trick of dancers is to use Curity brand lamb's wool to cover a blister. A wisp of lamb's wool is wrapped around the blistered toe, not tightly. Wrap it around a few times, then give it a couple of twists so the fibers intertwine and stick together. This protects the toe, and prevents blistering. It is also waterproof. Another trick was discovered by Jim Rumsey, trainer for the Florida State track team: Take a three-inch strip of elastic by Johnson and Johnson, and wrap it around the foot. Be sure it overlaps, and cut off the excess beyond the toes. The result is a "toe sock" that protects blistered feet.

Treat blisters immediately. Otherwise, you will favor the blister by adjusting your footstrike, even unconsciously, and altering your posture which may cause leg, knee or back injury. I sometimes run on blisters as though they don't exist, but if they cause me to alter my running form, I stay off them for a day or two. Two weeks before the 1976 New York Marathon, Lauri Pedrinan, our team's top woman competitor, told me she had injured her knee, and couldn't run without pain. After some questioning, I discovered that her knee began to hurt following a 15-mile training run during which she slightly favored a blister. The minor alteration in foot plant caused an abnormal strain on the knee. After resting a few days, she was able to run the marathon, but she had lost crucial days of training.

### Our Arch Enemy

The arches in our feet commonly bring pain and discomfort. One of them traces the underside and top of the foot, extending from just in front of the heel to the base of the first long toe joint. The "inner arch" (on the underside) is the one most often strained. The metatarsal arch across the ball of the foot, also causes problems. It is not a true arch but an off-weight arch that normally flattens under weight. Weight can be unevenly or excessively distributed and cause pain.

Tendonitis or capsulitis around the small bones of the foot

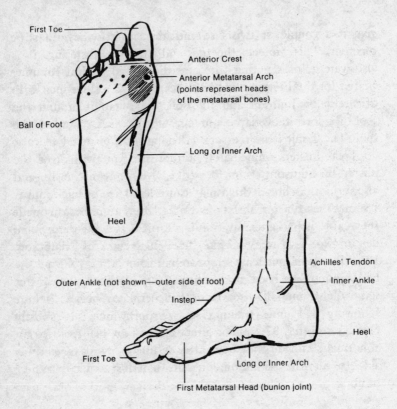

First Toe

Anterior Crest

Anterior Metatarsal Arch
(points represent heads
of the metatarsal bones)

Ball of Foot

Long or Inner Arch

Heel

Achilles' Tendon

Outer Ankle (not shown—outer side of foot)

Inner Ankle

Instep

Heel

First Toe

Long or Inner Arch

First Metatarsal Head (bunion joint)

**Anatomy of a Foot**

can make these arches painful or weak. This may be caused
by a weak structural foot which needs support. Often, flat feet
or feet with high arches both require support. Flatfootedness,
however, does not necessarily mean that the arch is flat. It can
be a condition in which weak ankles allow the foot to roll
medially, giving the appearance that the arch is flat. Not everyone with flat feet develops foot and leg injuries during run-

ning. According to Dr. Weisenfeld, the low arch may be normal.

Exercises to strengthen the muscles of the foot sometimes bring relief. Picking up marbles with your toes, rolling a Coke bottle under your foot, standing on a towel with your toes over the edge and then picking up the towel with your toes, all help. Walking barefoot regularly, especially in sand, also strengthens the muscles of the feet.

When exercise doesn't give enough strength to the muscles of the foot, arch supports may be needed. Commercially made arch supports (for all types of arch problems) and custom-made inserts or orthotics may relieve arch pain and other foot and leg injuries as well. Immediate treatment of arch strain consists of rest followed by gentle exercises.

My arches used to swell after running, and finally became so painful that I couldn't walk. A podiatrist sent me to a store to buy a pair of common, cheap supports, but the problem hardly lessened. Finally, he sent a mold of my feet to Dr. Schuster, who sent back custom-made arches. Not only did my arch problem disappear, but my knee pains also diminished. Many of our runners, however, have been relieved of arch pain after using Dr. Scholl's #610 arch supports.

### The Achilles' Heel

This is our body's vulnerable spot. The Achilles' tendon connects the powerful lower leg muscles to the heel. An injury to this tendon is painful and long-lasting. Dr. Schuster lists six major causes of Achilles' tendonitis.

1. The act of running tightens the calf muscles even more than normal, and most runners cannot dorsiflex their feet (bend them upward) to the ideal 10 degrees beyond the right angle. The result is added strain upon the Achilles' tendon.

2. Many runners, especially beginners, neglect warm-ups and stretching exercises. Tight, tense muscles and tendons are more susceptible to injury.

3. Many runners, especially beginners, run on the balls of their feet, which causes strain on the Achilles' tendon.

4. Bursts of speed by a runner who has not built up to it will strain the tendon, also.

5. Running shoes, especially those with low heels or that don't readily flex under the ball of the foot, are inadequate.

6. Runners with narrow Achilles' tendons have a higher incidence of tendonitis than runners with broader Achilles' tendons, Dr. Schuster has found.

There are other causes that may precipitate an attack of tendonitis. Any sudden change in footwear (thick heels to thin heels), running surfaces (soft to hard) or training pattern (flat terrain to hill work, endurance to speed, increased mileage) may trigger tendon strain. If you overtrain a fatigued body, or run on worn-down heels, or stretch with fast or jerky motions, or force a stretch beyond the first point of discomfort, you may harm your Anchilles' tendon. High-heeled shoes for women, and those funky platform shoes for men shorten the tendon. Earth Shoes and other similar brands with heels lower than toes may stretch the Achilles' tendon. This may help some people, but it may also strain the tendon in some cases. Sometimes, the problem is caused by a sharp bone cutting into the tendon, a condition which requires surgery. Finally, beginner runners must remember that their muscles are weak and tendons short. They need to be cautious, and work gradually on their running program.

Injury to the Achilles' tendon may take two forms: tendonitis or rupture. Tendonitis is marked by pain and stiffness during and after workouts, as well as tenderness to touch. It may lead to partial or complete rupture, which involves a tear in the tendon accompanied by pain and swelling.

In cases of normal tendonitis, treatment consists of soaking in ice or cold water to limit inflammation and swelling. Cold tap water running over the Achilles' is effective; or, pack the area in ice, or rub ice on it. Direct applications of ice as the foot is moved up and down for ten minutes immediately after running is a good technique. Later, heat should be applied before the workout and ice immediately afterwards until the injury has subsided.

Strain on an injured tendon may be lessened by placing heel lifts in street and running shoes. As much as one inch of surgical felt should be added under the heel. As the pain subsides the height of the heel lift is gradually reduced. People with chronic Achilles' problems may benefit from corrective inserts.

In the early stages of an Achilles' injury, stretching should be avoided. The injury developed in the first place because the tendon was overstrained. After a couple of days of rest, mild stretching, massage, heat treatments, ultrasound and whirlpool treatments may help. Drugs such as cortisone injections may be an immediate help, but can also be dangerous and contribute to a more serious rupture.

Slow down immediately at the first sign of Achilles' strain. This is one of the most dangerous injuries to run with because it can lead to a partial rupture, which in turn could lead to a complete rupture requiring surgery.

Hill work and speed work should be eliminated, and mileage limited until the symptoms disappear. If there is pain and stiffness, stop running altogether for two to ten days. Remember, this is one of the slowest injuries to heal. When training continues, running should be on flat ground, and easy. The pace should be slowed down at the first sign of pain.

There are some preventive measures that every runner should take. Stretching exercises for leg muscles and the tendon should be done before running to prepare the tendon for strenuous activity. Exercises done afterwards will keep the muscles and tendons from stiffening and shortening. Flexibility exercises should be done often. Walking barefoot or in flat shoes is also beneficial. Exercises that help stretch the Achilles' tendon include the Standing Hamstring and Calf Muscle Stretch (chapter 1), the Soleus Muscle Stretch and Sprinter's Position (chapter 6). You may also want to try the following:

- Sitting on floor, lean forward toward one outstretched foot, grasp your toes (if you can) and pull them toward you slowly. Keep your knees flat to the floor if possible.
- Stand on your toes on a two-inch board, step or curb. Slowly lower the heel below your toes, and hold. Repeat 2 more times.
- Build a slant board at an angle of about 15 to 20°, and stand on it as you watch TV, shave, etc. Jim Rumsey says that at Florida State this device significantly diminished ankle injuries and Achilles' tendonitis.

You should stretch the Achilles' tendon more than once a day. It should always be done before and after running. I often lean against the wall while waiting for an elevator, lower my heels off the curb while waiting for a traffic light to change, tug on my toes while talking on the telephone. I may look a little weird, but in New York, who notices! One day while waiting for a bus I leaned against the shelter doing my stretching and a couple of winos copied me for an impromtu fitness lesson.

### Shin Splints

Abnormal strain and stress on the muscles and tendons that lift your forefoot (dorsiflex) and control your toes often result in shin splints. These muscles and tendons absorb shock and stabilize your feet during foot plant. The angle at which the foot strikes the ground and the ability of the muscles and tendons to withstand the force indicates your susceptibility to shin splints. If you get them, you know it. Shin splints are a painful swelling of damaged muscles and tendons along the front of your lower leg between the two bones, the fibula and tibia; the pain occurs noticeably during running. Shin splints are common among beginner runners unaccustomed to the strain. I can determine the cause of at least 90 percent of their problems by asking three questions. Do you run on your toes? Do you lean forward when you run? Do you have good, well-cushioned shoes? When new competitors and veteran runners complain of shin splints, it usually means one of two things—either they have made dramatic shifts in their training programs, or they may have a strength-flexibility imbalance in the muscles of their legs.

Running style or training habits often cause shin splints. The following are to be avoided or corrected.

- Running on the balls of your feet and overstriding places strain on the muscles and tendons of the lower leg. Thick-heeled running shoes and heel lifts will help you land farther back on the heel at footstrike, and eliminate this problem.
- A forward lean of the body increases the strain on your leg muscles. Remember to run tall and concentrate on staying erect.
- A sudden shift from thick-soled shoes to thin, flat terrain

to hills, endurance training to speed work, soft surfaces to hard, short mileage to long, may cause pain in shins. Thick-soled shoes are important for beginners and anyone running on hard surfaces.

- Some runners need arch supports or custom inserts. Pain along the inside of the calf may be a second type of shin splint related to weak arches.

- Poor flexibility, muscle weakness and muscle imbalance between the front and back of the leg may cause shin splints. Tight calf muscles, weak arches and shortened Achilles' tendons also add strain to the shin area. Stretching exercises for calf, hamstring and Achilles' tendon are important, especially before and after running.

- Digging in with toes upon footstrike, and tension in the foot muscles during foot swing also strain the lower leg muscles. Shoes that fit snugly in the toes, or the addition of anterior crests under the toes may help prevent the former problem. The toes should also be allowed to "float" and relax during the forward swing.

- Bouncing on your toes on hard surfaces, stop-and-go running, and repeated pivoting should all be avoided.

- Sometimes tight clothing may cause the temporary symptoms of shin splints. Fritz Mueller, forty-one, 1977 American Masters Record holder for the marathon (2:27:25), got a scare just before the 1976 National AAU Masters Marathon Championship in Honolulu. He was slowed by shin splints that wouldn't go away. A week before the race he submitted to X-rays only to find no fracture, nothing. Finally, he discovered the cause himself. His sweat pants had elastic bands that were restricting the blood flow in his legs, perhaps resulting in shin splints symptoms. With looser clothing, the symptoms went away, but he had almost missed his trip to Hawaii. By the way, he finished second in 1976 (but won in 1977).

Dr. Sheehan recommends taking positive steps to reduce or prevent the occurance of shin splints. The following exercises are in addition to those for stretching the hamstring and calf muscles recommended in chapters 1 and 6.

1. Sit on a table with legs hanging freely over the sides. Flex the foot to lift a weight (a bucket filled with pebbles or a sandbag or other weight suspended over the top of the foot).

2. Attach a rubber bicycle inner tube to a board; slip your toes under the tube and lift them against it.

3. Turn the feet inward while standing and make a rolling motion.

4. Stand on the edge of a towel and curl the toes to pull the towel under the feet.

If you do fall victim to shin splints, it is best to rest a few days when the symptoms first appear. Running with severe shin splints may lead to a stress fracture. If the pain is severe and you are losing power in your legs, see a physician. Otherwise, here is the recommended treatment for shin splints:

- Rest the legs and elevate the feet as often as possible.
- Ice-massage the area after each run and before bed. (I have a favorite though unorthodox solution. Put a six-pack of beer on ice and go for a run. When you return, put the ice on your shins and drink the beer. Soon you won't feel a thing!)
- Add heel lifts, arch supports or anterior crests to your shoes. The latter are inserts that fit in the upper toe portion of the shoe, and are manufactured by Dr. Scholls (see Appendix: Runner's Aids).
- Strapping or taping by a knowledgeable athletic trainer or doctor may help.

- Cortisone pills may also clear up the inflammation but shouldn't be taken for more than three days. The drug Norflex, a muscle relaxant, can relieve pain and doesn't make you drowsy. Both are by prescription.
- Run slowly on soft, flat terrain within the limits of pain. Gradually return to normal training.
- Avoid recurrence by following the principles of prevention listed above.
- Surgery, as a last resort, may be needed to repair injured tissue.

### Pulling Your Leg

A variety of muscular aches and pains in the legs affect the runner. These include muscle fatigue, tension-related pain, cramping, and muscle strains and tears.

General leg muscle stiffness is common among beginner runners. So, too, is pain in the calf muscles from running on the toes and causing constant tension on the calf. This is why I recommend that beginners run much slower and for less distance than their hearts and lungs say they can. Leg muscles that haven't worked in years will rebel.

- Gradually improve your flexibility and increase your leg muscle strength.
- Build up running distance or time *slowly*.
- Run only in well-cushioned shoes, and on soft surfaces if possible.
- Stretch before and after workouts.
- Take plenty of hot baths to soothe the muscles.

When the experienced runner suffers from leg fatigue, it is generally due to overtraining. Therefore, the rules above also apply to him or her. All runners must stretch, to minimize leg fatigue, prior to workouts and afterwards.

A condition that I call "concrete legs" is a variation of leg fatigue. After my first marathon, I had to be carried from the stadium to the car. I couldn't move my legs. I had never run farther than 10 miles before that day. Eventually I recovered, and as my training increased, my legs became stronger and after races, the recovery was faster. With lots of help from my friends, and a bit of experimentation, I've discovered a way to minimize concrete legs, or other leg pain:

- Don't sit down immediately after the race, and don't cross the finish line and fall into a heap. Keep walking or jogging for a while, and stretch for 15 minutes. Continue stretching on and off throughout the day. Don't lie or sit in one position for long periods of time. Don't force the stretch, but do force yourself to stretch some, even when your body protests.
- Soak in a warm tub as soon as possible, and follow that with stretching exercises as often as necessary.
- Run the next day. Go slow and not too far, and it will help you recover.
- For the next few days, try short bursts of speed and a bit of hill work to "flush out" the waste products—lactic acid —in the legs.
- An increased pace with full leg stride at the end of a long workout will help prevent tightness.
- Applying various liniments before and after running to prevent or soothe muscle soreness can be of help. (Caution: Men, wash your hands thoroughly after using the "hot" liniments before going to the bathroom, or you may find yourself with a burning desire to soak in a tub of ice water.)

Leg cramping is also a painful experience. It usually occurs in hot weather, when the runner's body fluid reserves have been drained along with key minerals. Dietary deficiencies in potassium, calcium and magnesium can cause cramping. Other causes include tension, caffeine consumption and the lack of warm-up.

The beginner runner may get a charley horse—a pulled muscle, usually the hamstring muscle in the back of the leg. This is actually a strain or tear in the muscle. It occurs because the muscles are either too weak or too inflexible in the beginner, or imbalanced in the experienced runner. Sprinters have powerful thigh muscles and comparatively weak hamstrings. Distance runners have strong hamstring muscles and weak quadricep muscles. The beginner needs to strengthen his overall leg muscles to prevent pulls; the veteran runner needs to do special exercises for the quadriceps to balance leg strength and to prevent a thigh muscle pull.

A muscle that is suddenly jerked by a sharp action, or one that hasn't been properly warmed up, or is tight and inflexible will pull at its tendon or connection with the bone. The distance runner who is inflexible will often develop a hamstring pull near his or her buttocks. Stretching exercises (see chapters 1 and 6), are essential for minimizing hamstring pulls. At the same time, runners can hurt themselves while stretching if they jerk hard and fast, or force a stretch.

Hamstring pulls come with bursts of speed, or by jumping over obstacles. Cold weather also makes all runners more prone to pulls; they should warm up carefully and avoid speed work during these months. Running or walking on ice and snow may strain hamstring muscles that are unprepared.

If a leg muscle is pulled, ice should be applied as soon as possible. For forty-eight hours, the leg should be elevated if possible. Gentle massage, whirlpool, ultrasound and light exercise is the next step. Walking and swimming may be necessary before returning to running. Severe pulls should be referred to your physician.

### The Battle of Wounded Knee

Knee problems combine stresses or strains on the knee joint with the inability of the knee to handle the stress. Abnormal stress may come from the fact that your foot strikes the ground 5000 times per hour with the force of three times your body weight. If something in the supporting structure gives, the result is often pain, or the inability to run. Knee pain is the most common running injury. Dr. Schuster notes that 75 percent of his patients have some knee pain, although they may be in his office for some other reason.

The kneecap normally rides smoothly in a groove. It is attached to the large quadriceps muscle of the thigh, which is strong enough to pull the kneecap sideways if the angle of the pull is twisted. The result may be irritated cartilage, which is symptomatic of runner's knee, or tendonitis. A variety of factors may cause this faulty biomechanical problem.

When you have knee pain, avoid hill and speed work. Running with the toes consciously pointed slightly inward will help prevent the kneecap from moving out of place. Ice applied immediately after running and before bedtime reduces the pain. Ted Corbitt's favorite trick is to ice the knee before bed, and then place a damp cloth over it covered tightly with a plastic bag. As the moisture evaporates it keeps the knee warm and loose, and promotes circulation to the area to aid in healing. A similar benefit comes from wrapping the knee in flannel before retiring. Ultrasound and whirlpool may also help. Knee braces and supports are good temporary aids, but also tend to act as a crutch for muscles that need to be stretched and strengthened. It is often wise to bicycle or swim for a few days in order to keep the strain off a damaged knee.

A *Runner's World* survey indicated that more than 20 percent of all runners are sidelined with knee problems, and three out of four of Dr. Schuster's patients have injuries related to the knee. Our goal is to treat these injuries before they occur.

The following causes of and treatments for knee pain come from my own painful experience after injury in college, and information from the doctors who helped me return as a runner, Dr. Sheehan and Dr. Schuster.

- Structural instability of the foot. If you have a short big toe and a long second toe (Morton's Foot), weak arches or an unstable heel, you may be prone to knee injuries. With Morton's Foot, it is not the toe that creates the problem, but the metatarsal behind it. The toe reflects this abnormality. These foot imbalances can be helped with arch supports, heel cups, or custom-made inserts.

  Most runners have structurally weak feet that pronate (turn inward) or flatten while running, causing a tremendous torque action on the knee. I usually have my runners try the Dr. Scholl's #610 arch support first, and if that doesn't work or, at least begin to solve the problem, I refer them to a runner-podiatrist. Many runners are "saved" by commercial or specially made foot control products designed to neutralize the foot at impact.

- Short, tight calf and hamstring muscles and inflexibility in the supportive structures of the knee joint contribute to the problem. All the flexibility exercises in chapters 1 and 6 will help with knee problems. The following are also beneficial:

—Lie on your back, knees flexed. Slowly raise one leg overhead, grasping the leg behind the heel with both hands. Pull the straight leg toward your forehead. Hold the position; don't force it. Alternate legs.

—Sitting, place your right foot sideways on your left thigh, and gently apply pressure downward on the knee. Alternate.

—Standing, grab your right ankle with your right hand, and bending the knee, slowly pull upward behind you. Alternate.

—Standing, legs about 3 feet apart, toes pointed ahead. Now turn the left foot 45° outward and, keeping the knee locked, hands behind head, slowly lower your forehead toward the left knee and hold for 15 seconds. Do not force it. Alternate.

—Standing, place one leg on a chair or table at a comfortable height parallel to the ground. Push the heel downward, hold for 6 seconds, relax. Then lean your body weight forward, and feel the stretch. Repeat twice, and alternate legs.

• Weak quadricep muscles, or quads weak in relation to the hamstrings, can cause an imbalance which affects the pull on the kneecap and leads to pain. The solution is to exercise and strengthen the thigh muscles.

—Sitting in a chair, straighten the leg, and tighten it, holding the kneecap up. Hold for 10–20 seconds in isometric contraction. Repeat 10 to 20 times.

—Sitting on a table, lift any type of weight suspended from the legs, with legs straight, one leg at a time.

—Walk up several flights of stairs regularly.
—Walk in water emphasizing knee-lift.
—Hike or run on hills or in soft sand.

Dr. Weisenfeld notes that guards in basketball rarely get knee pain, which he feels is due to their running backwards a lot. He recommends, in addition to the above exercises, running backwards occasionally to strengthen the knees.

- Unequal leg length causes an unequal distribution of weight, and can cause knee pain. Heel lifts, even home-made with surgical felt, can relieve the imbalance. Custom-made orthotics may be necessary.
- Shoes must be well cushioned with a solid shank. Shoes with a "cutaway" under the arch are structurally weak, and allow the foot to pronate, twisting the knee. Watch the wear pattern on the soles of your shoes. If they wear down on the inside of the heel rather than the outside, you may need inserts.
- An uneven running surface may also twist the knee and bring damage. Avoid unevenness. Run on alternate sides of a graded road, being careful of traffic. Change directions, if possible, in a gym or indoor track to avoid running at a slant. Knee pain can result even from running along the slanted beach.
- Sudden changes in your running schedule may cause knee pain that may disappear when you ease off.

### My Aching Back

To determine whether you are a strong candidate for back pain, take these four simple tests. Two are from the Kraus-Weber Minimal Muscle Tests, the third is used by Dr. Richard Schuster in analyzing leg length discrepancies, and the fourth was developed by me after working with hundreds of people suffering from back pain.

*Test One: Abdominal muscle strength*   Lie on your back, knees flexed, both hands behind your head, heels as close to your buttocks as possible (held by a friend or heavy object). Roll into a sitting position. Incredibly, one out of every four people I test for beginner running classes or back classes cannot do one sit-up. My experience is that 10 percent of all runners cannot do sit-ups. You should be able to do at least 20 consecutive bent-knee sit-ups if you intend to run regularly. If your abdominal muscles can't support your erect body during running, then the pelvic girdle will tip forward, causing a swayback. The result is abdominal strain on the muscles and ligaments of the back.

*Test Two: Flexibility*   Stand with both feet together, hands together, and slowly lower your fingertips toward a point on the floor beyond your toes. Keep the knees locked, but don't force it! If you can't touch the floor, have someone measure how many inches distant you are, so that you can later measure your improvement. More than 85 percent of back pain sufferers in my classes fail this test.

Flexibility decreases with age, and with running, which strengthens—and tightens—calf and hamstring muscles. Yet flexibility returns with practice and exercise. Three years ago I was seven inches away from touching the floor, and now I can touch it with the palms of my hands. Regular stretching before and after workouts does wonders. Also, attacks of back pain and sciatica lessen with improved flexibility.

*Test Three: Unequal leg length*   Sit in a chair with both feet flat on the floor. Put a carpenter's level, or a flat piece of wood, across the knees. Major leg length discrepancies will be obvious. Unequal leg length places pressure on the lower back, and is a major cause of back pain among runners. It can be relieved with heel lifts or inserts to allow for the shortness of one leg and equalize the pressure at impact. However, Dr. Schuster emphasizes that if one leg is shorter than the other, but causing you no difficulty, it should be left alone.

*Test Four: Type A syndrome* The Type A personality is tense and jumpy. As a runner, he is recognized by his (or her) short, choppy stride, tense face and shoulders, clenched fists, high arm carry, and frequent compulsion for speed. As a result, he or she often suffers from back pain, and may need to learn to do relaxation exercises before running, and to run in a relaxed style at a slow to moderate pace.

Overcoming most back pain is merely a matter of flexibility and exercise. Studies show that more than 80 percent of all back pain is due to muscular weaknesses rather than pathological factors. Four basic types of people develop back pain:

- The sedentary, soft American who has weak postural muscles.
- The weekend athlete and the previous sedentary person who rushes into exercise without preparation.
- The experienced athlete who has developed a muscle imbalance by not strengthening his or her abdominal muscles, or stretching the hamstring and calf muscles.
- Tense people, whether sedentary or active.

If you suffer from back pain, you're not alone. More than 80 percent of all Americans are victims at some time in their lives. Within three days after appearing on a television show about back pain, I received 300 phone calls pleading for help. Sufferers are found everywhere. Both ultra marathon runners Gary Muhrcke and Dr. Norb Sander suffer from chronic back pain, as does Nina Kuscsik, a world class marathoner. Yet, with all the suffering, no one knows for certain what causes back pain. We do know, however, that overcoming most back pain can be merely a matter of flexibility and exercise.

In addition to the probable causes found in the four tests, there are several other causes that will concern runners:

1. *Poor flexibility* Stretching exercises for the hamstring and calf muscles will aid in limiting back pain. (See chapters 1 and 6.) Exercises in which you bend slowly forward, backward and to the side also loosen the back. The "Cat Back" exercise aids flexibility of the spine. "Hanging" from a bar for 30 seconds to 1 minute also helps stretch the back muscles.

2. *Weakness in key postural muscles* Abdominal strengthening exercises such as bent-knee sit-ups are essential. Next to sit-ups the best abdominal exercise is the basket hang: Hanging from a bar, you slowly raise the knees up to the chest and slowly lower them. Sucking in the "gut" and holding it for an isometric contraction is also good.

The gluteal muscles (rear end), erector spinae (back muscles along the spine), and the abdominals can be strengthened with two exercises: Lying on your back, tilt the pelvis back, tighten the buttocks and stomach, and push the lower back into the floor and hold; or, stand with your back against a wall, push your lower back towards the wall as you tighten the buttocks and stomach.

1. *Structural weaknesses* In addition to unequal leg length, structurally weak feet and back may cause back pain. Curvatures of the spine cannot be corrected in most cases, but the strength of the supporting muscle can be improved by exercise.

2. *Uneven footstrike* Running on a slant or in worn-out shoes is risky. Change direction on indoor track; alternate side of the road when outdoors.

**3.** *Impact shock*  With footstrikes between 5000 and 7000 times an hour, you need well-cushioned shoes.

**4.** *Running style*  Running in a constant forward lean will cause added strain on the back muscles.

**5.** *Pregnancy*  Additional pressure is put on the back during pregnancy because of the shift in weight distribution. The abdominal muscles are weaker after pregnancy. It is important to continue abdominal muscle strengthening both during and after pregnancy. (See chapter 8.)

**6.** *Obesity*  Men and women who are fat place a greater burden on their backs, especially if the stomach protrudes. A swayback condition may occur.

**7.** *Bad work and sleep habits*  Learn how to lift heavy objects. Don't lift with your back, but bend at the knees and allow your powerful legs, strengthened by many miles of running, to do the work. Sleeping on your stomach may cause a swayback condition, and strain the back. If you persist, place a pillow under your hips. Sleeping on your back may also cause problems, and placing a pillow under your knees will allow the lower back to flatten. Comfort is the key to sleeping correctly, but the preferred position is on your side, knees flexed—the fetal position. The bed should be very firm, and a bed board should be placed under the mattress. Dr. Kraus recommends a hard, horsehair mattress with no spring.

**8.** *Tension*  Back pain and tension go together. If you are going through a period of emotional tension, you may have to take it easy on your running. Something has to give; often it's your back.

**9.** *Sciatica*  The sciatic nerve is described by Dr. Sheehan as "the longest river of pain in the body." It begins in the lower back and extends all the way down to the ankle. Pain may occur in the back, hip, leg or even the ankle and the two lesser toes. It may be a numbing sensation or a severe pain shooting from the back down the leg. It is caused by a pressure on the nerve and can be the result of poor flexibility and weak postural muscles or a manifestation of a herniated disc. Not all leg pain is due to sciatica. Muscle pain sometimes mimics sciatica pain.

10. *Herniated disc*   Discs are located between each vertebra of the back and act as shock absorbers. If one is ruptured or damaged, it may be surgically removed and the bone fused together. Obviously, such an operation is a cure of last resort. By examining the possible causes for the stress on the disc, you may not need an operation.

11. *Student's disease*   Back pain may also be psychological. It is a well-known phenomenon, especially among medical students, that if you study a disease in great detail you begin to develop the problem yourself. I got back pain during an exhaustive study of that disease. Fortunately, I learned my lesson: I'll never do a paper on impotence!

If you've suffered back pain, you should rest a few days and return to running very slowly. Taking warm baths, as well as drawing the knees up to the chest, helps reduce a back pain spasm. Relaxation exercises, stretching exercises and gentle running are the next steps. Sometimes running intervals of fast bursts of speed will stretch out the muscles. Be sure to intersperse the bursts with slow jogging or walking.

Exercises can help a lot. A television executive I know was told he would have to wear a girdle for the rest of his life, or undergo a disc removal operation. He took a back-pain class, followed by a beginner's fitness class which emphasized exercise. He threw away the girdle, and told his sedentary, overweight orthopedic specialists where to go—go exercise. He's now running 5 miles a day and feels like a new man.

The National YMCA program, "The Y's Way to a Healthy Back," was developed by Dr. Kraus and Alexander Melleby. It is being offered at Y's across the country and is recommended for any runner who is experiencing back pain.

### The Thick Head

Overcoming stubbornness and stupidity may be a major problem. I've learned how to identify and deal with most major injuries, but I still get them because I often ignore early warnings. However, I'm less prone to injury than I once was, so perhaps I'm learning. Joe Henderson, editor of *Runner's World*, suggests becoming an "experiment of one," learning through experience and common sense. Bill Bowerman, former University of Oregon track coach, preaches "train, don't strain," and Dr. Sheehan says "listen to your body"—it will warn you when you're pushing toward injury or disease. To these great prophets of the running world, I can only add the warning: "Do as I say, not as I do." I'm still learning.

This chapter may seem to indicate that running inevitably leads to injury. It is true that, as runners, we are subject to injuries of a wide variety, but that doesn't mean we shouldn't run, only that we should be cautious, warm up and cool down carefully, and be alert to signs of injury or pain. By knowing what injuries are possible, we can better avoid falling victim to them. What signs are significant? What does pain tell us?

Here are other injuries I've had or heard other runners complain about. They are listed alphabetically, and the information here is not meant to replace a visit to your running physician.

## The Ankle

Ankle sprains are caused by structural imbalance, improper foot gear, rough terrain, and improper conditioning.

The typical runner's ankle sprain occurs when a sedentary, overweight person runs in thin tennis shoes. It also happens to the overweight runner, whose weight puts great stress on the ankles, and the beginner runner who has been pounding on weak ankles that become inflamed and painful. Women beginner runners are most prone to ankle sprain, and a surprisingly large number of them complain of ankle swelling. Californian runner-doctor Joan Ullyot calls this a "beginner's pseudo-sprain." It is not caused by stepping in a hole and turning the ankle, but by weak supportive muscles. These runners haven't been using their leg muscles much, and the muscles and tendons around the ankles have become weak and are easily strained or injured. Women's ankles are further weakened by wearing "high-fashion shoes"—high heels, pointed toes, which shorten the Achilles' tendon and hamstring.

Both men and women who begin running should wear well-cushioned shoes and work on the supporting muscles and tendons of their ankles. They need gradual strengthening, which can be done with exercises such as ankle circles (turning the ankle slowly in a circle), or walking on the sides of your foot. The ankles should always be loosened with these exercises prior to running. Swimming will also strengthen your ankles. Beginner runners should follow the Run-Easy Method that includes walking as well as running. Although ankle sprains are rare among veteran runners, the more experienced runner may suffer from a severe sprain that ruptures the tendons. But the most common sprain occurs when you've been running on uneven surfaces, especially during overtraining. As Dr. Richard Schuster notes, however, runners most often injure their ankles while they are walking because they are less alert to the change in ground surfaces than while running.

Once the damage is done, ice should be immediately applied to reduce swelling. The ankle should be taped or wrapped in an ankle support, and elevated. The elastic ankle supports should be worn all day until the swelling goes down. Later, whirlpool or ultrasound treatment and warm baths will aid in removing waste from the area. This may be followed by light exercises, but if the ankle hurts and is swollen, stay off it, even if that means using crutches for a few days.

Beware of doctors with needles and plaster. Cortisone injections may give temporary relief, but excessive injections can lead to joint destruction and perhaps tendon rupture. No more than one injection should be given per two months, according to Dr. Murray Weisenfeld. Other doctors believe that the best way to keep runners off their feet, even if they promise to be good, is to slap on a cast. This probably is not necessary.

My ankles were very weak. I was in a cast many times, although I still managed to play in a championship basketball game while wearing a shell cast and an oversized shoe. In fact, I officially became a road runner two days after getting out of a cast on my leg due to another ankle injury: I turned it playing Capture-the-Flag with a group of kids. The more I ran, I discovered, the stronger my ankles became. Previously, I would feel pain in my weak ankles just walking across a field. Running actually strengthened them, probably because of the twisting and turning of cross-country workouts.

Another ankle problem is caused by one of our ankles' best friends: our thick-soled running shoes. It's easy to turn an ankle in these shoes in the beginning, when you're not used to having so much rubber under your foot. It's also easy to turn an ankle in these shoes when running fast around corners.

Beware of speed work on tight-cornered indoor tracks. It may be better to use a thinner-soled racing flat.

### Arthritis

The cause of osteoarthritis is a mystery. But it is not attributed to exercise. The myth that running places a great strain on the joints, and leads to osteoarthritis is just that—a myth. Sedentary people are just as prone to arthritis as runners, maybe more so.

A study, "Running and Primary Osteoarthritis of the Hip," was published by some Finnish researchers in *The British Medical Journal* in 1975. It focused on 74 former Finnish record-holding runners whose average age was sixty-five and who had competed for an average span of twenty-one years. X-rays revealed osteoarthritis in only 4 percent of the athletes, compared to 8.7 percent among those in a control group of nonrunners.

Lack of use may contribute to the onset of osteoarthritis. Proper exercise apparently allows the joint fluid to circulate, which is necessary for the nutrition of the various components of the joints. Running may prevent the disease, but it cannot cure it.

Osteoarthritis should be diagnosed only by X-ray, not by complaint. Runners who have it may have to take a few days off when it becomes bothersome, and perhaps substitute swimming or cycling for their workouts. Aspirin may help. Heat also soothes. Also, a reasonable amount of movement of the affected joints may relieve the pain of osteoarthritis.

### Asthma and Emphysema

Many asthmatics are not allowed exercise by doctors and overprotective parents. In the fall of 1976, however, the New

York Lung Association developed a revolutionary exercise program for asthmatic youths. The result showed a noticeable gain in the amount of physical activity asthmatics could perform. Some doctors believe that physical activity alleviates asthma and emphysema symptoms by improving pulmonary circulation, liquifying and eliminating mucous plugs, and decreasing the viscosity of bronchial secretions. More important, perhaps, is the fact that exercise improves these patients' self-esteem and emotional well-being.

One beginner's fitness class included a group of five middle-aged women who had suffered from asthma most of their lives. They followed a running program with frequent walk breaks, and kept nasal sprays at hand in case of wheezing. They all found that they could breathe better because the muscles involved with breathing were strengthened by exercise. They also slept better at night.

On the other hand, the sedentary life often imposed on asthmatics seems to lead to obesity, high blood pressure, heart disease and other diseases of inactivity, which are far worse than the wheezing of asthma. Still, exercise-induced asthma attacks are a serious problem. Running in cold air, or when bothered with a respiratory infection, may make the individual more prone to an attack. Asthmatics should try to do interval walk-run workouts because prolonged running may induce an attack. Various medications, taken before and during running, may prevent these problems. Any exercise performed by asthmatics should be done under the supervision of an athletically minded physician. Dr. Norb Sander, for example, has also worked with asthmatics, and gets good results with asthmatic runners who inhale Chromylin Sodium prior to exercise. Again, check this with your physician. Other drugs may cause cardiac stimulation when combined with exercise, and should be watched.

Many world class athletes have been asthmatics, including several runners. With proper medication, they have competed with "normal" runners. American swimmer Rick DeMont was disqualified after he had won a gold medal during the 1972 Olympics, because he had used a forbidden "drug"—an asthma medication. But the controversy focused attention on the fact that asthmatics could exercise regularly and vigorously, and even win Olympic gold medals.

People with emphysema may also benefit from regular exercise, which improves the strength and efficiency of the cardiopulmonary system. Like asthmatics, sufferers of emphysema often are unaware of how much exercise they are capable of enjoying. They will also benefit from learning the technique of "belly breathing," which improves the efficiency of breathing.

### Athlete's Foot

Athlete's foot is a fungus which causes two types of eruptions. One occurs between the toes—the skin turns white and soggy, often peeling off and leaving red, raw patches. The other occurs on the sole of the foot, where small blisters cover the affected area. Athlete's foot can be more than a nuisance. It can itch and burn and cause severe discomfort, and left untreated, it can spread rapidly, causing large blisters, raw skin and swelling. It can make wearing shoes unbearable, and walking or running impossible.

It is most often caused by improper foot care, wearing sweat-soaked socks or tight, airless shoes that create a climate for fungus to grow.

Good foot care is the best defense. Feet should be washed

every night in warm water, dried thoroughly and sprinkled with anti-fungus foot powder. Fungus also feeds on dead skin tissue, so it's important to clean the skin regularly with a nail brush or pumice stone.

It is also important to wear clean socks every day, especially in summer. This means both your running footwear and your "civilian" apparel. Don't try to get another run out of a pair of wet, dirty socks. Since nylon socks and rubber footwear don't absorb sweat, they can also contribute to athlete's foot. Wearing sandals in the summer to allow your feet to ventilate and keep dry is also a good idea.

The myth is that athlete's foot can be picked up in the locker room. But I spend half my life walking in and out of locker rooms in bare feet, and have never had more than a minor touch of athlete's foot. Lucky? I prefer to think that the condition is more a matter of your health care for your feet.

### Ball of Foot

Pain in the ball of the foot may have several causes. Running too high on the toes, or running with thin-soled shoes can cause a bruise of the metatarsal bones. Morton's foot, a condition in which the second toe is longer than the first, and the first metatarsal bone is short, can cause the second metatarsal to accept an abnormal weight load. A large build-up of calluses can also cause pressure on the nerves in the foot, resulting in pain or a feeling of numbness. Improper weight distribution on footstrike results in pain, and sometimes even stress fracture.

A common remedy is to pad the ball of the foot heavily at the point of pain. Actually, the padding should go behind the painful area to take the weight off it. I had developed an excruciating pain over the metatarsal head below my second toe shortly before the Boston Marathon. The condition was instantly cured by Dr. Schuster, who merely added some extra padding to the inserts behind the painful area. Presto! I was running pain-free again.

If the problem persists, however, special orthotics should be prescribed to distribute the weight at footstrike. A delay in proper treatment could result in the development of a stress fracture.

### Blood in Urine

The first report of a runner's urine appearing bloody after "a severe run" was written by Dr. L. Dickinson of the Clinical Society of London; it appeared in 1894. Eighty-four years later, this occurrence, still largely unexplained, remains one of the most alarming and most mysterious of athletic ailments.

After a hard run, the runner's urine may indeed appear bloody. It may be blood, or hemoglobin from the destruction of red cells in the body, or myoglobin from the breakdown of muscle fibers during exercise. Don't panic. Stay calm, and collect a sample for your physician. Do this right away, because your next urine, says Dr. George Sheehan, may be "as clear as spring water."

Most likely, bloody urine is hemoglobinuria, which occurs in cyclical patterns. It comes and goes in athletes, and may be triggered by an allergy, exhaustion, or other factors. Frank Shorter, the Olympic marathon runner, has had episodes of bloody urine—and keeps on running.

One form of treatment is rest: The condition cures itself within forty-eight hours. Or, switch from pavement to grass running, use shoes with good cushioning and additional rubber or inserts, and practice a lighter footfall and a gliding style. Also, avoid extreme fatigue, and add vitamin C to your diet in substantial amounts. (See page 312.)

### Low Blood Sugar

Low blood sugar is frequently accompanied by feelings of drowsiness and fatigue. It may be a long-term condition (hypoglycemia) or only a temporary one, commonly called the mid-morning "blahs." By mid-morning your breakfast has digested and your blood sugar is low. This is the time when many people feel the need for a candy bar or cup of coffee with Danish.

But the best temporary way to raise your blood sugar level is with 10 to 15 minutes or more of exercise. This releases sugar from its storage spots in the muscle and builds up blood sugar.

Runners with hypoglycemia should follow a high-protein–high-fat diet, but should use high-carbohydrate dieting prior to long-distance efforts that may involve glycogen depletion. The runner with hypoglycemia should also be under the supervision of an athletically oriented physician.

### Chest Pain

Chest pain, especially upon exertion or shortly afterward, can be a vital warning of heart disorder. The chest pain, or angina, is caused by ischemia—a lack of sufficient blood flow for the heart's need. Angina attacks may be mild or severe, described either as "crushing pain, like an elephant sitting on your chest," or as a "mild discomfort or ache."

The pain may start in the middle of your chest and radiate to the shoulders, arms and even jaw, teeth and ears. Sometimes, the pain may appear in only one area, such as the left arm, and not in the chest at all.

Angina need not stop a person from running *if it has been stabilized*; that is, a predictable pattern of symptoms in relation to the patient's activities has been established over a period of time. Cardiac patients may take nitroglycerine tablets at the onset of anginal pain. Obviously, anyone with anginal pain should exercise only under close medical supervision.

Most chest pain in healthy people is not due to angina. We all have occasional twinges, aches and muscle spasms in the chest which are totally unrelated to the heart. Some pain is caused by your gastrointestinal tract, nerve pressure in the neck, gallbladder problems, ulcers and the like. Overbreathing or hyperventilation may also cause pain. So will soreness in the muscles around the breastbone.

I once questioned my own health when I developed a severe pain on my left side during three successive days of running. Then I remembered catching a sharp elbow during a basketball game. I was getting old. My ribs had been slightly bruised and were irritated by running, causing me to breathe deeper, and forcing the injured rib cage to expand and contract rapidly.

Chest pain shouldn't be taken lightly. We know of runners who have complained of pain and who then had positive stress tests indicating that they did, indeed, have heart disease. Obviously, having a heart attack is not the best, or safest, way of documenting the course of chest pain. See a doctor.

### Colds and Flu
Running can help you get rid of colds, but it can also weaken you to infection. It's possible for us to run right through colds that would level our unfit friends. When runners overstress themselves, however, they are very susceptible to the common cold; I'm most vulnerable during the two weeks after a marathon, or the pre-race build-up before one.

Exercise tends to break up the congestion of a cold. It also gives a psychological lift. But colds are a warning signal. Dr. Sheehan says, "I treat colds with respect. It is my feeling that they represent a breakdown of the defense system. The cold is an early morning symptom of exhaustion." There have been documented cases of sudden death in athletes who exercised heavily despite fighting a viral infection. If you have a cold, cut your mileage, slow down and run within the limits of your energy.

To avoid colds: Obviously keep warm, keep your head covered in cold weather, and don't stand around in wet clothing after a race or workout. Doses of vitamin C may also help fight colds and flu (see page 312).

Fever and flu are more dangerous. The body is in a weakened state. It doesn't need the additional stress of running, and it's best to rest completely, and then return slowly to a normal schedule. I once spent an entire summer bothered by flu, or perhaps a touch of mononucleosis. I was so intent on returning to my training program that I suffered three "relapses." It is wise to listen to your body, for your stubborn mind can lead you astray.

### Diabetes
Insulin is required by the body in order to store body sugars and to transport the blood sugar into cells for storage. Insulin is lacking in a diabetic, and must be injected or ingested. Also, the diabetic's diet must be regimented to maintain proper blood-sugar levels. During exercise the glycogen level is lowered and blood sugar drops. The diabetic athlete must take in sugar at regular intervals to keep from becoming weak and sick.

Diabetics have successfully competed in marathon running after gradually building to it. Initially, runs should not exceed 6 miles until a pattern of response has been determined. Diabetic runners should coordinate their diet, medicine and exercise under careful medical supervision. They need to be aware of the feeling of the onset of hypoglycemia. Dr. Norb Sander suggests that a diabetic carry a glucose solution in a small plastic squeeze bottle during all runs rather than take a chance on finding a supply along the route.

Diabetic runners may want to follow Dr. Sheehan's precautions: 1. Reduce insulin to half on the days of racing or hard training; 2. Eat a high-protein meal prior to running; 3. Keep sugar, in the form of candy or a sugar solution, near the practice area; 4. Maintain carbohydrate stores by eating a high-carbohydrate diet on easy-running days (every other day at first).

### Diarrhea and Constipation

Diarrhea and intestinal cramps may be caused by a wide variety of things—change in diet, especially to a vegetarian one; increased exercise; certain foods such as milk, wheat products, chocolate, nuts, raisins, fruits and vegetables. They may be caused by the onset of illness or the ingestion of new bacteria in a foreign country. Serious diarrhea will dehydrate your body, and may cause fever, uncontrolled bowel movements, fainting. These symptoms should be medically treated immediately.

Diarrhea from diet or nerves is less serious, and can usually be prevented or controlled by taking care with foods and training before a race or a long run, and proteins should be avoided. The worst possible combination would be a greasy hamburger and a glass of milk. The night before a race, eat carbohydrates. The morning of a race, fast if you can; if not, don't eat for at least three or four hours before the race (or long run). Always attempt a bowel movement before hitting the road. If you are planning a long run, or feel vulnerable, like the morning after downing lots of bad beer, be prepared by carrying along a wad of toilet paper. If the cramping becomes severe, stop and walk.

Don't try to hold off too long; sometimes you can get away with walking into a restaurant and asking for a bathroom, but you can't count on this solution. The best bet is to look for a hidden spot, and go! Constipation is rarely a problem for runners, but if it is, add bran to your diet because it acts as an "intestinal broom." However, do not eat bran before racing or a long workout.

Pre-race diarrhea is common, and it may even make us run faster. Bill Rodgers ran a 2:10:09 in the 1976 New York Marathon, only a few seconds off his American record. When asked what he thought about during the last few miles as he threatened the record, he replied: "I just wanted to get to the john."

### Groin Pain

Groin pain appears to be most common among women, perhaps because of their wider pelvic girdle. It often is coupled with limited rear foot motion and unequal leg length. According to Dr. Schuster, "Patient files seem to indicate that some groin pains are related to the inability of the lower ankle to move from side to side—particularly outward. The only other structures that can provide this kind of in-and-out control are the adductor muscles (which pull the leg inward) of the hip—hence the possibility of groin pain."

An insert or heel cup will stabilize the heel and limit the pain. Stretching and strengthening exercises for the adductor muscles that pull the leg outward should also be included in the treatment. Here are two exercises that may help:

To stretch the groin muscles, sit with the soles of your feet together and gently push down on the knees, holding the position. Repeat.

Lie on your unaffected side, with your back and leg straight, and suspend a light weight from your foot above the base of the ankle with the strap. Lift the leg about 12 inches, hold for one second, and return. Repeat several times, but don't continue if pain develops.

### Heel Pain

A heel bruise is generally caused by running on hard surfaces in shoes with thin soles. Running over sharp rocks and pebbles may also cause bruises, as will running too far back and too hard on the heels. A heel bruise may simply require a few days of not running to heal. Cushions under the heels will help you return to running sooner.

Heel bumps or spurs are more painful and can last longer. These are caused by pressure and friction over the top of the heel bone. Irregular movement of the heel bone caused by structurally weak feet, inflexible muscles, slanted running surfaces or worn-down shoes cause the irritation of the tissue (*plantar fascia*) that extends in a fan shape from the toes to the heel. The bursa (fluid-filled protective sacs) becomes inflamed, and the combination of bursitis and calcium deposits results in the heel bump. This bump is located between the skin and the tendon, or the tendon and the bone. Bumps may occur in the back of the heel where the heel bone and Achilles' tendon meet, or on the bottom of the heel. The pain actually comes from the inflamed *plantar fascia*.

Cortisone injections may give temporary relief. Sometimes surgery is necessary to remove excessive bone or irritated bursa. This should be a last resort. Of special danger is a heel bump that could cause a rupture of the Achilles' tendon.

A heel bump or spur on the back of the heel can be relieved by cutting out portions of the back of the shoe, and replacing them with soft elastic. On the bottom of the foot, the problem can be relieved by placing a one-inch thick strip of surgical felt under the heel, and cutting a hole around the area of the heel bump to take the pressure off it.

Dr. Sheehan recommends the following:

- Wear well-cushioned shoes with a good heel counter, high heel and solid shank.
- Use a Dr. Scholl's #610 Arch Support or have custom inserts made to eliminate the cause of the rolling action on the heel and foot. Sometimes just the addition of a heel cup to stabilize the heel is sufficient.
- Do flexibility exercises regularly for the calf and hamstring muscles.
- Run on grass or other soft surfaces, keeping away from speed and hill work.
- Apply heat to the heel before running, and ice afterward.

Recovery will take time. Rushing back into fast running or hard training after this injury would be unwise.

### Hip Pain

Hip pain is almost always caused by unequal pressure upon footstrike. Worn-down shoes, unequal leg length, slanted running surfaces and structurally weak feet are most often the culprits. The use of inserts, heel lifts, well-cushioned and evenly worn shoes, and staying away from slanted surfaces like tracks and graded, paved roads are the most frequent cures.

Sciatica, resulting from nerve pressure, can also cause hip pain. Stretching exercises are an extra benefit if sciatica persists. Osteoarthritis is another cause of hip pain, and can be partially relieved in its early stages with aspirin. Triggerpoints (see page 270) are also frequently found in the hip area. Many times, hip pain results from running while favoring another injury.

The following exercises will stretch and strengthen the key muscles of the hip:

1. Lunge position. Right leg in front of body. Lean forward on the right leg, bending at the right knees, left leg to the rear on its toes, stretched out straight. Do not bob. Hold position for 30 seconds to a minute, then reverse. Repeat several times.

2. Side lunge position. Hands on hips, extend your left leg sideways as far as you can along the ground. Stretch the left leg by resting on the inside of the left foot and putting maximum strength on the inside of the left thigh. Hold. Stretch for 30 seconds to one minute. No bobbing. Alternate legs, and repeat.

3. Stand sideways to a wall, one hand with arm outstretched to the wall for support. Allow hip closest to the wall to fall towards it. Do not move your feet. Hold for 30 seconds to a minute, then alternate sides and repeat.

### Jock Rash

Also known as "jock itch," this horror is similar to athlete's foot: it involves a fungus growing in a damp environment. Wearing clean, dry athletic supporters and bathing regularly are important. I've also heard of a drastic precautionary measure: Swab the area with vinegar; the acid creates an atmosphere in which the fungus cannot survive. Perhaps this method is indeed effective, but I've not tried it.

As a preventive measure, you might try one of the commercially available powders. Sprinkle a little on either side of your groin and along the crotch both before running and after showering. This will dry the area, prevent chafing, and soothe whatever rash may have begun.

If you have jock rash, your doctor will prescribe an ointment (or powder) to get rid of it. Follow his directions faithfully. My co-author recalls one soccer season in college when he and his teammates watched a football player in the locker room who had jock itch. The rash first took the outline of his athletic supporter, and then, ignored, it slowly spread down his thighs and up his abdomen until it covered an area—Shepherd swears it's true—almost two feet wide. The player had no trouble finding a shower after practices—or locker space.

Many men use powder and also wear "jockey shorts" or even nylon bikini briefs to prevent chaffing. Women, on the other hand, are turning from their nylon panties to cotton ones, which absorb moisture. Another preferred undergarment for men are "Speedo's" or similar brief swim trunks. European running shorts come with built-in supports. All of these garments should be washed after every run.

### The Stitch

*Runner's World* always refers to this as "the dreaded side stitch." And it is. The stitch is believed to be a spasm of the diaphragm muscle, which separates the lungs from the abdomen. It strikes the runner just as suddenly and painfully as a charley horse attacks the sprinter or the sedentary, middle-aged man or woman who tries to run hard without warming up. The stitch may, however, begin slowly, and gradually intensify. Sometimes it feels like a knife stuck deep into the bottom or upper side of the rib cage. It usually occurs on the right side.

There are several possible causes. Running on a full stomach makes one more susceptible, especially after having had milk or grain products, which disturb the stomach. An improper warm-up can lead to trouble as the body rebels against the sudden switch from inactivity. A stitch often occurs after the runner starts the race too fast and thus may be related to oxygen debt. Generally, faulty breathing is the primary culprit.

Beginner runners and veterans are both susceptible. A beginner is often tense; when his tensed diaphragm becomes stretched by the rapid breathing during running, a stitch may occur. Experienced runners sometimes breathe improperly, which can also stretch the diaphragm and cause a stitch, particularly late in a race.

How do you fight the dreaded stitch? An increased fitness level helps. As the beginner gradually improves his or her overall cardiopulmonary endurance, and the strength and flexibility of his or her abdominal muscles and awareness of pace, the incidence of stitching decreases. In fact, it rarely occurs again until the runner increases his or her pace or begins to compete—in other words, reaches another stage of running development.

To avoid stitches, beginner runners should carefully stretch all their muscles during the warm-up and perform a variety of abdominal exercises. They should concentrate on proper abdominal breathing, or belly breathing. Prior to running, beginners should walk, raising their arms high overhead and thrusting the stomach outward as they breathe in deeply, and dropping their arms, and exhaling through pursed lips as the stomach is sucked in. Running is started at a slow pace never exceeding the talk-test level. Between running intervals, repeat the walking/belly-breathing technique.

At the first sign of a stitch, walk slowly and repeat the breathing exercises. Emphasizing the belly-breathing technique helps the beginner runner adapt it to his or her normal running pattern of breathing. If the stitch becomes extremely painful, stop and grab the knee on the side of the pain and pull it to your chest for a few seconds, squeezing hard. This can be done while either standing or lying on one's side. This modified fetal position takes the pressure off the diaphragm, which is undergoing a muscle spasm; it's the same technique used to relieve pain from a back spasm.

Runners who experience a stitch in a race have more of a

problem. You can't just stop and do some exercises, although Tom Fleming did during one major race, and then went on to win. Most of us would find ourselves hopelessly behind hundreds of runners after only a few seconds' delay.

If you happen to be running the race of your life, the dreaded side stitch is especially annoying. More than likely you develop a stitch during a race because of a fast start, and tension. Dr. George Sheehan says that a racer who is tense and draws the stomach in while breathing places a tremendous strain on the diaphragm as he or she stretches the taut muscles very quickly and forcefully. Runners may also "trap air," which further stretches the diaphragm. Concentrating on something else, like the shape and movement of the runner—male or female—up ahead, may help. Dr. Sheehan suggests that we breathe out against slight resistance, even if we must groan. Listening to him and Ted Corbitt during a race is almost unpleasant. They moan and groan, these cagey ole aged fifty-plus running veterans, but they pass you by while you're grasping at your side. Super exaggerated belly breathing has worked for me. I'll breathe in very deeply and noisily and exhale deeply with a huge groan. This has two side effects: Everyone thinks I'm a little bonkers—which may be true enough—and, my noise-making startles runners about me, who then scamper ahead.

A more subtle on-the-run treatment for the stitch is to raise your arms overhead while breathing in deeply, expanding your stomach. As you lower your arms, exhale loudly and contract your stomach. Accompanied by a slowing of your pace, this may do the trick. Sometimes, however, you simply must stop and do some stretching exercises until the pain goes away. The ultimate treatment is just to tough it out and pretend the stitch has not happened, but there are few runners I know who can do this.

## Stress Fractures

A stress fracture is a partial or complete break of a bone. It usually occurs in one of the metatarsals in the foot, or in one of the shin bones. The exact causes of stress fracture are not known and sometimes a runner may even have one without noticing it. Runners with poor footstrike due to improper running style or foot instability seem to be more prone to stress fractures. So are runners who sharply increase their mileage or the intensity of their workouts. High school and college track coaches who really drive their young runners, particularly indoors, ruin many good athletes by pushing them into stress fractures. Even runners who have never had problems may suddenly find themselves with a stress fracture. This may be because bone is a metabolically active tissue, and stress fractures may occur during a period of momentary weakness.

The fracture comes on very subtly. At first it may seem to be a case of bad shin splints, but if the pain persists, X-rays should be taken. Sometimes, however, the fracture won't show up on an X-ray for two weeks or so, and if the pain persists, more X-rays may be needed. Often a magnifying glass must be used to locate the stress fracture on the X-ray.

Once diagnosed, it may keep you out of your running shoes for five weeks or more; or you may be able to do some running with inserts to properly distribute your weight. Otherwise, bicycling or swimming are good alternatives. Running on a stress fracture could result in a fractured bone and should only be done with the permission of a podiatrist or physician. The common treatment for any bone injury is to slap on a cast. This often is unnecessary, and can lead to muscle atrophy. An athletically minded podiatrist or orthopedist is your best friend when a stress fracture sabotages your running program.

It is possible to return to heavy training gradually after a stress fracture. Millrose AA runner Mike Cleary lost ten weeks of training due to a stress fracture of the shin bone, and within three months of resuming training ran his best times for 2:54 and 2:39 for the marathon. The key to his success was in keeping off the injury, and then gradually building his mileage back to normal. Often, stress fractures will reoccur. It is therefore important, after healing, to investigate the cause by having a thorough biomechanical evaluation by a sports medicine expert.

### Triggerpoints

Triggerpoints are local tender spots of degenerated muscle tissue in the skeletal muscle. They can produce severe pain or muscle spasm. The pain may radiate down the extremities, head, neck, and back. Runners are most susceptible to triggerpoints in the legs and back.

Triggerpoints may be caused by faulty running style or structural weakness that results in an abnormal strain on a particular muscle group, muscular imbalance produced by weak or stiff posture muscles, or tension. The pain may come and go, but becomes most intense during periods of emotional pressure.

I was a victim of triggerpoints. Actually, I was a victim of my inability to slow down and do one thing at a time. During the summer of 1976, I was running 100 miles a week, and feeling great. Then came graduate school, long hours of pressure at my old job, this book, the organization of the New York Marathon. I was in a self-spun web of pressure, and three weeks before the marathon, I broke down. My knee and back hurt in a whole new way. It wasn't pain from structural weaknesses or inflexibility. It was tension pain.

When I probed spots in the tendons above my knee, calf, hip and back, pain radiated from them. Dr. Hans Kraus ordered point massage twice daily. It was sheer agony as the masseur pressed deeply on the tension-knotted muscles. It almost worked. I ran the first 10 miles of the marathon pain-free and very fast, but it was hell from that point on.

The treatment procedure for triggerpoints is to inject an anesthetic (Lidocaine, Procaine or Novocaine) into the knot to break up the spots of degenerated muscle tissue. This is followed on succeeding days by electrical stimulation to relax the muscle. Absolutely no exercise or even prolonged sitting or standing are allowed during the treatments. Therapy is followed by a program of relaxation and stretching exercises, and a gradual progression back to a normal running schedule. I wasn't able to exercise for a month and a half, but I was able to return to competition. Treatment, however, only eliminates the symptoms, not the cause. The pain may very well return.

### Varicose Veins

The veins in the legs carry deoxygenated blood back to the heart. Since these vessels must conduct blood upward against the force of gravity, a series of valves is employed to prevent the backflow of blood. In people who sit or stand a great deal, the valves of the leg veins tend to wear out, and in time the high pressure of the long column of blood that they must support overcomes the elasticity of the veins' walls and valves. Thus, the veins are dilated and become "varicose veins." The tendency to develop varicose veins is largely, but not exclusively, hereditary.

Dr. Colin James Alexander hypothesized in *The Lancet* in 1972 that Western man's habit of sitting in chairs could be the major cause of varicose veins. Primitive people without chairs rarely suffer from the affliction. Chair sitting places a high and constant pressure on the vein walls. Rocking chairs, however, promote circulation. Sedentary life, therefore, may increase the normal dilation of the veins that comes with aging, and the veins become more sensitive to other factors like standing, pregnancy and tight clothing.

Medical studies show that people with varicose veins are bothered less if they follow an endurance conditioning program such as running. Running will not make varicose veins go away, but it will increase the strength of the supportive structures around the veins, and assist in the venous blood return from the legs to the heart. Actually, varicose veins may become more prominant as you run, but this isn't furthering the condition.

Superficial varicose veins are more a cosmetic than a medical problem. A surgical operation to strip the veins will improve the looks of the legs, but not aid in improving circulation. Sometimes surgery is necessary, however, if the condition becomes too painful.

Marathoner Nina Kuscsik often complained to her doctor about leg pains due to varicose veins, but the muscle tone of her legs from her marathon running hid the problem, and her doctor didn't think it serious. Not until she decided to have surgery, and was relaxed under the anesthesia did the true condition of her veins become evident.

Swelling is common after surgery. Nina was instructed to wear an Ace bandage on her entire leg for three weeks to promote circulation and prevent pressure over the incision. Oddly, she was also told not to bother with the bandage while running, which naturally improves circulation. She said, "So I was out there running four days after surgery, before the stitches were removed. I had no swelling at all!"

Runners with a tendency toward varicosity should sit with their feet up, wear elastic support socks to assist circulation, and avoid tight pants and socks.

# 12 THE HEART-LUNG MACHINE

What happens to your body when you run? At the center of your chest—indeed, at the center of your life—is your heart. It's an extraordinary muscle about the size of your fist that weighs 8 to 10 ounces, beats an average of 70 to 80 times a minute while resting, or about 4200 times an hour, 100,000 times a day, more than 36 billion times a year.

The heart is composed of muscle tissue different from any other tissue in the body: Cardiac muscle has its own distinct appearance under the microscope. The heart is also one of the best muscular structures of our bodies, ready to improve its condition if we exercise it in a proper manner. This muscle pumps your body's entire blood supply (about 5 quarts) through your vascular system in less than a minute; during exercise blood may travel through your arteries at speeds of 40 miles per hour.

The red cells in your blood carry oxygen to the muscles of your body, and return waste—carbon dioxide—to the lungs to be expelled. Exercise increases and enriches this exchange.

On either side of your heart are the lungs. These organs are light, porous and spongy in texture and highly elastic. Inside your lungs are microscopic air sacs called alveoli. The lungs contain millions of them, tiny and balloonlike. Here, your blood

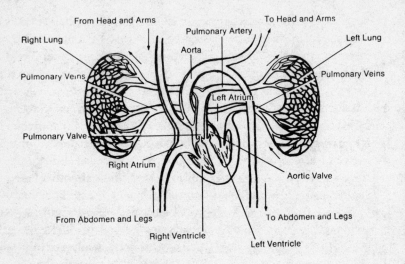

### The Heart-Lung Machine

becomes oxygenated. Each tiny alveolus is covered with a membrane wall one-cell thick. When air is breathed into the lungs, molecules of oxygen pass through the thin membrane of the alveolus (with its bronchi and bronchioles) to attach to the hemoglobin of red blood cells. The membrane is so small that each red blood cell must line up and pass through in single file to take in oxygen and give up carbon dioxide, water and other wastes.

These organs—the heart and lungs—nourish your body, give it strength, and help remove some of its wastes. During low levels of activity, the heart and lungs maintain a steady rate: 70 to 80 beats, 15 to 18 inhalations per minute. The lungs fill with between 200 and 350 milliliters of oxygen with each breath.

As you warm up prior to running, your heart rate increases. Your muscles begin demanding more oxygenated blood. Your heart begins pumping harder. It is a double pump. It consists of layers of muscles in circles and spirals that tighten, contracting blood out of its chambers (systole) and relaxing to let blood in (diastole). As its contracts, expelling blood, the heart shortens, shrinks and twists.

There are four chambers in this muscle: two at the top, called atria; two at the bottom, called ventricles. Each atrium is separated from the ventricle chamber below it by a valve; the right atrium and ventricle are separated from the left by a strong muscle wall. Each atrium is a holding chamber, each ventricle a pump.

Blood from your muscles, low in oxygen and dark red in color, arrives back in your heart by the veins; it flows from the right atrium into the right ventricle, which pumps it into the right and left pulmonary arteries, and through the bronchi and bronchioles. In the lungs, the exchange of carbon dioxide for oxygen by the red blood cells makes the blood bright red. It flows back to your heart through the pulmonary veins to the left atrium, which holds and passes it into the left ventricle. That durable pump ejects the oxygenated blood to your aorta, the body's largest artery, which branches and divides and reaches into all parts of your body. With every contraction, or beat, your heart receives back about 5 percent of the blood it has just rejected via the coronary arteries, for nourishment. Without oxygen, the heart muscle itself could not function.

The blood surges from the aorta to arteries throughout your body, then into arterioles and the smallest vessels, the capillaries, which carry blood to the individual cells. Here, oxygen and other chemicals are delivered, and waste like carbon dioxide collected. The blood begins its return trip to the heart by capillaries to venules to the veins.

As you finish your warm-ups and calisthenics, your heart is

driving blood through your arteries to meet the new demands of your muscles. With this greater flow of blood to your tissues, as you begin your run, there is a corresponding need for increased oxygen delivered and used by your body tissues. Your large arteries, as they always do, are expanding and contracting in rhythm to your heartbeat and pushing the blood along. Your smaller arteries are opening wider to get additional blood flowing to the active muscles. Your blood actually thins so it will flow better. This is why warming up is important: It lets the body's myriad functions begin, so that blood can increase its flow to your muscles.

Now, the metabolic process of your entire body is being stimulated. The cardiovascular system reaches into every distant cell, and your cells are responding to the demands that running makes upon them. The kidneys are activated to carry off the biochemical wastes of muscular work. The liver's enzyme system works harder to purify the blood and replace enzymes lost in running. Other organs begin producing young white blood cells. Blood flow to the stomach and intestines diminishes (one reason for not eating before exercising), while the blood flow to the skin and muscles increases sharply. The brain, lungs and heart are all being enriched and nourished.

As running becomes more vigorous, your blood pressure rises as the heart contracts and ejects blood (systolic pressure). Your body is demanding more oxygen; more blood must be pumped through the lungs, heart and arteries to the demanding muscles, and returned. Your heart increases its stroke volume, placing increased pressure on the walls of your aorta and the arteries themselves.

If you're in good condition, the systolic pressure will rise during your run, level off, and may drop slightly. Continued long-distance running may produce a second gradual increase.

Among people in good condition, the diastolic pressure during the relaxation phase of a heartbeat remains almost unchanged, or decreases slightly, during exercise; but among the unconditioned, it rises.

Exercises with heavy lifting may in some cases put a dangerous stress on the blood vessels and cardiovascular system due to the sudden increase and decrease in blood pressure. Gradual endurance exercise allows your arteries and capillaries to open for better circulation; opening causes a decrease in their resistance. The heart doesn't have to work as hard to get blood to those demanding muscles. Further, endurance training increases the number of capillaries in the heart and skeletal muscles, which brings even more oxygen to the heart and muscles, and helps remove waste products more efficiently. There is also evidence that endurance exercises like running actually lower blood pressure in hypertense people. Lowered blood pressure reduces the heart's need for oxygen.

In addition to increasing the rate at which oxygen is used by the cells, exercise also increases the rate at which carbon dioxide is formed. Changes in your breathing are essential, so that more oxygen is supplied and carbon dioxide is quickly removed. That exchange depends upon the rate and depth of breathing, the efficiency of your lung ventilation and the condition of your blood and circulatory system.

Now, you are running. Your brain is receiving stimuli demanding more oxygen for the muscles. It sends nerve impulses to your chest muscles, which increase the rate and depth of breathing. Your breathing has increased from 18 to perhaps 50 breaths per minute. The tidal volume of air has jumped from 10 percent of capacity to 50 percent; oxygen intake has gone up to perhaps 20 times what it was. With the increase in respiratory volume, lung ventilation—the exchange between alveoli and your bloodstream—also increases. You are now breathing in larger amounts of air, and making more efficient transfer of it to your bloodstream and muscles, including your heart.

In a single breath the average trained runner can process a full liter of air more than the untrained person. The maximum breathing capacity per minute may reach 40 to 50 more liters than the untrained person. Your lungs have become stronger, able to move air in and out at a faster rate. Your blood is carrying more oxygen.

Your training has also increased your heart's efficiency. It grows stronger, and pumps more blood with each stroke. A conditioned person may have a resting heart rate 20 beats per minute slower than an unconditioned person. That means that you may be saving as many as 10,000 heartbeats during a single night's sleep. Even while running, your heart pumps blood and oxygen at a much slower rate than the unconditioned heart, which may beat dangerously fast.

Some studies have shown that running also increases the number and size of blood vessels that carry blood to your body. It has enlarged your arteries, and made them more elastic, better able to expand and contract. There are more capillaries in your active muscles. Studies find, for example, that active children, as adults, have larger coronary arteries than their more sedentary peers. So do runners who train for marathons. *The New England Journal of Medicine* reported on the autopsy of the seventy-year-old Clarence De Mar, who almost all his adult life ran the Boston Marathon each year and was considered one of the greatest marathon runners ever. His coronary arteries were so enlarged that they couldn't possibly have been closed by atherosclerosis.

The key to your endurance is oxygen. Your body needs

oxygen for energy; it cannot store it. The lungs must bring it in and the body must deliver it to the organs or tissues that demand it. A runner's heart, grown in size and strength, pumps almost twice the volume of blood with each stroke (beat) than that of an untrained person. Moreover, myoglobin—the oxygen-binding pigment of muscle—has a strong affinity for oxygen. Exercise raises the levels of myoglobin to twice normal levels. This means that your muscles are better able to extract oxygen from the blood and also increase the amount of oxygen in the tissues. It may help delay the onset of lactic acid production, which causes fatigue.

As you slow down, and perform your cool-down exercises, other physiological changes occur. The rate and depth of your breathing return to normal, as do the heart rate and the stroke volume. As you become more fit, this process will take less time. An abrupt halting of all exercise after running can be dangerous because blood caught in the extremities may "pool" there. The muscles need a cool-down period to return the circulatory system to normal.

Some of the benefits of long, slow exercise to your heart-lung machine are well documented and not controversial. Jogging three times a week, 20 minutes a day, at aerobic levels, may reduce your resting heart rate on the average of 1 beat for every week of running up to 15 weeks. Post-exercise recovery rates should improve at about the same pace. Cardiac output and your stroke volume will also increase as a result of your training. That is, your ventricle will produce a more forceful contraction. The results, then, are fewer but stronger heartbeats. Hypertensive people have shown a tendency toward more normal blood pressure after running at least three times a week, over a 15-week period. Long, slow running also increases oxygen delivery to your brain, liver, kidneys, skin and genitals.

Here the controversy begins. There is a spirited discussion going on about whether or not running merely tones the cardiovascular and muscular system and improves the quality of life, or whether it actually prevents death caused by heart attack. Cardiovascular diseases are the major causes of death in men over thirty-five. Heart attacks rank number one, strokes, number three, and other blood vessel diseases, fourth. (Cancer is second.) Heart disease kills one of every ten people who die before age thirty-five, but one of every three over thirty-five.

The crucial question is whether or not vigorous exercise like running reduces the incidence or severity of heart attacks. There are few causes of coronary heart disease about which we can do nothing. We can control our diets to make them low in fat, we can lose weight, avoid stress, not smoke. And we can exercise.

There are several benefits of which medical science is certain. As we have discussed, vigorous exercise may improve your cardiovascular efficiency, lower blood pressure and modify blood chemistry. It may also lower your serum triglycerides, and better the ratio of high-density to low-density lipoproteins.

Your blood contains two fats essential to life: cholesterol and triglycerides. Cholesterol is naturally a part of your body; it is synthesized in the liver and nearly every tissue and organ. It is an indispensable component of cellular structure. But there is a sharp difference between the cholesterol your body produces and that ingested from foods.

When too much lipid (cholesterol/triglyceride) is in the blood, a condition called hyperlipidemia exists, and deposits form on the inner walls of the arteries. This reduces their diameter, and brings about atherosclerosis. It is thought that other fatty deposits on the arterial walls may cause the formation of a thrombus which would also block the artery. Exercise might prevent the formation of a thrombus or, because exercise increases the blood's clotting time, it may assist in dissolving one.

Recent research, however, suggests that the amount of cholesterol in the blood is not as important as the ratio of high-density to low-density lipoproteins, the protein compounds that transport the cholesterol in the bloodstream. Low-density lipoproteins (LDLs) carry cholesterol in their core, and are the major mode of transporting cholesterol into our tissues, where it may form an atherosclerotic plaque. This plaque of fats and other materials clogs our arteries and will limit or halt altogether the flow of blood. High-density lipoproteins (HDLs), on the other hand, clear away cholesterol from the tissues and return it to the liver to be excreted. It is not yet established as a scientific fact, but HDLs are also thought to remove cholesterol from the artery walls and prevent it from being deposited there, thus thwarting the atherosclerotic process.

Research in California and Scotland suggests that HDLs may protect against heart attack by interfering with the cell's taking in LDLs and by stopping this buildup of fatty deposits that cause hardening of the arteries and heart attacks. "The higher the HDL cholesterol level, the better off people seem to be," says Dr. William P. Castelli of the National Heart, Lung and Blood Institute. Other studies show that people who are highly immune to heart disease have high levels of HDLs in their blood, and low levels of LDLs.

Further, doctors know that LDLs can be lowered by reducing the intake of cholesterol and saturated fats in our diets, or by drugs. HDLs, some evidence shows, can be elevated by drugs, or diets rich in fish and low in cholesterol. Further studies are indicating that vigorous exercise raises high-density lipoproteins while lowering low-density ones.

The Stanford Heart Disease Prevention Program studied forty-one middle-aged California men who ran 15 miles or more a week, and a similar group of nonrunners. The runners had half the triglyceride levels of the nonrunners and slightly less cholesterol. But perhaps most important, the runners' blood contained almost half again as many high-density lipoproteins as the nonrunners. Some sixty-six-year-old runners had HDL levels comparable to those of a teen-age girl—the most immune group of all. In fact, women generally have higher levels of HDLs than men, which may account for the lower incidence of heart disease among them.

Studies are also showing that regular exercise will lower and stabilize your weight. Dr. Grant Gwinup of the University of California at Irvine put eleven obese women through a year's regime of vigorous walking. No weight loss occurred until the women could walk 30 minutes a day, or more. Then, during the rest of the year, all of the women lost between 10 and 38 pounds.

Most of us gain weight when we stop regular exercise, usually within a decade after we leave school. Few school programs develop exercise skills that carry over into adult life; even playing tennis once a week cannot be considered adequate. Consequently, most of us notice the first roll of fat by our late twenties. One pound of fat equals 3500 stored calories. If you are 20 pounds overweight, that means you've eaten and stored as fat 70,000 calories. If you had walked 10 minutes a day for 5 years, you probably wouldn't have gained any of that useless and dangerous weight.

Running burns as much as 100 calories per mile. Further, regular runners find that their weight drops to a steady level, and that regular workouts depress appetite. That is, the workouts, instead of increasing your demand for food, stabilize it.

Regular exercise can also help smokers quit. If you are still smoking, and trying to run, the next few paragraphs may—literally—save your life.

Smoking has been linked to cancer, poor nutrition, ulcers, increased resting heart rate, high blood pressure, and coronary heart disease. For one thing, tobacco smoke contains nicotine. If you took the nicotine from an average cigarette and injected it into your veins, it might kill you. Inhaled, you merely get the poison in smaller amounts, not immediately fatal.

Smoke from tobacco contains 500 to 600 known poisons. Among them are carbon monoxide, hydrogen cyanide (a respiratory enzyme poison), pyridine, phenols (known cancer-causing agents), aldehydes that irritate the lungs, acrolein (used in World War I as a gas), and seven different polycyclic hydrocarbons also known to cause cancer. This smoke, and its accompanying poisons, is absorbed by your lips, mouth cavity, throat, nasal passages and esophagus, and is drawn deep into your lungs. Nicotine, if swallowed, irritates your stomach and intestines. Chew a cigar, and your lips and mouth get poisoned; smoke a pipe and the tars from the stem are sucked into your mouth and throat.

Your body's nervous system alertly tries to combat these poisons. Saliva flows, your heart rate speeds up, your blood pressure increases. The peripheral blood vessels contract and the skin chills slightly. Your fingertips and feet may get cold, caused by the constriction of your veins from tobacco substances. Laboratory tests show that sometimes blood actually stops flowing in places like the fingernail fold—your fingers may die a little with each cigarette.

The constriction of your veins gives you a "slowed-down" feeling. Slowed circulation leads to the belief that cigarettes "calm the nerves." Actually, the body is undergoing terrific stress. Studies first performed in 1909 prove that one cigarette increases your heart rate by 20 beats per minute. This condition persists for about 25 minutes after you finishing smoking—about the length of time between cigarettes—and also increases your blood pressure. Yet your veins have constricted, and the heart now is being forced to pump harder to move blood through veins that are smaller.

Moreover, those small air sacs, the alveoli, so vital to the exchange of oxygen and carbon dioxide, suffer widespread destruction when you inhale smoke. At the same time, the small arterial blood vessels delivering blood to the lungs for oxygenation are narrowed. Now the heart is forced to beat still harder to get blood to your lungs where it absorbs oxygen from damaged air sacs. The smoke in your lungs adds to the heart's load, and the oxygen entering your bloodstream is not clean, but contains tars, nicotine, smoke compounds, carbon monoxide.

The heart strains in its effort to push blood through constricting vessels; the blood itself contains contaminants instead of vitally needed oxygen. If your arteries are partially blocked by cholesterol deposits, you're in further trouble. But at least now you understand some of the reasons behind the fact that if you smoke (and don't exercise) your chances of dying from a heart attack are twice those of the nonsmoking runner.

Smoking causes a multitude of other problems as well—to both smokers and nonsmokers. For example, a medical report in England indicates that the children of smokers have two to three times the incidence of pneumonia and bronchitis of children of nonsmokers. In 1975, the medical journal *Lancet* reported that after smokers and nonsmokers had spent an hour in a closed room, the nonsmokers ended up with more nicotine in their lungs than the smokers. Their healthier lungs and higher oxygen uptake capacity helped them absorb the greater amounts of nicotine.

Like running nonsmokers, newborn children have lungs that are also particularly receptive to nicotine in the air. One smoking parent exposes his child to 60,000 hours of "passive smoking" by the child's twentieth birthday. A long-distance runner with smoking parents, says Dr. Thomas Bassler, loses 6 minutes from his potential marathon time for each month of the first 6 months of his life spent indoors with cigarette smoke. There is even a noticeable difference between runners born to smokers in the months of spring and summer; they have a better chance because, as babies, they were more often outdoors and away from cigarettes.

Clearly, runners and other nonsmokers have a right—an obligation—to tell smokers to blow it in some other direction.

If you don't smoke, you exercise regularly (and aerobically) and enjoy all the accruing benefits we've discussed, what are your chances of suffering and surviving a coronary attack? One of the most outspoken enthusiasts for running is Dr. Thomas Bassler, who has aroused the medical profession by claiming, "The hard fact is that no marathon runner has ever died of coronary artery disease [atherosclerosis] confirmed at autopsy; nowhere in the world and at no time and including heart patients." Dr. Bassler argues that runners who train for and complete at least one marathon have "purchased" seven years of coronary-immune time. But he also admits that marathon runners have been known to drop dead of heart attacks caused by, among other things, heat stroke. And, marathon runners have had nonfatal heart attacks and atherosclerosis. There are, as Dr. Bassler's example indicates, no clear proofs that exercise protects. And the research itself contains well-documented contradictions.

One of the most comprehensive studies of cardiovascular disease and exercise was published in the April 1970, issue of *Circulation.* This study covered 12,770 men between the ages of forty and fifty-nine in seven countries—the United States, Japan, and in Western Europe. A review of this study in 1971 by the National Heart and Lung Institute Task Force reported that there was no difference in coronary-disease risk between sedentary and active men in this age category. "If physical inactivity is indeed a risk factor," the Task Force concluded, "it is of much smaller magnitude than hypertension, cigarette smoking, and elevated serum cholesterol."

A five-year review of two groups in west and east Finland, with high levels of activity and also high serum cholesterol, found that among the active men the rate of coronary heart disease was the same as that among sedentary men.

But before you sink into your easy chair and give away your running shoes, you might be interested in other research. In 1953, Dr. J. N. Morris of the Medical Research Council of London Hospital reported that London bus drivers who sat all day had 1.5 times as much heart disease and twice the coronary death rate as the bus conductors, who climbed up and down the stairs of the double-decker buses collecting fares. In 1956, however, Dr. Morris published a paper titled "The Epidemiology of Uniforms." When he examined the records of the uniforms issued to these London drivers and conductors, he found that the drivers had been consistently issued larger uniforms than the conductors. The fact that the drivers were fatter, not more inactive, may have caused their higher number of coronary attacks. Or, the thinner and less coronary-prone men may have preferred the more active work of conductor.

More conclusive support for exercise is found among workers in kibbutzim in Israel who were studied by Dr. Daniel Brunner of the Government Hospital at Jaffa. He reported that while the lives, diet, stress and other factors of these workers seemed identical, the sedentary workers had 2.5 to 4 times as much heart disease as more active workers.

A long-term study of San Francisco longshoremen, published in March 1975, reached similar conclusions. Once again vigorous activity was significant. Among the 6351 men studied over a twenty-two-year period, those who did the heaviest labor had a lower incidence of heart disease, and only one-third the rate of sudden death from heart attack than men in less strenuous work. The researchers concluded that vigorous exercise was "a critical factor in cardiovascular well-being, especially as it would prevent sudden death from coronary heart disease." They reported similar findings in a follow-up study in March 1977.

By far the most conclusive study on exercise and heart attack was reported in November 1977, by Dr. Ralph S. Paffenbarger, Jr. of the Stanford University School of Medicine. During a ten-year period, Dr. Paffenbarger questioned 16,936 Harvard University alumni aged thirty-five to seventy-five about their health and exercise. He reported that strenuous exercise, like jogging for at least three hours a week, has a "definite protective effect" against heart attack—even if the man has other medical liabilities like overweight or high blood pressure.

Furthermore, Dr. Paffenbarger found that as men exercise more, the risk of attack decreases. That is, men who expend fewer than 2000 calories per week showed a sixty-four percent higher risk of heart attack than those who were more energetic. Those who played "light" sports like golf, bowling, baseball or biking were no better off than those who were inactive. But men who walked regularly were better off than those who didn't, and men who exercised vigorously were better off than those who walked.

The study also held out hope for men (and women) who start to run long after they have left college. Dr. Paffenbarger concluded that active college students who stop exercising after they graduate have no more protection than their inactive peers. But men who, whether active in college or not, took up strenuous exercise later had a clearly reduced risk of heart attack.

As more data are gathered, other conclusions are becoming known. One area that supports the proposition that exercise protects against heart disease deals with men and women who have already suffered from heart attacks. Their rehabilitation offers some convincing arguments.

Since 1967, Dr. Terrence Kavanaugh, medical director of the Toronto Cardiac Rehabilitation Center, has been encouraging his post-coronary patients to exercise. The program includes no smoking, special diets and jogging; some also run marathons. Most of his patients run 3 miles a day in 36 minutes, five times a week if they are older than forty-five; those under forty-five run 3 miles in 30 minutes. The results are impressive. "We have a 1.4 percent-per-annum mortality rate from 1967 to last October [1976]," Dr. Kavanaugh told *The New York Times*. "In groups that don't exercise, the comparable rate is 6 to 12 percent. And we get those results with 780 patients—probably the biggest exercise coronary rehab group in the world."

By 1973, Dr. Kavanaugh's patients were so enthusiastic about running that eight of them trained for and finished the Boston Marathon. Now, more than twenty patients have trained for and finished a combined total of sixty marathons.

Dr. Herman Hellerstein of Case Western Reserve University, a co-speaker with me at the 1977 New York Lung Association dinner, is also an advocate of exercise for post-coronary patients, although he doesn't believe that running alone—without giving up smoking and eating a proper diet—offers much benefit. Dr. Hellerstein found in his experiments during the last decade that post-coronary patients who exercised regularly had much less chance of suffering a second, fatal heart attack than sedentary post-coronary patients.

While some of the conclusions are still being reached, most of us who run know it benefits the heart-lung machine. My fitness philosophy is that running may not guarantee you'll live longer, only that you'll live better. Jack Shepherd entered my beginners class out of shape and suffering from recurring premature atrial contractions (PACs) of his heart. Some days, when under stress, he would have as many as two dozen PACs that he could feel. Premature atrial contractions are not unusual in men over thirty-five, nor are they debilitating or indicative of heart disease. Within six months after he started jogging, Shepherd—who was keeping accurate records of his PACs— saw that they had diminished sharply; he suffered only two or three a day. Almost two years later, running 5 miles four or five times a week, he found that he had only one or two PACs *a month!* Under severe stress—such as an accident to his daughter—he found that he suffered no prolonged increased heart rate and no PACs at all!

In 1956, Jack Shepherd was a camp counselor at Camp Becket, a YMCA camp in the Berkshire Hills of Massachusetts. Dr. Paul Dudley White, then President Eisenhower's cardiologist, was an alumnus of Becket who frequently returned to the camp to extol the virtues of exercise. Dr. White would talk with small clusters of young Becket men, urging them to continue their exercise beyond high school and college. "If you want heart trouble," he later wrote, "be inert physically. The general warning to stop all exercise at forty seems to me to be ridiculous and more likely than not actually to lead to an increase in coronary attacks and hardening of the arteries."

Shepherd didn't pay much attention to Dr. White's advice until nineteen years later, when his heart gave him a warning. Luckily, for one runner, the results are conclusive and positive— and fun.

# 13 EAT, DRINK AND BE MERRY →

Runners understand that old cliche, "You are what you eat." They are forever in search of foods or vitamins that will increase their stamina, energy, strength and performance.

Diets promoted for runners, however, are confusing: Overload with carbohydrates? Favor the high-protein diet? Restrict sugar and salt intake? Drink beer to gain weight or strength? Swallow megavitamins plus protein supplements? Little wonder that one nutritionist says, with some exasperation, "American athletes have the most expensive urine in the world."

To understand what diet might be best for you, let's make several points clear. No one diet regimen is suitable for any large number of athletically active people. What works for one may not work for another. The best diet is also the most balanced and nutritious. Proper nutrition means that essential nutrients—carbohydrates, fats, proteins, vitamins, minerals and water—are consumed and used for optimal health. A runner's basic needs aren't very different from those of other healthy people. Finally, and most importantly, diet and exercise go together. Many people who start jogging do so because they are overweight, or they want to hold their weight in check. They may already know that unused muscle tissue becomes fatter—even though they may be eating less. No one can lose weight, and hold that loss, without exercise. Exercise increases your metabolic rate, and calories are burned up. The increased metabolic rate from exercise is sustained over a twenty-four-hour period; calories are burned up not only during active exercise, but also during the next day.

In fact, runners soon learn, if you exercise vigorously and regularly, you can ignore going on a diet. Your weight will stabilize. Food you eat will be burned up, nutrients absorbed more readily and efficiently.

Dr. Jean Mayer, a leading nutritionist at Harvard University, notes that when rats exercise moderately (less than two hours a day), they actually eat less than unexercised rats. When the rats exercised more than two hours a day, putting extra energy demands upon their bodies, hunger was indeed stimulated and food intake increased to match energy output. The same mechanism, Dr. Mayer theorizes, keeps the weight of humans who exercise regularly on a constant level.

"Diet and exercise go together," says Dr. Clayton Myers in his *Official YMCA Physical Fitness Handbook.* "If you diet without exercising, the result may be a thin weak person in place of a fat weak person. Muscle tissue that is not used will atrophy and proportionately become fatter even though the intake of calories has been reduced."

Statistically, when America's predominant way of life was manual labor, before the turn of the century, adult weights on the average remained steady. Since 1900, as we've become more and more sedentary, the average American caloric intake has decreased, but obesity has increased. Even our health charts seem to encourage us to be overweight! According to Dr. Irwin Stillman, the normal average weight for men over age twenty-five is 110 pounds plus 5.5 pounds for each inch over 5 feet. (A man 5 foot, 10 inches would weigh 165 pounds.) Women start at 100 pounds, and add 5 pounds for every inch above 5 feet. These calculations have become the subject of some debate. *Runner's World,* for example, has written that men and women should weigh at least 10 percent below these norms. Dr. Ernst van Aaken suggests 20 percent below. The way I figure weights of beginner runners during their fitness tests is to take four figures:

1. By using calipers, I obtain a body fat percentage;
2. The runner notes his or her weight at age twenty (or when last felt fit);
3. We look up his or her weight on the life insurance charts, and subtract 10 percent; and
4. I ask for a medical opinion.

I'll sum up these four measurements, and reach a reasonable weight goal. For more competitive runners I use another system. World class long-distance runners on the average weigh twice their height in inches or less. A quality runner should be within 10 percent of that figure. For example, the 5'10" (70") man should weigh 140 or less for world class status and 154 or less to be very competitive. The average fit man should be 16 percent fat (23 percent for women). The male competitor should be 10 percent fat or less. Studies of women competitors are yet to be made.

To be fit and maintain a healthy diet means discriminating between foods, understanding the basic value to you of carbohydrates, fats, proteins, minerals, vitamins, water and other fluids. All foods we eat contain some of these nutrients. They provide the body with heat and energy, the materials for growth and repair of body tissues. They assist with the regular body processes. Each nutrient has its own special function and relationship to the body. No nutrient is independent of others. We all need them, but the amounts we need vary according to age, sex, body size, environment, exercise level and nutritional condition.

Our cells obtain and use nutrients through the three-step process of digestion, absorption and metabolism. Basically, the foods we eat are broken down in the body to simpler forms, taken through the intestinal walls and transported by the blood to the cells. Because this process is important in helping you to understand the relationship between good nutrition and exercise, let's take a closer look at it.

## DIGESTION

Take a bite of food. Chewing breaks the large pieces into smaller ones. The salivary glands in your mouth produce saliva, which moistens the food.

A series of physical and chemical changes begins occurring along the entire digestive tract: mouth, pharynx, esophagus, stomach, small and large intestines. These changes gradually break down the food and prepare it for absorption from the intestinal tract into the bloodstream.

The chemical breakdown of food is caused by enzymes. Each enzyme can break down only a single specific substance: fat, carbohydrate, protein—and no others. Enzymes work in four areas: the salivary glands, the stomach, the pancreas and the wall of the small intestine.

That bite you took gets chewed, mixes with an enzyme, and passes to the pharynx and down into the esophagus. It is carried along by the slow and wavelike movement called peristalsis through the entire digestive track to the stomach. In the mid-portion of the stomach, your food is mixed with gastric juices containing hydrochloric acid, water and enzymes, which continue breaking it down.

After one to four hours—the time depends upon what you

ate—peristalsis pushes this mass, in a liquid form called chyme, out of the stomach into the small intestine. There is a specific order of departure—carbohydrates first, then proteins and then fats. Carbohydrates take the shortest amount of time to digest and fats the longest. You might remember this when considering what to eat before a race, and when.

Chyme enters the small intestine. If fats are present, the liver produces bile (stored in your gallbladder), and the bile separates fats into small droplets which pancreatic enzymes break down. The pancreas secretes a substance that neutralizes the digestive acids, and additional enzymes continue breaking down the proteins and carbohydrates. Undigested particles enter the large intestine and are eventually excreted.

## ABSORPTION

As the chyme is entering your small intestine, nutrients are taken up and passed into the bloodstream. Small fingerlike villi, which contain lymph channels, and tiny blood vessels called capillaries are the principal modes of absorption. Glucose is obtained from carbohydrates, amino acids from protein, and fatty acids and glycerol from fats.

The fats and fat-soluble vitamins move through the blood to the cells. Others go to the liver, where reactions produce material needed by individual cells. Others are stored, to be released later as needed. Water-soluble vitamins and minerals are absorbed into the bloodstream. From each, in its own way, the body begins obtaining strength for its multitude of functions.

## METABOLISM

In this stage, digested nutrients convert into material for living tissues, or for energy. This occurs in two phases, anabolism and catabolism. A great process of exchange takes place. Anabolism involves nutrient chemical reactions that aid in the construction or sustenance of body chemicals and tissues; this includes enzymes, hormones, blood, glycogen and other matter. Catabolism involves reactions in which tissues break down to supply energy. The metabolism of glucose, for example, supplies energy for the cells. It also forms carbon dioxide and water as waste products, which are carried from the cells by the bloodstream. Other sources of energy during metabolism come from the essential fatty acids and amino acids; amino acids provide essential material for the maintenance and repair of tissues, and for growth.

An extensive system of enzymes is vital to metabolism; they regulate its rate and generate thousands of different chemical reactions. Specific vitamins and minerals are essential for providing many of these enzymes.

This entire process may be interfered with by stress or anxiety; by eating while agitated, fatigued or hurried. But understanding the process helps us to understand the reasoning behind eating a balanced diet. It also helps us realize the absurdity in consuming the following:

*Junk foods*   These foods are any edible thing that contains no essential nutrients—except perhaps calories. Eating them creates two hazards: You ingest chemicals and unessential ingredients harmful to your body; and junk foods replace more nutritional foods that your body needs. Eating junk food is also an excellent way to put on fat—lots of it.

My friend Carl Eilenberg weighed 273 pounds when he was thirty-three; he was 5 feet, 10 inches tall and his waist was 46 inches around. His heart rate was 90, and his blood pressure 160/80. "I used to get out of breath just ripping open the pretzel bag or sucking up a milk shake," he says. "I'd skip breakfast, then down martinis, soup, sandwiches, fried clams, beer and banana splits for lunch. Well, sometimes I'd skip the soup. I'd eat crackers and popcorn after dinner."

Carl played golf on weekends, bowled once in a while, but never walked anywhere. "I honestly thought I was a pretty typical, reasonably healthy, in-shape adult male." Then he saw himself on television. "My head and neck looked like a watermelon. I was thirty, looked fifty. I was a big, fat slob, a very big fat slob."

He began running, a little at a time. He also cut the junk foods. Today, at forty-five, he looks more like twenty, and weighs 155. He has a pulse rate in the 50s, low-normal blood pressure, a greatly reduced cholesterol level, a much better home life. As he says, "Most important, I really like myself."

If you're in the junk food habit, try switching to Herbert Shelton's simple diet of fresh fruits, vegetables and nuts. Raisins, carrots, celery all taste delicious, especially after a run. Drink unsweetened fruit juices diluted with ice or water. You'll be decreasing calories and increasing essential nutrients.

*Sugar*   No other food has been so overemphasized in our diets. Sugar contains little of real value to your body (if you are already eating a balanced diet), yet it is consumed daily in large amounts by all of us.

White, refined sugar lacks nutrient value, and, in fact, requires vitamins (especially the B vitamins) for its digestion. In effect, sugar steals vitamins from your body for its digestion, and it interferes with some enzyme activity.

One myth states that sugar increases energy. Sugar actually decreases energy over several hours because it requires energy from your body for its assimilation. Pure sugar passes quickly through the intestinal walls into your bloodstream. Some runners think this is valuable because a quick energy burst is obtained. But this immediate sudden rise in blood-sugar level is followed by a dramatic drop in levels below your body's norm, which requires the ingestion of still more sugar, and thus the cycle begins.

Excessive sugar intake is associated with cavities, heart disease, stomach and bowel disorders, and cancer. A chocolate bar contains so many carbohydrates and fats that it should be used only as emergency rations. Honey, molasses, cane syrup and other sugar forms are just as rich as refined sugar, although they also contain traces of minerals.

*Salt* Sodium chloride, or salt, is found naturally in all foods, with higher concentrations in seafoods, carrots, beets, poultry and most meats. Salt also occurs naturally in the body's fluids. It works with potassium to regulate water balance within the body, and is involved with muscle contraction and expansion, and in nerve stimulation. Salt is readily absorbed in the small intestines and stomach, and carried by the blood to the kidneys where it is filtered out and returned to the blood as needed. Water in the human body is maintained with a precise level of salinity.

Obviously, deficiencies of salt are extremely uncommon. Most Americans take in on the average 3 to 7 grams a day, while The National Research Council recommends a daily sodium intake of just 1 gram per kilogram of water consumed daily. Too much salt may be harmful. In excess, it may cause potassium to be lost in the urine. Also, sodium retained in the body holds onto water, placing an extra load on the heart. A large salt intake is also related to high blood pressure, and other forms of cardiovascular and kidney disease.

High-sodium foods include smoked fish and meat, pickles, artichokes, sauerkraut, spinach and frozen vegetables processed with salt. Fresh vegetables are generally low in salt, as are fresh fruits. Junk foods like salted popcorn, potato chips, snack chips and pretzels contain high levels of salt. So, too, do organ, canned and kosher meats; bacon, olives, commercial salad dressings; cashews and macadamia nuts—which are also high in cholesterol.

Sea salt and coarse rock salt differ only in the amount of impurities in the product, not in the amount of salt itself. Going easy on salt is simple: Take the salt shaker off the dining room table.

*Coffee* Some medical studies indicate that more than 5 cups of coffee per day, caffeinated or decaffeinated, contributes to a higher incidence of heart attacks. Coffee is a stimulant, and causes hyperactivity and stomach spasms in many people. It should be cut back, or eliminated, from our diets. Runners may find that coffee causes diarrhea during races. And besides, it costs too much.

*Alcohol* Few areas are more controversial among runners and nonrunners alike than this one. Alcoholism is a major health problem in the United States (and other countries). Should runners drink?

Dr. Peter Wood of the Stanford Heart Disease Prevention Program argues that the idea that alcohol and athletics don't mix "is based more on the Puritan ethic than on substantial medical evidence." Dr. Ernst van Aaken told the New York Runner's Club at his 1976 lecture that beer is an important food. As a liquid, he told the thirsty runners, it ranks in importance only after water and definitely before milk. Beer, consumed in moderate amounts, supplies many essential vitamins and yeast. Dr. van Aaken suggested that runners should drink one beer for every 6 miles. I jumped up and asked if he was confused: Many of my friends drink 6 beers for every mile run.

The key to the use of alcohol is balance. Alcohol causes a

decreased oxygen uptake, reduced heat tolerance, muscle contractile strength, and impaired coordination. Most dangerous of all, alcoholic beverages constrict the arteries leading to the heart. This could be serious for a runner whose heart will require during exertion greatly accelerated blood flow and dilated—not restricted—arteries.

Still, Frank Shorter downed a six-pack of beer the night before winning the 1972 Olympic Marathon. Mike Cleary, who is a 2:30 marathoner, has this theory, "I go for a long run on Friday and then get wrecked that night. Saturday I'll just lay around holding my head and that evening I'll have four beers and then a pint of Guinness. On race day, I'm relaxed and raring to go!" Dr. Norb Sander, known for his drinks as well as his runs, tells about his infamous Irish teammate on the Millrose A.A., Jim McDonough. "The night before the Pan-Am Marathon Trials in Holyoke Jimmy downed thirty-six bottles of beer. The next day was brutally hot and Jimmy started off slow and then, as others dehydrated, he surged to finish second and qualify for the Pan-Am Games. He was in his forties then, too."

I know of several fun races sponsored by drinking establishments. Mike Cleary won the First Annual "Guinness with Oysters" race to kick off St. Patrick's Day week in New York City. He had to carry a pint of Guinness and a plate of oysters 1.6 miles from one pub to another, and easily won a free trip to Ireland. The *Long Island Press* reported, "Sure it's awkward for a runner to balance a mug of stout and a plate of raw oysters—throws the old rhythm off a wee bit. But for an Irish jogger with a crack at a free ticket to the Ould Sod, well it's as easy as finding a shamrock on St. Paddy's Day. . . . The Irish lad ran as effortless as a tippler hoisting his glass, smooth as a long, cool draft beer."

**Smoking** This is a major crime against your lungs, heart, digestive system—and family. Smoking is a killer habit.

As we detailed in the previous chapter, one cigarette contains five hundred known poisons. When a smoker inhales a cigarette, his or her heart rate quickens, blood pressure rises, the peripheral blood vessels contract, and the skin temperature drops. Nicotine and carbon monoxide in tobacco cause heart and artery disease. Tar collects in pulmonary passages, causing emphysema and cancer of the lungs. Smokers have a marked tendency to exhibit irregular heart rhythms, and run the risk of sudden death. In fact, the life expectancy of a fifty-year-old who has smoked a pack of cigarettes daily for thirty years is reduced by 8.5 years— almost a decade. Many runners have quit smoking. Jane Killion, an executive at Banker's Trust and a member of the Greater New York AA, gave up smoking as she became a more competitive runner, and is now a national class marathoner. She won the 1977 Orange Bowl Marathon in 2:54:03.

## WEIGHT

Food intake is measured in calories: A calorie is "the amount of heat required to raise the temperature of one gram of water one degree of centigrade." A pound of weight contains 3500 calories of energy. To gain a pound, you must take in and store that amount; to lose a pound, you must get rid of that.

All carbohydrates, fats and proteins contain calories; water, minerals and vitamins do not. The normal caloric intake is 18 per pound per day for men, and 16 for women.

As all of us know, it is easier to feed calories to the body than to burn them up. One chocolate soda, for example, equals a week-and-a-half's office work. Calories, in the form of fat, also build up easily.

This is one more reason why we need more, not less, exercise as we grow older. Dr. Ralph Nelson of the Mayo Clinic shows that a 154-pound man at age thirty who maintains a constant exercise level and eats the same amount will weigh more than 200 pounds by age sixty. To remain the same weight on the same amount of exercise, he must reduce his caloric intake by 11 percent. Professor Per-Olof Astrand states that "a person's weight should not increase after his or her twenties. Since muscular tissue declines [with age], a loss of a few pounds is actually good proof of no increase in fatty tissue."

Running is a high continuous energy burn-off: Some long-distance runners burn calories at the rate of 1000 an hour. Just by running and eliminating all sugar where you now use it, you might lose as much as 25 pounds a year. (Four extra teaspoons of sugar a day will add 5 pounds of fat a year, 52 pounds in ten years.)

Runners find that they can stabilize their weight and continue eating sensibly whatever they wish. We all need to eat carefully to maintain energy and to drink healthy fluids to preserve the body's balance. But what does this mean?

All of us need foods from the basic food groups: the bread-cereals, milk-cheese, meats (or cheeses, beans, peas, lentils, nuts), and vegetable-fruit groups (dark green and deep yellow vegetables, citrus fruits). These should give us our basic nutrients: carbohydrates, proteins, fats, minerals, and vitamins as well as water (or other fluids like vegetable and fruit juices). What do we need these for?

## CARBOHYDRATES

These are the energy foods. They supply the primary energy for all body functions and muscle exertion, and they assist in digestion and the assimilation of other foods. Carbohydrates regulate protein and fat metabolism. Fats, for example, require carbohydrates for their breakdown within the liver.

The principal carbohydrates are starches such as bread, cakes, potatoes, and sugar foods such as candies, preserves, syrups, or soft drinks. The starches require prolonged enzyme action before becoming simple sugar (glucose) for digestion. The simple sugars, like those found in honey and fruit, are easily digested and turned into quick energy. Cellulose, also a carbohydrate, is found in the skins of fruits and vegetables, and is largely indigestible although it contributes bulk for intestinal action and aids elimination.

Therefore, carbohydrates offer two sources of energy for runners. As snacks, the sugars and starches provide an almost instant energy burst because of the sudden rise in the blood sugar level from the glucose. But that level drops again just as suddenly, creating a craving for more sweet food and possibly fatigue, dizziness, nervousness or headaches. As stored energy, over a period of time, carbohydrates can gradually "feed" glucose to the exercising body. During vigorous exercise, such as running, those fat reserves are reconverted to glucose and burned as body fuel.

In addition, carbohydrates, by passing quickly through the digestive process, are easier to assimilate than other nutrients. They also provide a significant water supply when broken down, which is a benefit during hot weather.

On the other hand, carbohydrates are not essential for the sedentary person. The body can provide the carbohydrates for normal metabolism from stored fat. The National Research Council lists no specific daily requirements for carbohydrates because they are found naturally in the body as amino acids and the glycerol component of fats. All of us should be aware of research that shows that overuse of carbohydrates may contribute to atherosclerosis or bowel cancer.

## PROTEINS

These body builders help bone and tissue grow and repair. They are a major building material for muscles, blood, skin, hair, nails and the internal organs including the heart and brain. They aid in the formation of hormones that control growth, sexual development, the rate of metabolism, and they control the balance of acids and alkalines in the blood and regulate the body's water balance. Proteins form enzymes necessary for basic life functions, and antibodies that fight foreign substances in the body. Unused proteins are converted by the liver and stored as fat in body tissue.

Proteins are essential for energy, but how essential is still open to debate. During times of stress, as when running, the body needs to consume extra protein to rebuild or replace worn-out tissues. But does this mean that eating more meats, which provide complete proteins, is beneficial? Some doctors and runners claim that energy comes from mixing carbohydrates and fats, not proteins. For a full discussion of this theory and the practice called carbohydrate loading, see page 318.

The American Research Council's Food and Nutrition Board recommends 70 grams of protein every day for most adults. Many doctors feel this is too high, and recommend 35 grams, but most Americans now eat 118 grams daily, much of it in the form of concentrated protein in meats. The National Research Council suggests eating .42 grams of protein daily for every kilogram of body weight (to find kilograms, divide your body weight by 2.2; to find your protein amount, multiply by .42).

Most proteins contain a high level of fats, and some doctors now argue that eating a lot of meat is unhealthy. It takes too long for meat to pass through our digestive system, and the meat begins to decay. This, and other factors, may indicate why Americans, and other high meat eaters, are so subject to cancer of the colon. Vegetable proteins can be as nutritious as animal proteins. In raw form, fruits and vegetables are excellent sources. You can get your protein requirements from nuts, beans, whole grains and cereals, egg whites, milk, cheese, and some vegetables. For example, potatoes contain 2 percent protein of high quality. If you wish to avoid the high cholesterol levels of muscle meats, or are inclined toward vegetarianism, try shifting your diet toward nuts and grains. Whatever proteins you prefer, try cutting meat consumption way back, at least to the level of gram-per-body-weight recommended.

## FATS

This nutrient contains good news and bad news. First the good news. Fats are the most concentrated source of energy in our diet. They may contain 2.5 times the number of calories, when oxidized, than carbohydrates or proteins, although they break down more slowly. One gram of fat yields about 9 calories.

Fats aid in the absorption of the fat-soluble vitamins A, D, E and K. Fat deposits surround, protect and hold in place organs such as the kidneys, heart and liver. A layer of fat insulates the body from the environment, and preserves body heat. Fats also prolong digestion by slowing down the stomach's secretions of hydrochloric acid.

And now the bad news.

In 1977, Americans ate a record average of 56 pounds of fats in butter, margarine, cooking oils, shortening, lard, salad dressing and other fatty products. That doesn't include "invisible" fats eaten in foods like meat, cheese, milk, eggs, poultry, fish, grain products, even fruits and vegetables. Consumption of all fats is rising sharply, despite growing understanding that many fats and too much fat in our diets may be unhealthy.

Broadly, there are two types of fats: saturated and unsaturated. The saturated (with the exception of coconut oil) come largely from animal meats. The unsaturated, including the polyunsaturated, come from vegetables, and nut or seed sources such as corn, sunflowers, olives.

Saturated fats contain cholesterol. Doctors believe that we also manufacture cholesterol in the liver, adrenal cortex of the brain, skin, intestines, and testes. It is synthesized by the body and aids in the normal process of metabolism and it is necessary for the production of certain enzymes and endocrine secretions. It is found in all the cells of the body, but especially the liver, kidneys, brain and pancreas.

Triglycerides, as we noted in the last chapter, are formed in the breakdown of carbohydrates, and are probably just as dangerous to your health as cholesterol. Refined sugar is easily converted into triglycerides. Alcohol provides us with triglycerides and supplies empty calories and adds fat.

All fats get broken down in the small intestine. They contribute to high triglyceride and cholesterol levels, which can be killers. Without repeating the information of the last chapter, let's remember that these fats are the leading causes of atherosclerosis, or hardening of the arteries, and the clogging of the coronary arteries and the arteries going to the brain.

The average American diet is almost 45 percent fats. The National Research Council sets no recommended daily allowance for fats, but nutritionists suggest cutting fats down to 20 percent of our diets, which means cutting down or eliminating some of our tastier—though high in cholesterol—foods, such as spareribs, hamburgers, hot dogs, roast duck and goose, French fries, sausages, sweet potatoes and caviar. Some meats are higher than others: organ and glandular meats, hearts, kidneys, liver and sweetbreads all have high cholesterol contents; the highest is found in brains. Stay away from lobster; crab meat contains less cholesterol, shrimp less than crab, scallops less than shrimp. Trim all visible fat from steak. Also avoid all cold luncheon meats, all dairy ice creams (use ice milk instead), rich salad dressings, creamy soups, the yolks of eggs.

If this section leaves you feeling that there's no fun left, remember: cholesterol deficiency is unlikely to occur since the substance is stored naturally throughout your body; exercise stimulates the release of this natural, stored cholesterol, which (we forgot to tell you) is vital to the development of your sex hormones.

## MINERALS

These nutrients exist in most foods and in the body; seventeen are essential to human mental and physical well-being. They are constituents of the bones, teeth, soft tissues, muscle, blood and nerve cells, and are essential in maintaining the bodily processes, strengthening skeletal structures, the vigor of the heart and brain and nervous system. Minerals aid in warding off fatigue and cramps, and they maintain the body's delicate water balance. The following six minerals are of special interest to runners.

### Iron

Present in every living cell, iron combines with protein to make hemoglobin to transport oxygen in the blood from lungs to tissues. Iron builds up the quality of the blood and aids resistance to disease and stress. It also helps form myoglobin, found only in muscle tissues, which also transports oxygen to the muscle cells and benefits muscle contraction. The Food and

Nutrition Board says that women need twice as much iron as men, and from the age of thirteen through the late forties should ingest 18 milligrams per day, while men need only 10. Best sources: liver; then oysters, heart, lean meats, tongue, leafy green vegetables, dried fruits.

### Calcium

This is body's most abundant mineral. It works with phosphorus to build and maintain teeth and bones. It promotes the heart muscle and regulates heart rhythm (with magnesium), as well as the acid-alkali content of the blood. It assists in muscle growth and contraction, nerve transmission and the passage of nutrients in and out of cell walls. Best sources: milk and dairy products, bone meal, oranges, eggs.

### Phosphorus

This mineral often works with calcium. It plays a role in almost every chemical reaction within the body, helping the body use carbohydrates, fats and proteins for growth, cell repair and energy. It stimulates the heart and muscle contractions. It also helps tooth development, kidney function, and nerve impulse transfers. Foods rich in proteins are also rich in phosphorus. Best sources: lean meats, fish, chicken, eggs, whole grains, seeds, nuts.

### Sodium

Sodium aids fluid balance in blood vessels, arteries, veins and capillaries, intestinal fluids surrounding the cells, and bones. With potassium, sodium regulates the body's water balance, the acid-alkali combination in the blood, muscle contraction and expansion, nerve stimulation. It also keeps blood minerals soluble, preventing them from building up as deposits in the bloodstream. It improves the health of the blood, purges carbon dioxide from the body, aids digestion. Sodium also helps produce the hydrochloric acid in the stomach. Best sources: seafoods, poultry, meats, carrots, beets and kelp; but sodium is found in all foods.

### Potassium

Assists sodium in the ways mentioned above. It also aids in the conversion of glucose to glycogen, which is then stored in the liver. It helps with cell metabolism, enzyme reactions; it stimulates the kidneys to eliminate body wastes, and it nourishes the muscles. Best sources: green leafy vegetables, oranges, whole grains, sunflower seeds, mint leaves, potatoes (especially the peelings), bananas, cantaloupes, apricots, plus the juices of oranges, grapefruits and prunes.

### Magnesium

This mineral stimulates the essential metabolic processes by activating enzymes that break down carbohydrates and amino acids. It aids neuromuscular contractions and regulates the body's acid-alkaline balance. Magnesium helps the body absorb other minerals, and the C, E and B-complex vitamins. It helps bone growth and heart and nerve functionings. It may also help regulate the body temperature. Sufficient amounts of magnesium are vital to the conversion of blood sugar into energy. Best sources: fresh green vegetables, unmilled wheat germ, soybeans, figs, corn, apples, oil-rich seeds and nuts.

## VITAMINS

Natural vitamins are found in plants and animals as organic food substances. Because our bodies cannot synthesize vitamins (with a few exceptions), we must supply them with our diet or with supplements. Basically, their only function is to help enzymes. Vitamins help to regulate the metabolism of our bodies, to convert fat and carbohydrates into energy, and to form bones and tissues. There are about twenty active vitamins in human nutrition, but we will only discuss a few of the most important ones—Vitamins A, the B-complex, C, D, E.

### Vitamin A
Little is known of this vitamin's specific influence upon physical performance, although it is added to a lot of foods. It does aid in the growth and repair of body tissues, and it promotes strong teeth and bones, the formation of rich blood, and helps maintain good eyesight. It reduces our susceptibility to infection by protecting the mucous membrane of the mouth, nose, throat and lungs. It also protects the lining of the digestive tract, the kidneys and bladder, and it promotes the secretion of gastric juices necessary for the proper digestion of proteins. Best sources: fish-liver oil, carrots, and green leafy vegetables such as beet greens, spinach and broccoli.

### Vitamin B-complex
The B-complex vitamins, of which there are thirteen, provide the body with energy by converting carbohydrates into glucose. They are also essential to the metabolism of fats and proteins. They may be the single most important factor in the health and normal functioning of our nervous system. The value of the B vitamins is long and impressive. They aid in easing postoperative nausea and vomiting resulting from anesthesia, with heart abnormalities, barbiturate overdoses, migraine headaches. Yet the B vitamins are lacking in many American diets.

All of the B vitamins—except B-17—are found naturally in liver and whole-grain cereals, but brewer's yeast is the richest natural source of the B vitamins.

*Vitamin B-1 (Thiamine)*, by its link to carbohydrate metabolism and lactic acid utilization, increases a runner's caloric use during endurance performance. A high carbohydrate diet requires more B-1 than most diets and exercising athletes on a high-carbo loading should take at least 2 milligrams daily. It is vital for the breakdown of carbohydrates into glucose, which is oxidized by the body to produce energy. It is also known as the "morale vitamin," because of its relationship to a healthy nervous system and positive mental attitude. Thiamine is also thought to help prevent the buildup of fatty deposits on the arterial walls. Best food sources: brewer's yeast, seeds, wheat germ, nuts, blackstrap molasses, germ and bran of wheat, husk of rice. The portion of all grains usually milled away to give the grain a lighter color and finer texture contain vitamin B-1.

*Vitamin B-2 (Riboflavin)* works with enzymes to break down carbohydrates, fats and proteins. Perhaps most important to runners, riboflavin aids cell respiration. It works with enzymes in using cell oxygen, and it also helps with good vision, hair, nails and skin. B-2 is not stored in the body, and therefore must be supplied regularly in the diet. Best food sources: liver, tongue and other organ meats; richest source is brewer's yeast.

*Vitamin B-6 (Pyridoxine)* is important to the runner because it facilitates the release of glycogen for energy from the liver and muscles. It also helps maintain the balance of sodium and potassium in body fluids, and produces antibodies and red blood cells, and it aids in digestion by helping produce hydrochloric acid and magnesium. Best food sources: meats and whole grains.

*Niacin* also assists the enzymes in breaking down and using fats, carbohydrates and proteins. It is effective in improving circulation and in reducing cholesterol in the blood. It is present in most foods, but best food sources include: lean meats, poultry, fish, peanuts and brewer's yeast.

*Vitamin B-12* is the only one in the B-complex that contains vital mineral elements. It cannot be made synthetically, but must be grown in bacteria or molds. Like other vitamins, it is essential to the normal metabolism of carbohydrates, fats and proteins. It is of value to the runner in that it provides some long-term relief for fatigue, and is an anti-anemic. Best food sources: liver, kidney, fish and dairy products.

### Vitamin C (Ascorbic Acid)
A controversial vitamin, its use has been linked to everything from preventing colds to preventing cancer. Maybe Dr. Linus Pauling, who advocates vitamin C for cold prevention, is right, and maybe not. I do know other doctors who take it to ward off colds, and a lot of people—runners and nonrunners alike—swear that vitamin C protects them against illness and injury, and speeds recovery.

Man, apes and guinea pigs are the only creatures that need this vitamin. It prevents and relieves scurvy, and is necessary for the connective tissue in the skin, ligaments and bones. It also facilitates the formation of connective scar tissue, helping to heal wounds and burns, and it aids in the forming of red blood cells. Some medical studies indicate that vitamin C fights bacterial infection, and reduces the impact on the body of some allergy-producing substances. Others believe that the lack of vitamin C may be a cause of stroke begun by breaks in the capillary walls where clots form.

Vitamin C takes two to three hours to be absorbed, and most of the vitamin not used by the body is passed out within four hours by urine and perspiration. Under stress, the vitamin passes through the body faster. Ascorbic acid is readily absorbed from the gastrointestinal tract into the bloodstream. The body's ability to absorb C is reduced by smoking, high fever, inhalation of DDT. Drinking excessive amounts of water also depletes the body's vitamin C, and cooking in copper utensils destroys the vitamin C in foods.

Some medical authorities believe that vitamin C is important under all stressful circumstances, from illness to competitive running. Tissues require more vitamin C during vigorous exercise. The sex glands, too, develop a greater need for vitamin C with increased exercise; if you're overdoing it, they will draw vitamin C from other tissues, causing a depletion.

Runners should take plenty of vitamin C. The recommended daily dosage is 500 mgs a day. I take 1 gram a day (1000 mgs), or 2 to 3 grams when a cold is coming on.

The best food sources include most fruits and vegetables. Natural vitamin C supplements are prepared from rose hips, acerola cherries, green peppers and citrus fruits. Vitamin C in natural form, some doctors feel, is superior to that in synthetic.

### Vitamin D

This is a comparatively unknown vitamin that aids both in the absorption of calcium from the intestinal tract and in the breakdown and assimilation of phosphorus, required for bone formation. Without it, bones and teeth will not calcify properly. It is also valuable in maintaining a stable nervous system, a normal and strong heartbeat, and normal blood clotting. It helps in fighting fatigue. Best food sources: fish-liver oils.

**Vitamin E**

This vitamin plays an essential role in muscular performance, especially the cardiac and skeletal muscles. It increases the endurance and strength of these muscles by letting them function with less oxygen. By causing dilation of the blood vessels, it helps increase the flow of blood to the heart. It inhibits formation of blood clots, aids in bringing nourishment to cells, strengthens the capillary walls, protects red blood cells from destruction by poisons like hydrogen peroxide in the blood. In an ointment, vitamin E promotes healing and lessens the formation of scars. It helps regulate menstrual flow. It also protects against many environmental poisons in air, water and food, and especially protects the lungs and other tissues from damage by polluted air. Runners may appreciate this effect. Dr. Gabe Mirkin, a medical advisor to *Running Times* magazine, recommends 200 mgs the day before competition, but only then. Some doctors and nutritionists believe that E has a role in increasing male and female fertility, and in restoring male potency. Best food sources: raw seeds, nuts, soybeans, wheat germ oil.

## WATER

This vital "food" is often overlooked in value. But water is responsible for and involved in nearly every bodily process: digestion, absorption, metabolism and elimination. It is the primary transporter of nutrients throughout the body. It also helps maintain normal body temperature, and is essential for carrying waste material from the body.

Nearly all foods contain water that is absorbed by the body during digestion. Fruits and vegetables offer a source of chemically pure water that is 100 percent hydrogen and oxygen.

The average adult body contains about forty-five quarts of water, and loses about six pints (a quart and a half) daily through normal excretion and perspiration. The rate of loss depends almost entirely upon the level of activity and the environment: the range may be from one quart up to ten quarts in the desert.

To replace lost water, our diet may give us several pints, we may drink several pints, and the body may create a pint in the oxidation of food through digestion and metabolism. Most of us do not drink enough water; it is impossible to drink too much. Water itself will not add on pounds although it is retained in the body as required by the precise balance within the tissues. Fat people retain water because of their fat tissues. Most doctors agree that anyone exercising regularly should drink at least a quart of water a day.

## FASTING AND VEGETARIANISM

Neither one of us fasts regularly, nor are we vegetarians. But in researching this chapter we encountered arguments from other runners against eating meat, and for fasting. Dr. van Aaken, for example, believes that the runner's body is capable of "living off its own resources" for extended periods, and thrives on it. Some runners fast for periods up to two weeks, ingesting only pure water or fruit and/or vegetable juices. We would suggest trying some fasting only after consulting with your doctor.

Vegetarianism is a complex issue. Some vegetarians eat no meat at all. Period. Others, the ovo-lacto vegetarians, exclude all flesh foods: meats, poultry, fish. But they do eat eggs, milk and cheese. A major cutback in all meats would probably be a sound idea for every American, runner or nonrunner. Non-meat sources of protein are easily found (nuts, soybeans, whole grains, etc.) and are basically better for you. Vegetarians have sometimes gone too heavily for exotic diets that ignore some elementary essentials, especially the minerals and vitamins. Heavy meat eaters are going in the other direction.

But what is a good runner's diet? Basically, we have found the balanced diet best. Too much emphasis upon one aspect—carbohydrates over proteins, for example—can cause as harmful an imbalance as the present average American diet heavy on meats and fried foods. We also make the following suggestions:

- Cut out all white sugar (and all brown, "raw" and "kleen-raw" sugars, which are merely disguises). Use honey (but very moderately) and fresh fruits for sweeteners.
- Eat only 100 percent whole-wheat products. "Unbleached white flour" is almost as bad for you as ordinary white flour; it can gum up your stomach and intestines.
- Cook vegetables lightly. The Chinese have developed this to a culinary marvel. Eat raw salads together with cooked vegetables. Try a little lemon juice on them for flavor (and vitamins).
- Eat little beef or pork. The more of these meats you can cut out of your diet, the better. Substitute fish and chicken (cutting away the underlayer of fat in chicken). Try eating more vegetable proteins and whole grains; try complementary proteins like rice and beans, peanut butter and legumes. They are low in cost and cholesterol.
- Cut out all soft drinks, all hard liquor. Be moderate with beer and wine. Drink more water, and add vegetable and fresh fruit juices. Use little coffee, and drink herbal teas.
- Eat only when hungry, and eat less than you need. Wheat germ, yogurt, brewer's yeast, desiccated liver (if you can stand it), and vitamin C are good daily.
- Avoid all junk foods and prepared, processed foods. Read all food labels, and avoid chemical additives.

Eat wisely—and you will run well.

# 14 FOOD AND DRINK FOR RACING

Americans originated eating on the run, and perfected the art of indigestion. All of us know we shouldn't eat and run.

Still, some joggers persist. I was one of them: I once ran 6 miles only half an hour after downing a couple of hamburgers and a beer. First came terrible stomach cramps, and then diarrhea. I learned my lesson in the bushes alongside the running path. Other foods upset your stomach on the run: milk, raisins and other fruits, coffee (stimulates the bowels). Avoid these before any run, and especially before a race.

Every runner has his or her own digestive problems. As a rule, we should not eat before running, yet some runners eat heartily and still enjoy their run. If in doubt, leave it out: don't eat and run. Also, don't eat the wrong things at the wrong time, and don't eat too much too late.

Many runners insist upon eating a solid meal the morning of a race to give them strength during a long run. Dr. Ernst van Aaken notes that "no one ever got fast by eating." His theory is that runners shouldn't eat 12 to 24 hours before a race because they have already stored all the fuel they need. I believe that the need to eat before a race is psychological. We have been brought up in a society that promotes the full stomach. Some chicken in every pot. Runners equate eating with energy. In fact, I do not eat 12 hours before competition. To me, running "hungry, lean and mean," fasting the twelve hours before a race, means that I'm able to direct more energy towards performance and less toward digestion or other bodily needs. But you must determine what is best for you and your body. To help you do that, let's look at the carbohydrate-loading diet, and a few variations.

## CARBOHYDRATE LOADING

Not too long ago, college track stars would eat steak the night before a big meet. So would the football team. The theory was that protein was needed for strength. Today, the theory of carbohydrate loading has replaced the big steak.

Dr. Per-Olof Astrand, the Swedish physiologist, has been a leader in the research on carbohydrate loading. Dr. Astrand believes that protein foods—the big steak—play no immediate role in the energy production of a runner. He argues that energy comes from a combination of slow-burning fat stored inside the muscle—"trained-on fat" not "eaten-on fat"—and glycogen, a product of carbohydrate foods. By regularly fasting and/or going for long runs of two hours or more, the runner utilizes this source of energy, which adds strength in the late stages of a race of at least 15 miles. Glycogen is stored in muscle, and limited in supply. It is also the major source of energy during high intensity effort. When the glycogen reserves are depleted late in a race, performance may decrease from fatigue.

When I ran a 50-mile race, I had the experience of running through four stages of energy: initially, a normal stage of adrenalin flow (I had to hold myself back); then settling into my pace; and third, at about 20 miles, I felt a period of adjustment where apparently my body was switching over to my stored glycogen packed in during carbohydrate loading. Finally, at 30 miles, I felt as if I were in the "land beyond," almost unaware of where I was, and my body was adjusting to the fat for energy for the long run effort. The last 5 miles were totally euphoric, with a strong sense of accomplishment.

Dr. Norbert Sander describes the principle behind the carbohydrate-loading diet:

There is some evidence in recent experiments that when fatigue sets in after more than two hours of constant effort glycogen in leg muscles decreases to virtually zero levels. After these stores are again replaced, the muscle tends to overshoot and glycogen is soon built up to a level greater than the normal resting one. On practical terms, if one can remove all the glycogen from his or her muscles and then suddenly replace it prior to a marathon, he or she would be starting with extra energy, giving added strength later in the race. Trials with long-distance skiers and runners have shown that in most cases tested competitors did objectively better in prolonged effort over two hours when the pre-race glycogen storage diet was carefully followed. It is important to note that from a scientific viewpoint the trials are too small and limited to be completely accepted at this time, and it is recommended that the diet only be used three or four times a year.

How does the carbohydrate loading diet work? The standard carbo-loading schedule consists of three phases. First, the runner goes for a long run of two or three hours about seven or eight days before a race. This drains the glycogen reserve. Secondly, the runner keeps his or her glycogen level low by eating high-protein, low-carbohydrate meals for three days. The next three days are the carbohydrate phase. For three days the runner eats mostly carbohydrates and builds up his energy reserves. Normal caloric levels should be maintained; overstuffing with food is not necessary, and, in fact, could be counter-productive. Follow the same training guidelines that Dr. Sander gives next.

As I mentioned, I've used this diet, and entered races full of energy and ready to fly, so it does have psychological value at least. But I've also found the depletion part of the cycle to be nerve-wracking; I've become very irritable and, I felt, susceptible to disease.

Dr. Sander, who won the 1974 New York City Marathon for the Millrose AA, recommends a modified diet that begins five days before a marathon. Here is what he recommends:

*Tuesday and Wednesday:* Aiming toward a race on Sunday, take a long run of two or three hours the first day to remove glycogen stores. After running, eat no carbohydrates for 48 hours, only protein and fats—fish, beef, pork, green vegetables, tomatoes. No fruits, bread, corn, chicken, sugar, milk. For fluids drink water, but do not drink coffee or tea, Gatorade or beer.

*Thursday–Saturday:* Begin your high-carbohydrate intake. Eat potatoes, bread, spaghetti, sugar, fruits, ice cream, pancakes, beer, cakes, etc. Continue until Saturday evening, and then eat a light pre-race meal, if you are accustomed to it.

### Training During the Diet

*Tuesday–Wednesday:* The only long run during this brief training period comes on Tuesday. On Wednesday, train lightly; a feeling of extreme fatigue may prevail and a 5- to 9-mile workout will be adequate.

*Thursday–Saturday:* As little effort as possible should be expended while storage is taking place. On Thursday, run an easy 4 to 5 miles with between six and eight 30-second accelerations. Friday and Saturday, take an easy 3 to 8 miles with no other effort. Some runners may prefer to take one or both days off.

Dr. Sander adds, "The above program is still speculative, but empirically the results have been promising. It is no substitute, however, for a solid background of preparation, decent sleep, and, in my opinion, a strong mental attitude prior to and during 'The Classic Distance.' "

Carbohydrate loading is still controversial. It works for some runners, but with others the results are inconsistent, or even dangerous. In some cases, leg cramping, angina (chest pain), abnormal EKGs, and kidney problems have been associated with carbohydrate loading. Moreover, no research exists about the long-term effects of loading.

Still, for some of us, it works. I loaded in dedicated fashion for my first two sub-three-hour marathons, and felt great. Later, I "loaded" on beer the night before a 50-kilometer (31.1 miles) race, and despite no effort at carbohydrate loading, I finished very strong.

Bob Fitts, a noted marathon runner and physiologist, states that the results are almost as good if you skip the potentially dangerous and nerve-wracking depletion cycle. He suggests going for a depletion run four or five days before the race, and then loading right away. I've been following this technique with success, and would recommend it for the beginner marathoner. Only the experienced runner, who is attempting an all-out performance, should even consider the full depletion-loading program. Dr. George Sheehan best sums up this conservative approach, "It isn't healthy to fool with Mother Nature."

## EATING AND DRINKING ON THE RUN

As a college runner I was always told to eat honey and Hershey bars before a race for quick energy. Salt tablets were part of the training diet during hot spells. And soccer and football coaches were adamant about not allowing athletes to drink water during workouts. The myth was that drinking and exercise would cause stomach cramps.

We've learned a lot since those days. For one thing, thirst quenchers such as Gatorade and ERG have been discovered to give quick energy and replace important minerals lost during sweating. We've also learned a lot about salt and potassium losses. Physiologists are still studying the effects of eating and drinking on the run, and runners are experimenting with their own bodies.

Drinking on the run is of more concern than eating. Prevention of dehydration and heat stress certainly takes precedence over carbohydrate replacement, especially on hot days. You can die from heat stroke during a race, but not from hunger. According to *The Runner's Diet:* "Calories only burn up at a rate of about 100 per mile in a distance run; this means it takes 35 miles to lose a pound of flesh. On the other hand, a pound of flesh may *drain* away in as little as 2 miles; on hot days, the pace may be faster yet." [Emphasis added.]

There are three basic reasons for drinking and eating on the run. By eating sweets or drinking sugar solutions, glucose (used for energy) is supplied to the body, offsetting that lost during exercise, especially late in a long run. Also, as you run, your body temperature rises as body fluids are depleted. This loss dehydrates the body, and can cause serious damage to your circulatory system. Drinking fluids during a race prevents this dehydration.

Third, important minerals and chemicals known as electrolytes (sodium, potassium, magnesium) are lost through the pores in perspiration. Fluids containing these minerals can be ingested before and during the race to replace those lost.

Many runners carry dextrose tablets with them during a long run, or have friends pass them candy bars. The most common form of adding carbohydrates on the run is by drinking one of the packaged drinks, such as Gatorade or ERG, every few miles. These are often handed out at special drinking stations along the route. You may also want to follow the example of my teammate Jerry Mahrer, who pins a bag of jelly beans to his shirt for energy during a race. Perhaps it works, perhaps not. As long as he *thinks* it works, it does. However, there are *caveats* in these practices. According to Dr. David Costill, a physiologist at Ball State University, carbohydrates taken immediately before or during running do not reach the muscles in significant amounts for at least twenty to thirty minutes after ingestion. He suggests eating carbohydrates before the run, and supplementing at frequent intervals.

Other experts feel that there is no scientific evidence for eating dextrose tablets, candy bars, jelly beans, honey or what have you as you tire during a race. Since it takes twenty to thirty minutes for benefits to occur, there is no immediate "lift." This is a controversy that remains unresolved. During my first Boston Marathon in 1974, a little girl handed me half a banana popsicle late in the race. The "lift" I got from that (probably psychological) will never be adequately explained by physiologists.

Sugar, some medical people feel, can be an enemy during a race. Even small amounts in a drink can slow down the absorption of fluids from the stomach. Sugar interferes with the quick passage of water into the circulating blood, where it helps combat dehydration and overheating. Dr. Costill states, "You need a fluid which will get out of your stomach quickly. Cold drinks tend to empty faster than hot ones. When sugar has been added, the water tends to remain in the stomach longer. Since Gatorade is 5 percent sugar, it would seem to be less commendable than drinks which are closer to water in content and effects. The main thing to remember is to concentrate on the water content." Plain water, reports show, vacates the stomach as much as 50 percent faster than a sugar solution. This could be a critical factor in preventing dehydration and heat disorders on a hot day.

Dr. Costill researched this problem with national and world class runners during the 1968 Boston Marathon and the 1968 U.S. Olympic trials. He found two types of dehydration: acute and chronic. Acute dehydration occurs during a run and hurts performance, but the fluid losses are usually replaced soon afterwards. Failure to replace lost liquids, however, during consecutive days of training may produce an accumulated fluid loss known as chronic dehydration. Let's remember that some runners' body temperatures may increase during long runs on hot days from the norm of 98.6° F. to as high as 106° F., which is extremely dangerous if prolonged.

Dr. Costill has made several observations concerning acute dehydration. Rectal temperatures of runners were 2 degrees (F.) cooler when the runners drank fluids during a two-hour run, than when they did not. Drinking a special glucose solution provided the muscles with greater amounts of sugar for energy and allowed runners to recover more rapidly after the run. In general, a weight loss of 2 percent or more of one's body weight by sweating affects performance. A loss of 5 to 6 percent affects health. A weight loss of 5 to 7 pounds is not uncommon during long runs. A runner may lose about 3 or 4 pounds per hour during a marathon, but he or she can only remove about 1.8 pounds of water from the stomach in the same period. Obviously, regardless of how much a runner drinks, he or she cannot keep up with the weight loss from sweating. Thus, a runner will dehydrate twice as fast as he or she can replace fluids during a race, and will finish dehydrated. For this reason, it is important to drink fluids after running as well.

Dr. Costill also believes that chronic dehydration is an important condition that is frequently overlooked. He says, "Large body-water losses incurred on consecutive days may cause an accumulated weight and fluid loss. We generally rely upon our thirst to control body fluid balance. Unfortunately, this mechanism is far from accurate. In laboratory tests that required about eight pounds of sweat loss, we found that thirst was temporarily satisfied by as little as one pound of water. Total replacement of body weight may take several days unless the runner forces himself to drink more than is desired."

Chronic dehydration lowers a runner's tolerance to fatigue, reduces his ability to sweat, elevates his rectal temperature and increases the stress on his circulatory system. Obviously, these factors sharply reduce a runner's endurance. "Probably the best way to guard against chronic dehydration," says Dr. Costill, "is to check your weight every morning before breakfast. If you note a two- or three-pound decrease in body weight from morning to morning, efforts should be made to increase your fluid intake. You need not worry about drinking too much fluid, because your kidneys will unload the excess water in a matter of hours."

All commercially prepared drinks for runners are designed to replace lost fluids, electrolytes and glycogen. These "electrolyte replacement drinks" contain sodium chloride, potassium and calcium, among other things. These, plus magnesium, are lost by runners, and need replacing. Dr. Kenneth Cooper has tested 750,000 volunteers for loss and replacement of fluid electrolytes. Of the four components, he found that sodium chloride may be the least important, and magnesium the most. Marathon runners show no significant loss of sodium chloride during races, but heavy losses of magnesium.

The most widely consumed prepared drinks are Gatorade, ERG, Sportade and Bike Half-Time Punch. All are designed to replace fluids, electrolytes and glycogens during activity. They are mostly water, with salt, potassium and sugars.

Gatorade was the first, and probably remains the best known. It was invented to quench the thirst of football players at the University of Florida. It is low on essential potassium, very sweet, and often sits in the stomach, causing problems. At the finish of the 1974 Boston Marathon, I spewed a green stream of this stuff, which hadn't been absorbed by my body, at the runner I had just beaten in a ferocious stretch run—*Love Story* author Erich Segal.

*Medical Times* has tested three of these drinks—not ERG— and found that their salt content causes potassium loss, which could be dangerous. Potassium depletion is often found in large numbers of heat strokes. *Medical Times* also reported that all three drinks had similar sodium contents, approximately the amount found in a glass of milk. Potassium was highest in Sportade, about five to ten times that in Gatorade and Half-Time Punch. Yet Sportade had only about half the potassium found in whole milk or orange juice. (Gatorade and Half-Time Punch had less than that found in a can of beer.) Sportade and Half-Time Punch had twice the carbohydrates found in Gatorade. All three contained less calories and carbohydrates than fresh orange juice.

In fact, *Medical Times* discovered that none of the three exercise drinks rated as well as orange juice or milk in replacing body fluids lost in running. Fresh orange juice was rated best of all, although it is low in sodium. Milk contains sodium and potassium, but fewer carbohydrates or calories than orange juice.

Dr. Costill believes "The commercialization of products such as Gatorade and ERG is aimed at convincing us we are losing valuable nutrients in our sweat. This is not really so because most nutrients are easily replaced in the runner's normal diet. Salt loss from a race or heavy workout can be compensated for by the kidney's decreasing the amount of salt lost through urine. Potassium loss is generally so small it can be replaced by drinking a glass of tomato juice."

Runners, as we've mentioned, can come up with a variety of concoctions of their own making that satisfy their needs. Some prepare a half-and-half solution of orange juice or tomato juice and water, and I suggest diluting most drinks with water, especially the sugar solutions like Gatorade. I know one runner who feels that a few ounces of cold coffee give him a "lift" late in a race. Frank Shorter has popularized the use of de-fizzed Coke. Dr. George Sheehan, never one to buy something off the shelf, put together his own homemade concoction for marathons—fresh orange juice in a weak salt solution.

Runner-chemist Bill Gookin invented the most popular drink among marathon runners, Gookinaid, or ERG (Electrolyte Replacement with Glucose). It is available in powdered packets. ERG is really "synthetic sweat," a balance of water, essential minerals and sugar. Gookin arrived at his still-secret formula by analyzing his own sweat lost through running, and then approximating the lost electrolytes in his drink.

Drinking fluids during long workouts is important even in cold weather. You may have to use your imagination to find something, but chewing snow or munching icicles is one solution. On a hot day, I'd advise bringing something with you (if you can). Jack Shepherd sometimes carries his son's Army canteen when he runs in Vermont, and because it bounces and interferes with his running rhythm, puts it in shady grass half-way along his route. Many runners suck ice cubes on a hot day but be careful not to choke on or swallow one accidentally. Also, the location of drinking fountains should be part of your pre-run course mapping. Sometimes the faucet in a sink at a gasoline station is the only source.

On some brutal days in Central Park, where water fountains are frequent, I stop as often as once a mile to drink water, and pour it over my head, down my back and stomach. It's a good idea to pin a dollar or so to your clothing, so that you can buy a soda if you must. Nina Kuscsik and I stopped twice during the steaming hot 1976 Holyoke Marathon, and split a Pepsi. The runners who passed us couldn't understand why we were sitting on the curb drinking a soda and chatting away, but it proved to be the "pause that refreshes." Nina went on to win the women's championship, and we passed many runners who had snickered at us.

In spite of any precautions drinking during a race can still be a problem. Be careful. On a cool day you can drink too much; on a hot day it's impossible to drink too much. Most runners try to grab a cup of liquid and throw it down fast, as they run. This is difficult to accomplish, and tough on your stomach; it may also spoil your rhythm more than stopping altogether for a moment. You probably won't have time to examine the fluid, either. More than once I've grabbed a cup of water to douse my head, and a cup of Gatorade to drink, and reversed the procedure. Warning: Gatorade stings the eyes and feels sticky dripping down your face. Another warning: During the 1977 Boston Marathon—a hot day for runners, but a cool 80° for spectators—I was looking for water but only found people offering orange slices. Citric acid can upset the stomach, especially when you run, and I was looking for fluid replacement, not a thirst quencher. Orange slices are a welcome quencher, but the fiber can be a problem. Finding water, even during such a popular marathon, may prove impossible.

The easiest way to drink on the run is to use a plastic squeeze bottle with a nozzle that fits into your mouth. You can control your intake, and you don't have to worry about spilling a drop. Of course, you need someone to hand the bottle to you, trot alongside, and take it back. Many runners, including me, find that the best method is to stop completely, and walk a few yards until finished drinking. The pause can be as refreshing as the drink, and, you may lose less time overall than if you had continued running slower while drinking. Bill Rodgers amazed everyone when he did this several times while leading the 1975 Boston Marathon, but he went on to win in an American record time of 2:09:55. Speaking of fluids, in the 1977 Boston Marathon, Jerome Drayton of Canada, the winner, complained because the only official drink available along the route was Gatorade, which evidently makes him ill. So be sure you can drink what's offered on the run, or bring your own.

It is also important to know, as I've said before, that cold fluids absorb faster than warm or hot fluids. If possible, have your friends who hand the fluids to you keep them on ice. For some runners, cold liquids cause stomach distress, so be careful.

Here are some concluding rules about drinking on the run that you might want to keep in mind before your next race:

1. Drink early and often, not just when you get thirsty. Thirst isn't always the only indicator of your need to replace fluids, especially on hot days.

2. Discover for yourself which fluids work best for your body. You might run several long workouts (over a period of weeks) as though they were races, consuming the fluids some-

one hands you on the run. This enables you to discover which fluids are best for you, how you can most easily consume them, and how often you need to drink.

3. Drinks that supply glucose and electrolytes can help performance, but on hot days, lots of plain water is essential in order to help keep the body from overheating.

4. One pint of fluid should be consumed about 10 minutes before the race (or long workout) so the body will be prepared to sweat. Up to half a pint should be consumed at 10- to 15-minute intervals on hot days.

5. Drink plenty of fluids throughout the day after a long run or race to replace the fluids lost.

Hooray for the postrace six-pack of beer!

# 15 STRESS AND TENSION

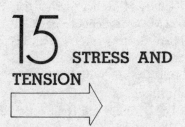

Stress is essential to life, but a cause of death. It sweetens victory, and defines defeat. It relieves boredom. It helps us maintain life, resist aggression and adapt to changing external influences. It may be pleasant or unpleasant, damaging or helpful. Its effect, especially its negative impact on our bodies, may be long lasting, even occurring after the stressful event has ceased.

Stress is everywhere in our daily lives. We may feel its characteristic signs immediately after someone's car nearly collides with our own, or both before and after an important business conference, speech, appearance, event.

What causes stress? Geographical change, social readjustment, a sudden surprising occurrence. Work is a major source of stress. Reaching a long-sought-for position, for example, and feeling inadequate for it, can raise blood pressure. "Stress," says Dr. Hans Selye, Director of the Institute of Experimental Medicine and Surgery, and author of *Stress Without Distress* and *The Stress of Life*, "is essentially the wear and tear in the body caused by life at any one moment."

There are various kinds of stresses: emotional (from a family argument, the death of a loved one), environmental (from excessive cold or heat), and physiological (caused by an outpouring of the steroid hormones from the adrenal glands, which are extremely sensitive indicators of stress).

Drs. Thomas H. Holmes and Richard H. Rahe, psychiatrists at the University of Washington Medical School, have attempted to list stressful events. These doctors interviewed 394 men and women and asked them to rank—using marriage as equivalent to 50 units on their scale—a series of life events. They then devised a "social adjustment scale" of stressful events. After compiling their scale, Drs. Holmes and Rahe found that stressful events had specific physiological impacts. Their scale places death of a spouse as the most stressful event we experience. Corroborating this, the doctors discovered that widows and widowers were ten times more likely to die within the first year after the death of their husbands or wives than all other people in their age group. Divorce, the next most stressful event, had a similar effect. The doctors found that divorced people, in the year following their divorce, had an illness rate 12 times higher than married people. Divorce now strikes one third of all married couples.

What does this mean to us? Changes in our lives, whether good or bad, cause stress. And stress itself, whether good or bad, may impair the way we live, work and feel. Stress changes us physically, and may cause a variety of medical ills, some imagined and some very real, painful, even lethal. Each period of stress, Dr. Selye says, especially from frustrating, unsuccessful struggles, leaves some irreversible chemical scars. Dr. Selye and other medical authorities believe that most diseases are the result of too much stress. Dr. Ernst van Aaken agrees that stress places a severe burden on our bodies, with specific sequential reactions. When we become burdened beyond our stress tolerance, we become ill, or we develop emotional problems, or we suffer the physical breakdowns of athletes.

What actually happens to a human being under stress? Imagine that you're facing a deadline. The boss comes in and tells you what you've done so far is awful, that you'd better get the job finished, in good shape, on time. This may cause stress; your body prepares for action. The stressor excites your hypothalamus (a brain region at the base of the skull) which produces a substance that stimulates the pituitary gland to discharge the hormone ACTH (adrenocorticotrophic hormone) into the blood. ACTH induces the external, cortical portion of the adrenal glands. Signals begin rushing out to all parts of your body. Adrenalin pours into your bloodstream. The adrenalin increases your heart rate, sometimes to a rapid pounding. Your blood pressure quickly rises. The heart demands more oxygen, and there is an increase in respiration. (Obviously, if you smoke during stressful situations the constriction of blood vessels caused by the ingredients of the cigarette add additional, sometimes fatal, physiological stress to the heart.)

Now, your heart is pounding, your blood pressure is up, your palms, armpits, stomach or back may be sweating. Blood sugar provides emergency rations for your muscles. You and your body are ready to act. However, too often in our society, instead of taking action or fleeing—the fight-or-flight reaction of our ancestors—we merely sit and seethe.

Research in the early 1900s by Dr. Walter B. Cannon at the Harvard Medical School showed that animals used this physiological change to act. When a wild animal fought or ran, it consumed this energy; its muscles later relaxed, its heartbeat slowed and returned to normal, its blood pressure dropped and its breathing steadied. The constant suppression of this natural sequence puts an unnatural strain on our bodies. Our failure to respond with physical action to stress is the main cause of tension. Many Americans lead lives without regular exercise; their underexercised muscles never get a chance to get rid of tensions. The constant imbalance between stress and the lack of exercise underlies hypokinetic disease. The results are tension and injury.

The impact of stress upon our bodies is measurable. When some people become upset, they vomit or get diarrhea. Others may suffer from psychosomatic diseases, such as migraine headaches, which can be extremely painful.

Stress takes its physiological toll. Our emotions affect our muscles; and our muscles reflect our emotional problems. Repeated tensing of the muscles results in loss of length of contracture. When a shortened muscle is forced to stretch, it cannot. It may react by going into a spasm, or by tearing. And muscle tension causes other problems.

Take back pain. According to Dr. Hans Kraus, the internationally known back specialist, back pain occurs because Americans are underexercised and overtense. Our crowded cities, the rush to work, our jobs and striving, the pressures of our daily lives make us overstimulated and overirritated. We constantly face the fight-or-flight syndrome, and do nothing about it but seethe. Our muscles, Dr. Kraus believes, are tensing for action and not being used for anything all day long. Our underexercised and overirritated life today is especially bad for our children. They are even less active than their parents. They watch a lot of television; as they sit before the screen they are both tense and motionless. Their predicament—tension and inaction—almost symbolizes our daily lives. Not surprisingly, Dr. Kraus has found that 60 percent of American children cannot perform the six basic Kraus-Weber tests that measure minimal physical fitness.

Some headaches, for example, may be caused by tension in the occipital muscles in the back of the head, and the frontalis muscles in the forehead. Neck pain may be caused by tensing of the trapezius muscles, which reach down to cover the shoulder blades, and the rhomboid muscles. Lower back muscles are also prime targets, as are, less frequently, the legs, thighs and arms. The result of such tension is a series of common ailments: tension headaches, aching stiff necks, lower back pain. The latter, in fact, is epidemic. In Chapter 10, we discuss this problem and suggest exercises for it. The YMCA offers classes to help people relieve lower back pain. This program was developed by Alexander Melleby and Dr. Hans Kraus. They have found, as other researchers have, that lower back pain is rarely caused by organic disease, but by muscles that are weak or tense, or both. Obviously, regular exercising would alleviate much of the problem.

Tension also works on our bodies in ways that we are unaware of. In a well-known study about heart disease and behavior patterns, Drs. Meyer Friedman and Ray H. Rosenman of Mount Sinai Hospital in San Francisco examined some 3500 men during a four-year span. They broadly divided the behavior patterns they found into two types: Type A and Type B. The Type A man was aggressive, ambitious and success oriented. He talked fast and was always on the run to meet deadlines; he competed against himself. Type B was a calmer man, working at his own pace, and under little stress.

"Type A" runners are also easily recognized. They carry their tensions visibly during a workout, running with tight face muscles, tight and high shoulders, and short, choppy stride. Very often, this type of runner will power by you going up a hill, and you will pass him on the downhill as you open your stride and guide along. The Type A runner, I've observed, is often a successful man or woman who works hard and believes that he or she has to run hard. They run, in part, as an escape from environmental pressures. They are usually too busy to warm-up, stretch and begin running slowly before beating their bodies into the hard, paved roads. They also think cooling down is for other runners, and risk serious injury by foregoing that series of exercises as well. Tight calves and hamstrings as well as back pain are often the penalty they pay for running this way.

Not surprisingly, Drs. Friedman and Rosenman found the Type A man to have 2.5 times more heart attacks than Type B. They also discovered that, among other things, emotional stress and nervous tension play a relevant role in coronary heart disease. John Hunter described coronary disease, and later suffered from it, "I am at the mercy of any fool who can aggravate me." The Type A man is also good at aggravating others.

Stress causes other diseases. Anger, fear and anxiety—all forms of stress—contribute to hypertension (high blood pressure), which can lead to heart attacks or strokes. Our stress-filled lives may also generate peptic ulcers, skipped heartbeats, even mental illness or suicide.

Medical research also shows that physically inactive people have high neuromuscular tension, higher levels of blood pressure, higher pulse rates, less vital breathing capabilities, and lower andrenocortical reserve.

Stress and tension and their symptoms can be greatly relieved, if not eliminated altogether, by learning to relax and by exercising regularly. Jogging or running, which allows the release of mental and physical tensions, can prevent stress. The easy run lets the mind wander. The feeling, if not the fact, of emotional release takes place. Research shows that running gives runners a sense of well-being and enhances creativity. A conference of the New York Academy of Sciences concluded in 1976 that long-distance runners tend to be more independent and emotionally stable and less anxiety-prone than their non-athletic counterparts.

Dr. William Glasser, author of *Positive Addiction*, suggests that jogging 1 mile three times a week results in increased self-confidence and greater imaginative powers. In his work, Dr. Glasser reports that the lonely runner, like the lone meditator, drains off tensions and releases negative emotions. Few runners can run and worry.

Dr. Selye identifies "the sense of aimlessness" as a serious stress on our modern lives. Most people, he notes, "just give up and drift from day to day, trying to divert their attention from the future by some such sedatives as compulsive promiscuity, frantic work, or simply alcohol." Dr. Selye believes that one's ultimate aim should be "to express ourselves fully, according to our own lights."

Running gives people specific goals, often replacing aimlessness with a sense of purpose, of being in charge. It gives a sense of being in control of one's life, and offers continuity. In a life of irregular meals, late meetings, missed planes and trains, running offers a constant, sure, pleasurable event. If you run at the same time every day, that time is sacred, and your life becomes regulated. You are giving yourself a time of relaxation, pleasure and peace.

There are, of course, stresses in running. The person exposed to stress throws up defenses to it. If the stress comes in small quantities and regularly, the body may adapt. But if the doses are too heavy, the body cannot cope, and exhaustion, ailments or injuries may result. The trick is to learn to relax and stretch, to train enough to build, but not to injure.

Tom Osler, a former national 50-mile champion, lists some danger signs when our stress burden is becoming excessive:

1. Mild leg soreness.
2. Lowered general resistance (sniffles, headaches, fever blisters).
3. A washed-out feeling, or an I-don't-care attitude.
4. Poor coordination (like general clumsiness, tripping, poor auto driving).
5. A hangover from a previous run.

To overcome stress—even the stress of exercise—one must do several things: identify the stressor; learn to relax, possibly with meditation or yoga; exercise regularly in a gentle manner. "The more we vary our actions," Dr. Selye says, "the less any part suffers from attrition." The ultimate goal is to keep our organs, muscles and brains fit.

We cannot—and Dr. Selye and others argue that we should not—avoid stress. Stress is part of life, a natural by-product of all our activities. What we must avoid is allowing stress to make us ill, weaken our resistance to disease, or kill us. We need to control the stresses we face, not the reverse. But how?

## RELAXATION

The ability to relax improves with training. Medical studies show that relaxation exercises can reduce tension and distress. Most importantly, they reduce high blood pressure and heart rates resulting from stress as well as muscle tension. They help to "break" muscle tension which frequently causes injury. Also, relaxing prior to exercising helps stretch tense muscles; a relaxed muscle stretches more easily. Third, relaxation exercises reduce muscle strain and soreness after workouts.

Meditation and yoga are two of the best forms of pre- and post-exercise relaxation. Experiments show that during meditation there is a marked decrease in the body's oxygen consumption, respiratory rate, and heart rate. Studies at Harvard indicate that by meditating some people can dramatically lower their blood pressure. As we will see in chapter 16, meditation before, during and after the run is reaping a wide variety of benefits for its adherents.

There are several well-known methods of relaxing and meditating; we will describe here a few that runners have tried with success.

### Autogenic Training

Devised by Dr. H. H. Shultz, a German neurologist, these six mental exercises should be practiced several times a day until you can elicit them at will.

In a quiet room, lie down, close your eyes and

1. Focus on a feeling of heaviness in the limbs.
2. Focus on the sensation of warmth in your limbs.
3. Concentrate on your heart and its slow beat.
4. Focus on controlled breathing.
5. Concentrate on feelings of coolness on your forehead.
6. Concentrate on total relaxation of the whole body.

### Progressive Relaxation

After twenty years of investigation, Dr. Edmund Jacobson published a book about relieving skeletal muscle contraction, which he believed caused or aggravated anxiety and related diseases. The idea is to lie on your bed, assume a passive mental state and calm "uncontrollable" tensions by relaxing controllable muscles. For every minute that you keep larger muscles relaxed, other smaller ones let go as well. Even tiny contractions of the muscles are avoided to achieve deep relaxation.

### Transcendental Meditation

One of the most widely practiced forms of meditation, TM became popular in the 1960s when the Beatles, Mia Farrow and others practiced it. TM is a controversial form of meditation requiring lessons at a qualified TM center, and a large fee.

### The Relaxation Response

This popular meditative technique employs the traditional four components of meditation coupled with some reassuring medical findings about reduced blood pressure. It was devised by Dr. Herbert Benson of the Harvard Medical School. The four components:

1. Find a quiet environment, which will help you concentrate.

2. Employ a mental device to shift your mind from the external, stress-filled world to your inner, peaceful world. Such a stimulus may be a sound, word or phrase repeated silently or aloud; or gazing at an object. "Mind wandering" is a major obstacle here.

3. Assume a passive attitude. This includes not worrying about how well you are performing.

4. Be comfortable. Some people sit in the cross-legged "lotus" position. Dr. Benson warns, "If you are lying down, there is a tendency to fall asleep."

Runners at Harvard's Thorndike Medical Laboratory, and Dr. Benson, developed a variation on these four components. Shepherd has tried them and thinks they're fantastic and beneficial if you get into some of the running meditation in chapter 16.

- Sit quietly in a comfortable position, close your eyes, and deeply relax all your muscles. One method Shepherd uses is the yogic massage: Begin by gently rubbing your head, and move slowly to every part of your body including fingers and toes. Keep the muscles deeply relaxed.
- Breathe through your nose. Try some yogic breathing

here: In one nostril and out, then in the same nostril, but out the other (block the first with a finger), in that nostril then out the first. Continue for several minutes, alternating nostrils. Then as you breathe out, silently say the word "one." Continue for twenty minutes. You may open your eyes to check the time, but don't use an alarm. When you finish, sit quietly for several minutes, first with your eyes closed and later with your eyes open.

- Maintain a passive attitude. Permit relaxation to occur at its own pace. Ignore all distracting thoughts. Continue repeating the word "one." Do not worry about whether or not you are achieving a deep level of relaxation.

### Yoga

After you've been running for a while, let's say a year or even sooner, and are increasing your distance and looking for new warm-up and cool-down exercises, yoga may appeal to you. If it already does, you're ahead of us.

Yoga is widely used among athletic teams. In baseball, the Kansas City Royals, St. Louis Cardinals, Philadelphia Phillies and California Angels practice it. In football, the New England Patriots, Pittsburgh Steelers, Denver Broncos, New York Giants and other teams teach yoga for stretching and relaxation. Among the many college teams, Georgia Tech's Bulldogs have the well-known Arden Zinn instructing them in yoga. Jean-Claude Killy, the skier, and his French teammates practiced yoga 30 minutes a day in training for the Olympics and European championships. Their coach, Honore Bonnet, says, "The purpose is to liberate the mind and relax the body."

Yoga is a good answer to a lack of flexibility. The stretching is gentle, smooth, nonpainful and achieved over a period of time. "Stretching by bobbing or bouncing," writes Dr. Herbert

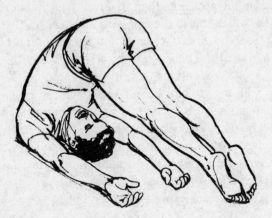

**Halasana**

de Vries, the U.S.C. physiologist, "invokes the stretch reflex which actually opposes the desired stretching."

It is difficult for a book to teach yoga, since it is a spiritual as well as physical exercise. But there are yoga positions that may benefit runners. Here are several we like. Most of them will be difficult to perform at first but with consistent, unforced practice, they can be mastered.

*The Plough (Halasana)* On your back, arms forward on the ground, slowly lift your legs and inhale; raise your hips and back and bring your legs all the way over your head until your toes touch the floor behind you. Bring legs slowly back to floor, and rise into a sitting position. Then slowly lie back down.

Variations: In the Plough, stretch your legs as far apart as possible. Or, bring your knees down to your ears.

*Forward Bend (Paschimothanasana)*   Sitting on the ground, back straight, legs together straight out in front of you, raise your arms as high overhead as possible, stretching your spine upward. Inhale deeply, exhale and lean forward catching your toes (if possible). A supple runner or reincarnate can hook his fingers around his big toe, and bring his head to his knees, elbows on the floor.

*Knee Stretch (Bhadrasana)*   Sit, and press soles of feet firmly together. Place hands on knees, and gently push them to the floor. Pull heels as close to your crotch as possible, clasp toes, and bend forward until your head touches (or almost touches) the floor.

*Deep Lunge (Sirangusthasana)*   Stand, legs wide apart, hands clasped behind back. Bend your left knee, and lean forward over it, trunk bending and head pressing down. Try to bring your forehead all the way down to your toes. Hold for half a minute and repeat to the other side.

*Forward Bend (Padahasthasana)*   Stand, inhale and raise your arms high overhead, arching slightly to the rear. Slowly bend down, exhale, legs straight, bring hands to heels and head to knees. Hold for several seconds. Inhale while straightening.

Variation: Clasp hands behind back, bend from waist, bring head down slowly to one knee and then the other, stretching sideways.

Try sitting in the lotus position: Bend right leg and place the foot on left thigh; draw the ankle in towards the groin. Fold the left leg over it onto other thigh. Keep back straight. Place hands, palm out, on knees.

If you are troubled with back problems, don't try doing The Cobra or The Bow. These, and some other yoga positions, may be harmful to your back and sciatic discomfort.

**Bhadrasana**

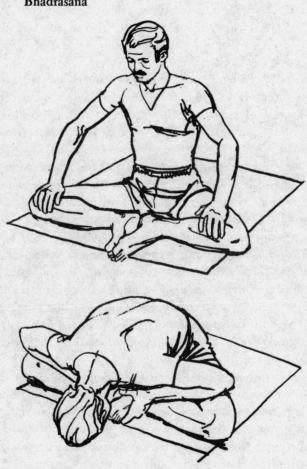

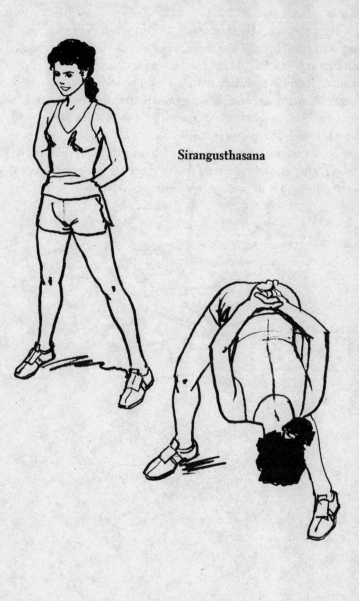

**Sirangusthasana**

Try some of these yoga positions as substitutes for your regular stretching. (But remember to do the full amount of stretching exercises.) One reason we emphasize varying warm-up and cool-down exercises is that they are so important we don't want them to become boring or repetitious. Substituting yoga is fun. Remember to continue the deep breathing, and to breathe with the yoga exercises, too.

So, run after warming up with meditation, relaxation (or yoga) and stretching. Run loose, because running is vital to your emotional as well as physical health.

# 16 RUNNING INSIDE YOUR HEAD

John Donahue is forty-three years old, and works for a contractor in Rochester, New York. He runs 5 miles almost every day. Like a lot of other runners who have gotten into shape and run regularly, Donahue is a running addict. He began running to lose weight but he continues because of his head. "After about 35 or 40 minutes," Donahue told a reporter, "it seems as if all sorts of tension is relieved. It's almost like floating. . . . I am more mentally alert after I run. Things are more noticeable, clearer—imagine lots of cobwebs, that you have just cleared away. Problems can be sorted out a lot easier afterwards."

Dr. George Sheehan, the cardiologist and marathon runner, talks about "the third wind" and his "peak experience" when he is "completely at peace with things" and becomes "quite creative, almost poetical" while running.

Dick Traum, the New York businessman who runs with an artificial leg, says, "I really enjoy the opportunity to organize my thoughts away from business interruptions. Sometimes I just 'tune out' for hours and release tension. It takes about a half hour to completely unwind, at which time I feel very high, as if I were running without any effort whatsoever."

Running also helped Mary Beth Byrne, a financial librarian

in New York and a member of the Greater New York AA, to find time to think about a change in her career, and to sort through her attitudes toward her work. "Running helped me find more satisfaction in my work. It gave me the courage and strength to make several major decisions. I found new challenges at work and was happy that it was not more demanding than it is because now I have time to run a lot. If I had made the career change I had been contemplating, I would have had very little time for running.

"I have found that running allows me to think of positive things, and to solve problems. I can think things through on the run and later I can make a better decision. Sometimes I just go blank. I feel great freedom—sometimes just looking at the trees and scenery, and not thinking about anything at all. It has been a very personal thing for me, allowing me to be more optimistic. The act of running combines body and mind in a way that is very satisfying."

Joe Henderson calls the experience "meditation on the move." And it is. If you are running more than 5 miles a day, more than four days a week, you may have experienced it: the flow of movement, the second wind, the creativity, the euphoria, the "third wind" and the meditative high. Dr. Sheehan calls running at this level "the opening of the creative side of your brain." It doesn't always happen, but when it does, he says, "I seem to see the way things really are. I am in the Kingdom."

Ian Thompson, the world-champion long-distance runner, told the London *Sunday Times* on June 30, 1974: ". . . E. M. Forster wrote a story about rowers in which he said they reached a state of transcendentalism which was the goal of every sportsman. You lose a sense of identity in yourself, you become running itself. I get this in training. I only have to think of putting on my running shoes and the kinesthetic pleasure of floating along, the pleasure of movement, starts to come. I get a feeling of euphoria, almost real happiness. It's an unvicious circle; when I am happy, I am running well, and when I am running well I am happy. . . . It is the platonic idea of knowing thyself. Running is getting to know thyself to an extreme degree."

Dr. Thaddeus Kostrubala started running to strengthen his heart and to lose 60 pounds. As he got into shape, he realized that not only was his body becoming firmer, but also his mind was sharper and more creative. A psychiatrist in San Diego, Dr. Kostrubala began treating some forms of emotional disease with therapy that included running. His patients began running up to an hour a day, three days a week, followed by group therapy. He has already returned a paranoid schizophrenic to school, and helped a heroin addict kick his habit. "I've never experienced this kind of success in psychotherapy before," he says.

Dr. John H. Greist, a University of Wisconsin-Madison psychiatrist, is studying the effect of jogging on clinically-depressed patients. During a ten-week running program for eight patients, six found relief from depression by walking, jogging or running two to seven times a week, both alone and in groups. Most recovered from their depressed state, Dr. Greist says, within three weeks of running, and have maintained the recovery.

Dr. Herbert De Vries, a physiologist from Los Angeles tested patients who experienced strong anxiety and tension. One group was given tranquilizers. The others went on regular vigorous walks. Dr. De Vries found that those taking the 15-minute walks on a regular basis were calmer; that is, the exercise had a greater calming effect than drugs.

There may be scientific evidence for this. Drs. Paul Insel and Walton Roth of Stanford University in California have found that running relaxes a tense body. Deepest relaxations come after voluntarily increased muscle tension. And recently, the New York Academy of Sciences concluded that men and women who run long distances are more emotionally stable, less anxiety-prone and more independent than nonrunners.

In 1973, *Psychology Today* magazine studied the effects of running on behavior. It found that people who began running tended to *become* more imaginative, self-sufficient, resolute and emotionally stable. They might not have been that way before they started running, but running helped them change their behavior. As Dr. William Glasser, author of *Positive Addiction*, says, running also gives us a wide range of emotional supports, including "increased self-confidence and even increased ability to use one's imagination, which of course makes life much more enjoyable." Dr. Glasser argues that "for those who get into running and do it on a regular basis, something builds up which is akin to an addiction. That is, if the runner doesn't run, he feels nervous, upset, anxious, tense—a tension which is relieved only by running his prescribed amount of time."

Perhaps the most dramatic argument comes from Dr. Malcolm Carruthers and his British medical team, who found that men and women who exercise vigorously released greater levels of the hormone epinephrine. This hormone, Dr. Carruthers reports, is "the chemical basis for happy feelings," and even just 10 minutes of strong exercise "doubles the body's level of this hormone, destroying depression—and the effect is long lasting."

Long, slow running can, as Dr. Kostrubala writes, "produce an altered state of consciousness. A non-ordinary avenue of perception does seem to open up." The experience is often like a dream, but remembered by the runner and there to be mulled over after the run. Dr. Kostrubala, himself a marathon runner, is very clear about what we runners are experiencing. "The slow long-distance runner experiences a part of his unconscious." His or her running also achieves "an altered state of consciousness that can be called a kind of Western meditation."

Dr. Kostrubala, in a magazine called *The Physician and Sportsmedicine*, writes that during "the first 20 or 30 minutes [of a run] you feel rotten, fatigued, shot down. Some in depression will actually cry. The draining feeling is emotional, not physical. That sense of depression disappears in 30 minutes. . . ,

"Almost as consistent is the 'runner's high' that occurs 30 to 40 minutes after starting. It's a distinct euphoria with feelings of excitement and enthusiasm. This is why most of our group runners supplement the dosage with independent running.

"I call the period of 40 to 60 minutes the 'altered state of consciousness' that must be similar to the catalytic experience of drugs or religion that allows us to alter our lives from within. It's an opening to the unconscious. . . .

"The thought process is altered. Problems become irrelevant or annoying, and are let go. And, like some inner consultation, a random jumble of ideas flashes through the field of consciousness."

There is, of course, the need to "listen to your body." Dr. Kostrubala, and other runners, recommend that if running doesn't begin to feel good after 30 minutes, you may want to stop. There are usually distinctive stages in running inside your head. The first 30 minutes may make you ask, "What the hell am I doing here?" Mild euphoria may start after 30 minutes. Tensions may drain away. The rhythmical sound of your breathing, or the rhythm between your steps and your breathing may lull you. Ideas flash in and out of your mind from the periphery of your consciousness. After an hour, a form of meditation, in which colors and thought patterns will flow through your awareness, may take effect. Robert Merrill, the opera singer, told reporter Valerie Andrews, "I just listen to my legs and feet, turn everything off, and my mind becomes very clear."

There are many ways to achieve this state of mind. Several doctors are studying the effects of yoga, meditation and running. The Esalen Sports Center offers some offbeat ways of relaxing and getting into the meditative mood for running.

Joe Henderson, author of *The Long-Run Solution,* suggests five steps, which are good general rules for running as well as for reaching a meditative state. First, he says, start your run without an end in sight. It will take 20 to 30 minutes to pick up the flow, and by then you'll know how much you can do. If the run goes badly, stop and try again tomorrow. Next, any running is better than none at all: "Even a trickle of running adds something to the pool of fitness." Third, let the pace find itself. You will usually run along the edge between comfort and discomfort. Fourth, run for yourself; don't look ahead or behind. And fifth, run for today, don't compete with yesterday or tomorrow; take pleasure in less than being best.

There are certain things that will inhibit or facilitate "penetration into one's inner world" while running. On the negative side:

- Competition, or the obsession with running miles.
- New surroundings, which focus your attention outside your body, rather than within. Some runners disagree, and argue that new surroundings take your mind off your run during those first, often uncomfortable 30 minutes.
- Other people and the yakketty-yakking of group runs; valuable for fun and sociability, group runs are out if you wish to reach a meditative state.
- Conversation, with someone else or with yourself, will misdirect your concentration; some runners like to talk to

themselves to pass through stages of their runs. Don't talk, either to yourself or others.

By avoiding these four circumstances during a run, and by running at a steady, non-tiring pace, and letting your mind spin free, with ideas flowing through it like water down a mountain stream, you can encourage the meditative state.

Dr. Leonard Reich, a New York City psychologist and runner, says, "I tell my friends cryptically that I try not to think about anything. In fact, I concentrate on clearing my mind of all thoughts so as to become receptive to the activity in which I am engaged. I call this 'meditative running.'" The first step, Dr. Reich suggests, is to "focus oneself in the present, to become aware of the here and now. This means to be receptive, to open awareness to all internal and external stimuli, to allow all the forces in the immediate situation to have equal attention."

Some runners sit and chant a mantra—a repeated word or sound—and then run. Others relax, begin running, and meditate on their steady breathing or the sound of their feet. Dick Buerkle, an Olympic distance runner, hears a steady beat as he runs, and sometimes the beat takes the form of a song with his feet pounding out the rhythm. He also likes to tie bells on his runnings shoes for a meditative sound. Other runners perform math computations, and still others seek meditative trances, almost becoming hypnotized like the Tibetans who run for 24 hours at a speed of 7 minutes per mile in a trance state achieved by meditation.

There are several ways of entering such a meditative state. Dr. Kostrubala recommends an "inner-directed attention" upon parts of your body: legs, back, feet; and your sweating and breathing. He also finds that saying over and over a childhood prayer like "Mathew, Mark, Luke and John, bless this bed I lie upon" sometimes works. Counting is also excellent; use numbers like a mantra by counting to 100, or, says the running doctor, "just count until you're silly with numbers."

The following are some methods to try for reaching meditation on the run, and since I believe running should be fun, I've included some wild ideas.

Sit quietly and alone near your regular running path. Close your eyes, or focus them on the ground immediately before you. Concentrate on your breathing. Count your breaths: Count 10 exhalations; start over and count 10 more. Do this for 15 minutes. Now, start walking. Focus on your feet hitting the ground. Listen to your breathing. Focus on your body. Begin a slow shuffle, and then a slow run. Bring the meditative state into your running by counting breaths, steps, or by repeating prayers, a mantra or numbers. After 30 minutes, let your mind wander free. Let ideas, fantasies, colors, smells flow through you. Be receptive, open to internal and external stimuli. And, as Dr. Reich stresses, "make your body rhythm so graceful that it enters the rhythm of the universe."

Another run, for men and women in good condition, might follow this pattern: Meditate alone in a field until ready to run. Stand, keeping your eyes half-closed, run slowly, and accelerate to surge. Open your eyes as you increase your speed. Then slow down, and return to a meditative position; rise, and run again.

The latter method is utilized by several west coast runners who have added meditation between sets of runs or before and after each workout.

We know, from medical studies, that one of the most inhibiting factors in muscular activity is the production of lactic acid in the blood. Lactic acid escapes from the muscles to the bloodstream when the oxygen supply is inadequate. *Scientific American* published medical reports that show that 10 minutes of meditation may reduce lactic acid in the blood equal to the reduction caused by 8 hours of sleep. Meditation before running, therefore, could have a profound effect on muscle strength. (For some standard meditation techniques, see chapter 15.)

Mike Spino of the Eslalen Institute, and James Hickman, a San Francisco research psychologist, have devised several mental exercises that are both meditative and helpful in preparing runners for running. One of the best is called a "witness meditation," which is designed to move you from a sitting into a running meditation.

First, you assume the standard Zen sitting posture, fingers curled, the left hand in your right palm, thumbs touching gently. Place your hands in your lap, and close your eyes. Breathe deeply into your abdomen. Proceed gently and slowly, and relax. Inhale deeply, filling the cavity, and as you exhale, release tension. After two minutes or so, switch and breathe deeply into the upper chest and lungs. Fill the upper chest. Exhale slowly and relax. Inhale and exhale in long draws, relaxed and rhythmical. After another two minutes, combine the two: inhale, filling your abdomen first and then your chest. Exhale from the chest and then the abdomen. Inhale, filling the abdomen and then chest; exhale from the chest and then the abdomen.

Spino and Hickman suggest that you next "visualize a light about the size of a halo directly over your head," and while inhaling slowly "draw light from this halo into the body." This "light" should relax and calm you. As the light fades from sight, you have "a personal energy source."

If this is too much for you, move to the next step from the rhythmical breathing: the "Zen walk." This helps you carry "the contemplative state of awareness into movement." Walk around a circle, slowly making contact with the ground, first with your heel and then toe and then gradually increasing to a faster walk.

Stop, look at a spot on the ground, "breathe into the spot." Now, "picture yourself as a primordial person," begin shuffling at a slow pace and then, in a "state of concentrated awareness," slowly begin running. Here, you might incorporate Dr. Kostrubala's ideas for meditating on the move.

This exercise with all these separate steps and ideas won't appeal to some runners, but my co-author Jack Shepherd thinks we all ought to have at least one crazy run every week. Mine is what I call an "Animal Run." I'll just run like a wild animal, full of speed and fury, with abandon, often alone, although sometimes with a fellow animal who takes turns pushing the pace. These runs strengthen my body and sharpen my mind. I think "guts" all the way through the run, and fantasize about my memories of one of my greatest heroes—Steve Prefontaine. I can still see him running beyond his limits on mental stamina alone with his agony mask hiding his joy for exceeding his threshold of pain, and when I play "animal" I pretend I'm as tough as he.

I believe a sense of euphoria comes with three types of runs, the meditative high from running alone at a reflective pace; the competition high of running fast at the edge of our physical limits; and the "high" of running with friends, of fellowship.

We are just beginning to understand the relationship between running and meditation. The so-called "primitive" peoples may be our ultimate teachers. The Tarahumara Indians in northern Mexico live in the mountains and run slowly from house to house, village to village. During workdays, groups may jog 30 miles or more, and on weekends, 150 miles.

Australian aborigines track kangaroo by slowly jogging with them until the animals are exhausted. The famous Bushmen hunters of the Kalahari Desert in Africa jog after eland for distances of more than 20 miles, and remain fresh. A group of Hopi

Indians traditionally ran 10 miles before dawn to their fields, worked all day, and ran 10 miles home. It is not surprising that some of these—the Tibetan runners, the Hopi—were meditative people. None counted miles, aerobic points, or time per mile. They ran out of desire, or the need to obtain food; it was part of their lives.

Now that running is part of your life, expand it. There are many ways, at many levels, to achieve meditation on the move.

For me, Dr. Sheehan sums it up best: "For every runner who tours the world running marathons, there are thousands who run to hear the leaves and listen to rain and look to the day when it all is suddenly as easy as a bird in flight. For them, sport is not a test but a therapy, not a trial but a reward, not a question but an answer."

# 17 WHERE TO RUN WHEN YOU'RE ON THE RUN: TWENTY-ONE CITIES

Carl Eilenberg, the radio announcer, travels as much as any of us, maybe more. "The first thing I pack," he says, "is my running stuff. Then, if there's any room left, I take my civvies. I've made a real personal commitment to myself to run every day, regardless of where I am."

Whatever the reasons for traveling, at one time or another almost every runner will be alone in strange cities. Happily, running is a gregarious as well as healthy activity. Most runners like nothing better than new runners to accompany them on their daily rounds. If you are a runner and you travel on business or pleasure, you have spent your last lonely days out of town. There are brothers and sisters out there jogging in parks, along canals and lakes and the ocean, through rain forests and along country roads, or even in motel parking lots and city streets. This chapter will detail what's available in our major cities, but Carl Eilenberg has the best advice.

"Live a little—explore!" he says. "Some of the very best runs I have had have been explorations. Just get dressed and take off. Decide how long you want to be out, and after you've covered half the time, turn around and start back." Eilenberg has gotten lost several times, and suggests that you remember the name

and approximate location of your motel or hotel. One em-
barrassing weekend, before broadcasting the Syracuse-Navy football game, Eilenberg trotted out from his Holiday Inn near
Bowie, Maryland, and took off. It was a magnificent fall day,
and he felt as though he could run forever. "I got lost," he
admits. He stopped to ask a man sleeping in a car. "I'm lost,
where am I?" The man eyed his T-shirt and fancy jogging
shorts, and replied, "You're in the United States of America,
son." When Eilenberg told him he wanted to get back to the
Holiday Inn, the man asked, "Holiday Inn One, Two or Three?"
Eilenberg didn't know.

So, learn to pick out landmarks on your run that will help
get you back. Eilenberg has one other helpful suggestion: Get
reliable information about distances. While in Virginia during
the football season, he decided to run from his motel to Monticello, Thomas Jefferson's home. He asked several people, and
they all agreed the round trip would be 15 miles. Eilenberg
started out at seven-thirty but didn't reach Monticello until
nine, and the man at the gate told him the distance was 11
miles—one-way! Halfway back, he hailed a cab, and when he
pulled up to the motel, Carl found the entire Syracuse University football team, coaching staff and press corps standing at
the entrance. "The boos, jeers and catcalls persisted for weeks."
Not only that, he had to borrow seven dollars for the fare.

Most runners like to run outdoors. But in really bad weather,
it is good to know where you can run indoors if you wish.
Three good sources of information for either type of runs are:

## THE ROAD RUNNER'S CLUB OF AMERICA

This nonprofit organization, founded in 1957, promotes running
as a sport and healthy exercise. It also hosts weekly running

events for all skill levels. There are more than 100 RRC chapters in the United States with 30,000 members. Many chapters publish regular newsletters and race schedules. Five regional vice-presidents can supply any runner with information about local running contacts. A list of club officers, chapters and publications will be found in the Appendix.

When writing to the RRC (or any running club) be sure to enclose a stamped, self-addressed envelope. It helps them save expenses and promptly answer a large volume of mail. Don't forget to thank them for their help—they're all volunteers.

## THE NATIONAL JOGGING ASSOCIATION

Hometown joggers have the best, and latest, word about where to run when you're traveling. Oregon, for example, that hotbed of joggerdom, has more than 250 miles of bikeways and foot paths (paid for by one percent of its highway funds) that runners enjoy. The N.J.A. keeps contact with perhaps 10 million American joggers. They can tell you whether or not your destination has one of the country's Road Runner's Club chapters, and provide information for advice on the best local running places. Write: The National Jogging Association, 1910 K. Street N.W., Washington, D.C. 20006 (202-785-8050).

## THE YMCA

Despite its name, this organization is co-ed. There are thousands of YMCAs located throughout the United States, and overseas. You don't have to be young, male or Christian to be welcomed at any YMCA. They are open to everyone. Many have indoor tracks readily available (for a small fee); many are banked and padded for comfort. Some Y's have developed outdoor running paths, and will direct you to them.

A YMCA membership card is good at any Y in the country for a limited number of visits. Most Y's accept one-day guests anytime. Many Y's also offer rooms for the night, which include the use of the facilities.

Before leaving home, if you plan to use a Y, remember to toss in a combination lock with your running gear. It's also a good idea to telephone the Y when you arrive. Some stagger their gym and track hours. In wet and wintery weather, any indoor track is likely to be crowded. If you can stagger your hours to an off-peak time (other than before 9 a.m., during noontime, or from 4 to 6 p.m.), you might find more room on the track.

When you first arrive in a city, inquire about jogging at the front desk of your hotel; ask whether any running clubs exist in the city (other than those listed here). Sometimes, you'll get pleasantly helpful replies (and sometimes not!). One psychological obstacle to running is getting from your hotel room to your running course. Jogging suits are so fashionable now that wearing one through a hotel lobby—even the lobby of the posh Mark Hopkins in San Francisco, the Hay-Adams in Washington, or the Pierre in New York City—presents no problem. Returning may elicit small displeasures—one doorman once tried to make Jack Shepherd use the service entrance—but most hotels have elevators near exit doors, or in garages. A little scouting beforehand helps.

Whatever you do—wherever you go—get out and run. Once while struggling through a lazy run along the Central Park Reservoir, I was joined by a slightly-built, bearded jogger. We started talking. He was visiting the city and wanted to know where to run. He also wanted company. His shuffling pace was even slower than mine. After half an hour of pleasant conversation I found out who he was: Tom Derderian, a national class

2:19 marathon runner who was in town to watch his wife, Charlotte Lettis, perform in the National AAU Indoor Track Championship.

Explore while you run. While attending a conference in La Crosse, Wisconsin, I ran a different direction every day. I crossed the muddy Mississippi River into Minnesota, checked out a local state park, and discovered cow paths through local farmlands. I even ran up an imposing three-mile cliff overlooking the city, and then looked down at the land I had conquered. In Montreal, during the 1976 Olympics, I visited all the city's historic sites—by jogging. In Ventura, California, I frolicked along the ocean for miles of sunrise euphoria, and ran again in the evening exploring the endless paths through the foothills where two-time National AAU Champion Garry Tuttle trains in peace.

There are some words of caution for the traveling runner. Dr. William L. Haskell of the Division of Cardiology at Stanford Medical School suggests, "It's wise to back off a bit from your usual [running] schedule. If you've gone suddenly from a moderate climate to a hot and humid one, the demand on your cardiovascular system, of course, is going to be greater. The same is true when going to a cold climate. Or to high altitudes: the Colorado Rockies, a place like Aspen." At 8000 feet, Dr. Haskell says, there is a decrease in oxygen availability of 15 percent compared with sea level.

Also, be alert to changes in running surfaces. As the chapters on injuries made clear, such a change can lead to problems. If you've been running on a padded track surface or grass, running on asphalt or concrete will pound aches into your legs and knees.

But don't be discouraged. Get out there and explore. Despite his disorientation, Carl Eilenberg offers some good advice for businessmen and women on the run: "A large part of the fun I have running is trying to figure out, during very busy days, when I'm out of town, what time and where I'm going to get my hour's worth in.

"Also, I have set a goal for myself (beyond a lifetime of pleasurable running). Before I leave this world of Addidas, Nike, Heartbreak Hill and Jock Semple, I plan to run at least five miles in every one of the fifty United States. So far I can count nineteen."

## RUNNING AROUND TOWN

Whatever your goals, here are some favorite running spots, and cities:

### Atlanta

This is the "Running Capital of the South." Atlanta runners congregate at Phidippedes, owned by former Olympian Jeff Galloway.

Best runs: The downtown hotels are within two miles of Piedmont Park, with its woods, streets and golf course, and mounted police are around to protect joggers from nonjoggers.

Emory University, not far from Piedmont, is surrounded by neighborhoods filled with runners. Morningside and the Emory areas are favorites. Try the university's quarter-mile track, open to runners year round.

In Southwest Atlanta, Adams Park offers hilly running over a trail used by high school cross-country teams. In the north-west, just off I-75, the Atlanta waterworks features two 1.2-mile courses that follow small lakes.

For a steep, 5-mile run, try Stone Mountain, fifteen miles west of Atlanta. The running path begins near the main parking lot.

Atlanta also offers a very popular "Peachtree" 10-kilometer run, held during the steamy July 4th weekend.

Running contacts:

YMCA (Downtown Branch), 145 Luckie St., NW, Atlanta, Ga. 30303; (404-525-5401).

The Atlanta Track Club, C/O Billy Daniel, 1760 Dyson Drive, NE, Atlanta, Ga. 30305.

### Baltimore

Downtown visitors have several options. The Central YMCA on Franklin Street has a splendid elevated and banked indoor track. Or, you might want to take the historic run: Charles Street to Fort Avenue to Fort McHenry, a 6-mile run to the birthplace of the Star-Spangled Banner, with excellent views of the harbor.

Best runs: For hills, try Loch Raven Reservoir, over the city line on Loch Raven Blvd. From the parking lot near the dam to Dulaney Valley Road is about 3.5 miles. The toughest run in town is Satyr Hill, not far from Johns Hopkins University.

Herring Run Park offers a 1.35-mile flat course around Lake Montebello. The city's bicyclists and joggers work out on a two-loop, two-mile cross-country path through hills and woods. The park's athletic fields also offer a flat, measured mile loop, broken into 100 yard distances for those wishing to do interval work.

Running contacts:

Every Sunday afternoon at two the Towson Branch of the YMCA sponsors a 1- and 2-mile Run for Your Life. (John Paletar, 301-256-1088).

The Baltimore Road Runners are also active on weekends throughout the year. They run 2 to 22 miles every Saturday morning at eight o'clock from the Loch Raven Dam. The start is actually in the lower Dam parking lot, one-third of a mile off Cromwell Bridge Road (301-668-3766).

The YMCA Central Branch, 24 Franklin St., Baltimore, Md. 21201; (301-539-7350). The Towson Family YMCA Branch, 600 W. Chesapeake Ave., Baltimore, Md. 21204; (301-823-8870).

### Boston
Home of the Bean, the Cod, and the Marathon.

Boston is a runner's town, and features the world's most famous runner-bartender, Tommy Leonard. You can find him at Eliot's Lounge (Bill Rodgers' hangout), just around the corner from the finish line in Boston. In 1977, Tommy held a carbohydrate-loading party for runners the day before the Marathon, and a glorious day-night after-the-race party. I think I remember something about that. Bill can also be found at his sports store on the course of the marathon at Cleveland Circle.

Best runs: The most pleasant runs may be along the Charles River. One, from the Prudential Center to Harvard University campus and back is about 10 miles. On the Cambridge side of the Charles is a wide path that is paved, flat and scenic. It is often filled with joggers. You can pick your distances by running along the Charles and looping across one of the many bridges.

Some distances: from Science Park to Watertown Square, 17 miles; to Eliot Bridge, 10 miles. At this bridge, turn to Fresh Pond, which *Runner's World* describes as "perhaps the most ideal running site around Boston." Run along Route 3 from the river. The paved path becomes 2.5 miles long by including the hill overlooking the parking lot. Distance markers are painted on the pavement.

Running from downtown hotels may be a problem. There is Boston Commons or the waterfront (Atlantic Avenue–Commercial Street), both pleasant during the day. Also, the park along the Charles on the Boston side by the Storrow Memorial Highway.

Long-distance runners who don't qualify for the Boston Marathon might want to pay homage to the infamous Newton Hills. Commonwealth Avenue in Newton covers three of the notorious four. Follow Lake Street to Newton Lower Falls; the return run totals 11 miles.

If you're on Cape Cod in August, try the scenic 7-mile run in Falmouth. In 1977, more than 2000 runners made the trip.

Running contacts:

The Huntington Avenue Branch of the YMCA has an indoor track at 316 Huntington Ave., Boston, Mass., 02115; 617-536-7800.

The Road Runners put out *Yankee Runner* that covers New England. Write: Rick Bayko, 19 Grove Street, Merrimac, Mass. 01860; (617-346-9664).

The Greater Boston Track Club, Bill Rodger's outfit, knows every path in the area. Try Bill Squires, 16 Crosby Road, Wakefield, Mass. 01880.

Women runners might want to check out the Liberty Athletic Club, which trains one of the top women's running teams in the U.S. Write—of all things—a man: John Babington, 4 Washington Avenue, Apt. 12A, Cambridge, Mass. 02140.

### Chicago

The Windy City offers some fine runs along Lake Michigan. Best runs: Lake Shore Drive, which follows the contour of the lake, is unmatched during warm weather. Between Foster Avenue Beach and the Museum of Science and Industry stretches 20.9 miles of sidewalk and path. Pick your distance and go running.

From most hotels around the Loop, a warm-up jog or brisk stroll to McCormick Place brings you to the Drive. From the University of Chicago, the Midway takes you directly to the beach.

There are also good parks and tracks. Riis Park, on Fullerton in the northwest section, holds races both winter and summer. There is a 400-meter cinder track. The fieldhouse, at last report, has working showers. Calumet Park, near the Indiana border, has a 4-mile loop and a lake view, while Washington and Jackson Parks near the University of Chicago have shorter loops. Both of these parks, however, should be avoided after dark. Stagg Field, near the university, offers a 440-yard Tartan track plus a larger oval track open for workouts between April and November.

Running contacts:

Lawson Center YMCA has a track at 30 W. Chicago Avenue, Chicago, Ill. 60616; (312-944-6211). The Tower YMCA (6300 W. Touhy, Niles, Ill. 60648; (312-744-8515)) also has an active fitness program.

The Mid-West Road Runners contact is Dick King, 500 So. Drexel, Chicago, Ill. 60606.

### Dallas

Everybody runs in Big D, the home of Lt. Gen. R. L. Bohannon, M.D., president of the National Jogging Association, and Dr. Kenneth Cooper and his Aerobics Center.

Best runs: The Aerobics Activity Center at 12100 Preston Road has a track, marked in tenths of a mile, which explores a landscape of willows and crepe myrtle. Visitors must be accompanied by a member, and there is a small charge. The center is open Monday through Saturday, 5:30 a.m. to 9:30 p.m.; (214-233-3842).

Every day, at noon, joggers leave the downtown Dallas area for workouts. One favorite run starts at the Downtown YMCA at 12 p.m., and covers up to 8 miles along Turtle Creek Boulevard. You may run as much of that distance as you wish.

Weekends, runners favor the shores of White Rock Lake in Highland Park. Races and workouts usually begin in The Big Thicket, and the path, except for two miles, closely hugs the shoreline.

Running contacts:

The Downtown Branch YMCA is located at 605 North Ervay, Dallas, Texas 75201; (214-743-3251).

The Cross-Country Club of Dallas is at 6891 Avalon, Dallas, Texas 75214.

### Denver

Talk about hills!

Denver rests on the eastern slopes of the Rocky Mountains. It's called "The Mile High City," and runners from closer-to-sea-level areas should get acclimated by being on the site for at least a week before starting out. Also, the sun can be stronger at this altitude, although city planners have planted Denver's parks with a variety of shade trees, a blessing to runner and stroller.

Best runs: Downtown Denver offers City Park along 17th Street between York and Colorado. The distance here is about 2.2 miles. Or, try Washington Park at Downing and Virginia Streets, which has a 2.2-mile paved road dotted with drinking fountains. To the west, Sloans Lake includes a 2.9-mile sidewalk course, the longest run in the Denver park system.

Denver runners will gladly show a visitor some 46 miles of paths from the suburb of Littleton through Denver to Aurora, on the east side. This is the Highline Canal; in Littleton and Aurora the running clubs have kept the trail alongside the canal clear.

For hilly workouts, try the Arapahoe Loop. This 5-mile run in Littleton will challenge the best. Begin at Arapahoe High School (at University and Dry Creek Roads), head west to Broadway, south to County Line Road, and east. A turn at Mount County Line will bring you back to Arapahoe High School.

Running contacts:

Central Denver YMCA, 25 East 16th Ave., Denver, Colo. 80202; (303-861-8300).

The Denver Track Club, C/O Pat Conroy, 901 Kearney, Denver, Colo. 80220; (303-377-4718).

Rocky Mountain Road Runners, C/O Buzz Yancey, 129 Washington #5, Denver, Colo. 80203.

Gar Williams, former RRC national president, 6555 High Circle, Morrison, Colorado 80465.

### Detroit

Home of the American motor car, Detroit is also a good place to use your legs to get around.

Best runs: Along the Detroit River, four miles from downtown, Belle Island offers three courses: the perimeter of 5.3 miles and AAU certified; a 5000-meter road course; a 1-mile loop. The courses are on pavement, with dirt paths running alongside.

Five miles north of downtown is Palmer Park with 4- and 5-mile courses. These paths are not well marked, however, and the runner might do well to run in Sherwood Forest, an elegant suburb, one block beyond.

In Chandler Park (at Edsel Ford Freeway, and Conner) a cinder path attracts joggers who run a figure-eight pattern with each loop counting 1.5 miles. Two miles north of downtown, Wayne State University has a 1.1-mile-per-lap track.

Running contacts:

The Belle Island Runners are 150 people who enjoy weekend jogs around the island, about 7 miles. Contact Dr. Edward Kozloff, 10144 Lincoln, Huntington Woods, Mich. 48070.

For indoor running try the YMCA Downtown Branch, 2020 Witherell St., Detroit, Mich. 48226; (313-WO 2-6126).

**Hawaii**
These islands have excellent temperatures and winds for running.

Best runs: There is lots of good running around Waikiki. The Ala Wai Canal is about 1.2 miles long. Near Mount Tantalus is a 10-mile loop, 5 miles up and 5 back, with great views of the Pacific. There is also a 1.7-mile loop around Kapiolani Park at the Kuhio end of Waikiki Beach, past the zoo. If you continue on, going up around Diamond Head crater, which includes the park, you'll cover 4.8 miles, with more long views of the ocean.

Kapiolani and Ala Moana Parks, cared for by the city, have running paths. You may want to start at the bandstand in Kapiolani and head out towards and over Diamond Head (following Kapiolani Blvd.-Diamond Head Rd.-Kahala Rd. to the golf course and back to the bandstand). That's 8 miles.

The Honolulu Marathon Clinic has maps with good running

routes and miles marked on them. Contact Mimi Beams at the clinic, a member of the Greater New York Athletic Association who moved to Honolulu.

On the other islands—Maui, Kauai and Hawaii—you can run anywhere.

Running contacts:

Road Runners Club of Hawaii: Col. Thomas J. Ferguson (Ret.), 4191 Halvpa St., Honolulu, Hawaii 96818; or The Mid-Pacific Road Runners, C/O Gordon Dugan, 704 Ainapo St., Honolulu, Hawaii 96825.

## Los Angeles

This is another runner's city. There are parks, and beaches along the Pacific Ocean, and lovely weather. The only drawback is the smog.

Best runs: Near downtown, Griffith Park offers hilly roads and 40 miles of bridle paths. Or, try the beach at Santa Monica, or the sidewalks overlooking Redondo Beach. San Vincente Boulevard, which offers a grassy stretch for 6 miles, is a favorite with LA joggers, who ignore warnings that the worst air pollution is found along highways.

This city also has excellent outdoor tracks. U.C.L.A., the University of California at Irvine, Long Beach State, Pierce College and Mt. San Antonio College have grass fields and good tracks. Santa Monica City College (near the beach) is a good meeting place for joggers of all ages.

One rule: Never jog on the freeways. Also, to avoid the worst smog hours, jog in the early morning or on weekends.

Running contacts:

The YMCAs are very active in Los Angeles, and two good ones are The Hollywood YMCA, 1553 N. Hudson Avenue, Hollywood, California, 90028; (213-467-4161). Or, West Side

Family Branch, 11311 La Grange Ave., Los Angeles, California 90025 (213-477-1511).

### Miami
Running in the summer is a trial here, but the other three seasons offer good weather.

Best runs: The bayside bike paths in Miami's Coconut Grove, the University of Miami campus and Miami-Dade Community College South. On Key Biscayne, the road from Crandon Park to Cape Florida Lighthouse (about 2.5 miles, some of it dirt) is a good run. Also, a bike path follows the contour of the beach for almost two miles. Birch State Park and Holiday Park in Fort Lauderdale offer good runs.

Running contacts:

The Road Runner's Club in Fort Lauderdale is very active, C/O Dennis Tunks, 731 Northeast 61st Street, Fort Lauderdale, Florida 33334.

The Downtown Branch YMCA, 40 Northeast Third Avenue, Miami, Florida 33132; (305-374-8487).

### New Orleans
There are long, isolated runs available along Lake Pontchartrain, and short jogs in City Park. But most runs in this gracious southern city begin at or pass the Gernon Brown Gymnasium at Harrison and Marconi Avenues. Here, too, begins the famous Mardi Gras Marathon.

Best runs: From the flagpole in front of the Gernon Gym, jog along Marconi toward the lake, left on Robert E. Lee Boulevard, right a mile later to West End Boulevard (which becomes Lakeshore Drive). Here, you can run for 15 miles, or shorter distances, by watching the painted markers and turning back when you wish. Saturday mornings, this course is crowded with local runners.

In downtown New Orleans, try Audubon Park on St. Charles Street across from Tulane University. On River Drive, just beyond the zoo, an "S (3)" painted on the pavement starts a 3-mile course that borders the park. Or, take Riverside Drive between Audubon Park and the Mississippi River, and follow it to the levee along the river.

Running contacts:

The New Orleans Track Club, C/O George Green, Apt. 100 N, 300 Ridge Lake, New Orleans, Louisiana 70001.

### New York City

Be prepared to run with the famous and beautiful: Robert Redford, Joey Heatherton, Jerry Stiller, Donna De Verona, Joseph Heller, Jackie Onassis, Paul Simon, Spencer Haywood all work out at one of the city's YMCAs or in Central Park. Dustin Hoffman trained for and filmed *Marathon Man* around the park's popular reservoir. Mohammed Ali likes to run there as well—"floating like a butterfly."

Best runs: There is an unbelievable assortment. On the East Side of Manhattan, walk or jog to the East River promenade, which begins just north of the Queensboro Bridge at 61 Street, and run along the river north to Carl Schurz Park, home of Gracie Mansion, the mayor's official residence. Twenty city blocks equal one mile.

If you are staying near Central Park, you have every kind of running challenge at your door. Weekends and holidays year round, and summer weekdays from 10 a.m. to 4 p.m., as well as certain summer evenings, the interior roadway of the park is closed to cars. Joggers can run the complete loop, of 6 miles, or shorter loops of 5 miles by taking the cut-off at 102nd Street, and 4 miles by taking both the 102nd & 72nd Street cutoffs.

The park's reservoir between 86th and 96th Streets offers two paths. The upper cinder oval that borders the reservoir itself is 1.5 miles. The lower, softer bridle path covers 1.6 miles. Between 5 and 7 p.m. the reservoir area is filled with talkative runners. It's a social affair, which centers around the 90th Street and Fifth Avenue entrance. Here, too, on Saturday mornings, you'll usually find me teaching a Road Runner's Club beginners class starting at 10 a.m. We generally have more than 200 beginner and intermediate runners out there ready to go.

Other runs in Central Park include the Oval, just above the pond by Belvedere Castle (a weather station) and Shakespeare-in-the-Park Theater at 82nd Street. Distances are marked on the pavement; a dirt path parallels the hard surface. In the evenings, the view of lighted Midtown Manhattan is unequalled.

Another Manhattan park with a good run is Riverside Park, on the upper West Side along the Hudson River. There is an outdoor 220-yard cinder track at West 72nd Street in the park, which is popular with runners like Arnold Spellon and author Kitty Lance. A longer run begins at 72nd Street and follows the upper promenade for 5 miles to the tower of Riverside Church, which you can see in the distance. One section of this run is marked each quarter mile by paint on the wide sidewalk.

On Wednesday evenings at 6:45, the Road Runner's Club and the Greater New York AA sponsor a group run that begins on West 63rd Street between Broadway and Central Park West. We usually meet under the YMCA's awning and jog over to Riverside Park at 72nd Street, and follow the Hudson to the George Washington Bridge. That's 13 miles. You can run with the group as far as you wish, but the run usually ends back on

West 63rd, where everyone heads over to Martin's Bar for 45-cent draft beers.

Also from the West 63rd Street Y, head into Central Park and run on the cinder bridle path which joins the one at the reservoir, a distance of about 1.5 miles. Other Y's in Manhattan are just as well located. The Vanderbilt Y on East 47th Street is a short jog from the footpaths along the East River Drive. Like the West Side Y, the downtown McBurney Y on West 23rd Street has an indoor track, or you can run from the Y to the West Side Highway which is closed to cars until a plan to rebuild is decided upon. From 23rd Street a 6-mile run along the highway would take you south to Battery Park and back. (Stop in to see McBurney member John Weiss at *Runner's World*, a nearby runner's store, for advice about shoes and running from a local marathoner.)

Other runs include the paths in Brooklyn's Prospect Park, a 5-mile cross-country trail in Van Cortlandt Park in the Bronx, Queen's Alley Pond Park, and Staten Island's Clove Lake Park. All are excellent running spots, although a bit far from midtown hotels.

Running contacts:

The New York Road Runner's Club hosts more than 100 races a year, including the nation's biggest marathon and women's race: the New York City Marathon in October; the 10 kilometer "Mini-Marathon" in late May or early June. Contact Fred Lebow, President, New York Road Runners, P.O. Box 881 FDR Station, New York, New York 10022; (212-595-3389).

The West Side YMCA has an indoor, padded track, 23 laps to the mile; 5 West 63rd Street, New York, New York 10023; (212-787-4400). The Vanderbilt Y is at 224 East 47th Street, New York, N.Y. 10017; (212-PL 5-2410). The McBurney Y,

215 West 23rd St., New York, N.Y. 10011; (212- CH 3-1982).
The YM/YWHA also has an indoor track at 92nd Street and
Lexington Avenue (212-427-6000).

### Philadelphia

In the movie *Rocky*, Sylvester Stallone jogs through this
city and ends up sprinting up the steps of the Philadelphia Museum of Art at dawn. It's a poignant scene, and Philadelphia
joggers recognized it also as almost impossible: The total run
would have covered almost 30 miles.

Still, the best runs are found around the Schuylkill River
(pronounced Sku-kill) or in Fairmount Park. One of the  finest
runs in Philadelphia follows the Schuylkill in Fairmount. A
5-mile course starts near Belmont Plateau; it is hilly and tough,
and about 15 minutes from downtown. Near the Art Museum
along the Schuylkill, follow the East River Drive. Joggers can
run on either grass or pavement.

To follow some of Rocky's route, try The Parkway from
Center City out toward Fairmount Park.

In downtown Philadelphia, an ideal all-weather track is the
University of Pennsylvania's Tartan oval at Franklin Field. Take
South Street to 34th to reach the field.

Running contacts:

Central Branch YMCA, 1421 Arch Street, Philalelphia,
Pennsylvania 19102; (215-569-1400).

The Mid-Atlantic Road Runners Club, C/O Joe McLihin-
ney, 908 Cottman Street, Philadelphia, Pennsylvania 19111;
(215-342-7600).

### Pittsburgh

Although Pittsburgh is a sprawling city, the visitor is seldom
more than 10 minutes from a good run.

Best runs: Downtown, the Golden Triangle YMCA holds a daily run at noon. Route: From the YMCA to the Mononga- hela River Wharf to the confluence of the Monongahela and Allegheny Rivers, upriver along the Allegheny, down the east bank encircling Three Rivers Stadium, returning across the Fort Duquesne Bridge. The Y is close to the William Penn and Hilton Hotels. Call 412-261-5820 for that day's run.

There are also 36 parks in Pittsburgh with running paths. One run is in the North Hills around North Park Lake, exactly 5.1 miles. Joggers meet there most mornings. University of Pittsburgh joggers like the 10,000-meter bike trail in Schenley Park. The park is primitive, much as it was when the French and Indians fought there more than 250 years ago. There are also excellent trails in Frick Park near the outer edge of the city.

Running contacts:

Golden Triangle YMCA, 304 Wood Street, Pittsburgh, Pa. 15222.

The Greater Pittsburgh Road Runner's Club, C/O Stuart Levy, 818 MacArthur Drive, Pittsburgh, Pa. 15228; (412-341- 4141). Or, the Allegheny Mountain RRC, C/O Shirley Mc- Daniels, 721 Vallevista Avenue, Pittsburgh, Pa. 15234.

### Portland/Eugene

Oregon has as many runners as raindrops—and it rains a lot there. Eugene, home of the late Steve Prefontaine, is the earth's center of jogging. The University of Oregon runners there fill pathways and roads, as do the Oregon State joggers at Cor- vallis.

Eugene claims the title "Jogging Capital of the World." The University of Oregon track meets are standing-room-only affairs filled with knowledgeable, enthusiastic spectators. Jim

Ferris, men's coach of the Greater New York AA, and a former U. of O. trackman, claims that "the town explodes with runners" of all ages and abilities.

Best Eugene runs: The bike path along the canal; the Alton Baker 10,000-meter wood chip path called "Pre's Trail" after Prefontaine. There is also good running in Hendrix Park, and along the streets of Eugene, in Laurelwood golf course outside town, or at the U. of O. track, which is open 24 hours a day. For local information, check in at The Athletic Dept. at the Eugene Mall, where you'll find some of our top runners.

Portland offers some fine runs within easy reach of downtown. Best runs: Duniway Park, on the foot of the West Hills near SW Fifth Avenue. A bicycle path leads into the hills for about 3.4 miles; the grade is steep and a good workout. Bonus: the trail is paved, the route overgrown with ferns, trees, grass and bushes. The Willamette River winds below, and on clear days—a rare occasion—you can see Mt. Hood.

Mt. Tabor Park on the east side of Portland covers 200 acres on the site of an extinct volcano. Forest Park, a little farther out, is a 7000-acre preserve with some 30 miles of cross-country paths.

If you have a car, try Seaside over on the Pacific Ocean. There, the Trail's End marathon and a 7-mile beach run are held in February and August. Or, drive twelve miles northwest to Sauvie Island, where the Willamette flows into the Columbia River. This flat agricultural island and waterfowl flyway features a 12-mile loop road, the site in November of an annual Island Marathon.

Running contacts:

Portland YMCA, 831 SW Sixth St., Portland, Oregon 97204; (503-223-6161).

The Oregon Road Runners, with 500 members, is very active. Contact Ken Weidkamp, 14230 SW Derby Street, Beaverton, Oregon 97005.

### St. Louis

If you are planning to meet anyone in St. Louie, Louie, be sure to pack your running shoes.

Best runs: Forest Park, near the Kingshighway hotels and across the street from the Chase Park-Plaza Hotel, offers the best paths. It is also within a jog of the St. Louis YMCA.

Forest Park is four miles west of downtown. The asphalt bicycle path loops in a 10-kilometer arch past fountains and lagoons, up steep hills, alongside playing fields and the St. Louis Zoo. A fork allows the runner to follow the J. F. Kennedy Forest route (6.53 kilometers) or stay outside (6.2).

In the suburbs, try the Tartan track at Florissant Valley Community College. Next to it is a 1.4-mile course with a steep hill. In University City, Heman Park has a 1.5-mile path. On the Illinois side of the Mississippi, the annual River Run in November features 10 miles of grey, misty views between Principia College in Elsah to the Alton city limits.

Running contacts:

The St. Louis YMCA Track Club runs a March marathon over the 1904 Olympic course, and includes a 10-kilometer race and a 1-mile fitness run. Contact the St. Louis YMCA Track Club, Downtown YMCA, 1528 Locust St., St. Louis, Missouri 63103; (314-GE 6-4100). The Y also has an indoor, banked oval track, 26 laps to the mile.

The Road Runner's Club may be reached through Jerry Kokesh, 1226 Orchard Village Drive, Manchester, Mo. 63011.

### San Diego

The variety of San Diego is exciting: flat beaches, steep hillsides, rugged canyons, green parks and bayside marathon courses.

Best runs: Balboa Park is almost in the center of San Diego. Runners meet there to work out on either the grass or paved running paths. Another favorite route is Rosecrans Street to Cabrillo Monument Drive to the monument itself, which juts into the sky along the Pacific Ocean. This is a great sunset run. Or, try the beaches at Coronado; the crescent view is unsurpassed anywhere.

Workouts are also popular along the magnificent, steep, winding hills of La Jolla (pronounced La Hoy-ya) north of the city. Beyond La Jolla, a long beach stretches for 20 miles; runners may pass nude bathers, hang gliders and other California fauna. Hills and altitude training await the serious runner to the east of San Diego, where Penasquitoes Canyon contains a tough 22-mile marathon course. The Laguna Mountains, an hour's drive, reach 6000 feet and offer unlimited paths and roads for mountain running.

Running contacts:

Bill and Donna Gookin are excellent long-distance runners. She teaches women runners; he invented the famous runner's drink, ERG. Contact them at the San Diego Track Club, 5946 Wenrich Drive, San Diego, California 92120.

Downtown YMCA, 1115 Eighth Avenue, San Diego, California 92101; (714-232-7451).

### San Francisco

This city has more hills than Rome, and cable cars to climb them. But there are also flat places to run, if that's your preference, and for a unique run, the lovely Golden Gate Bridge.

Best runs: One of the best in the West begins with a cable car ride. From the major hotels, take the Hyde Street cable car, which passes the St. Francis Hotel and within a block of the Hilton, Mark Hopkins and Fairmount Hotels. At Hyde Street, where the cable car ends, run in either direction. Van Ness and the end of the Municipal Pier is 1.25 miles one way, past outstanding restaurants, stores, maritime museums and fishing boats. Or, for the best run, turn west to Marina Green Boulevard, and follow the lush grass toward the Presidio. By jogging through Crissy Field, you cover 2 miles and reach the Golden Gate Bridge, which you can run across on the fenced sidewalk (1.5 miles round trip).

Or, from the same cable car stop, try the flat run to the Ferry Building 2 miles away. Continue to Third Street, and run by the dockyards toward Candlestick Park and the Cow Palace, 10 miles from the start.

There are also paths in Golden Gate Park, which is four miles by a half-mile wide, and reaches to the Pacific. A 5-mile AAU certified course circles Lake Merced near the ocean, south of Golden Gate Park.

For hill work, you've picked a good city. Try running from the Maritime Museum to California Street and return—up Nob Hill. (If you are staying at the Hopkins or Fairmount Hotel, you can run from your front door.) Or, run 1.5 miles to the Coit Tower. Twin Peaks, to the southwest, offers a steep mile with a sweeping view of city and harbor.

Running contacts:

The Dolphin-South End Running Club (DSE) is led by the barrel-chested, sixty-five-plus legendary Walter Stack. They run every Sunday morning, and turn out runners by the hundreds. Awards are made annually on a point system: one point for every mile of racing; one point for every 20 miles of training.

The DSE, C/O Walt Stack, 321 Collingwood St., San Francisco, California 94114; (415-647-9459).

One of the largest running clubs on the West Coast is the West Valley Track Club. Contact Jack Leydig, P.O. Box 1551, San Mateo, California 94401.

Also, the Bay Area Road Runners Club, C/O Bill Flodberg, 12925 Foothill Ave., San Martin, California 95046; (408-683-2810).

### Seattle

This city offers mountains, lakes, the sea and wonderful running companions.

Best runs: One includes Lake Washington Drive, which covers 3 miles between the original Floating Bridge and Seward Park. On clear days, Mt. Rainier and the Cascade Range are visible. To extend your run another 3 miles include Seward Park Peninsula by following the beach road. The path is paved, with dirt alongside.

Or, begin at the University of Washington on Union Bay, and follow two options: Either run south to the university's Arboretum, which includes several miles of dirt paths through woods and bird sanctuaries. Or, follow the Bert Gilman Trail, converted from an old railroad line, west along Lake Union. This trail follows the ship canal through park areas, fishing boat marinas and railroad tracks to Puget Sound—a distance of 3 miles.

At the locks, you might want to continue toward Ft. Lawton and Discovery Park, a route with running trails that follow high bluffs. One road descends to the beach and a mile of variety.

Great Lake, north of the University of Washington, may be Seattle's best known running spot. A paved path course 2.8

miles traces the lake's shore. There are rest rooms and a nearby zoo.

Running contacts:

The Pacific Northwest A.C., C/O Bill Roe, 2557–25th Avenue East, Seattle, Washington 98112; (206-325-3167). The Seattle Downtown YMCA has an indoor track at 909 Fourth Avenue, Seattle, Washington 98104; (206-MA 2-5208).

### Washington, D.C.

This is a jogger's city. Runners line the major roadways and follow paths through their favorite parks every day. The only drawback is the fact that, in summer, Washington steams.

Best runs: Loop the Tidal Basin during cherry blossom time. This short run of about 1 mile starts at the Lincoln Memorial and follows the Ohio Drive to the D Street Bridge, and return. To lengthen the run, lap the basin and follow Ohio Drive into East Potomac Park to Hains Point. A loop around the park, with splendid views of the Potomac, is about 3 miles.

The most famous run follows the old C & O Canal. Joggers may enter the towpath at 34th Street NW, just below M Street in Georgetown. The path follows the canal for about 5 miles; on its left side (leaving Washington) are mile markers. Horse-drawn passenger barges make daily trips along the canal in summer.

Washington has more than 47 miles of bike paths, and some of these offer good and safe running, too. From a downtown hotel, Rock Creek Park may be reached by public transportation (or a short run). Or, hill work may be preferred along Embassy Row on Massachusetts Avenue. Follow Massachusetts to Westmoreland Circle, about 3.5 miles and up some tough hills.

During winter or after dark (when the parks are unsafe),

runners can try the Central YMCA, with its banked, rubberized track (25 laps to the mile). This Y also hosts the annual Cherry Blossom Classic, a 10-mile run that coincides with the Cherry Blossom Festival every April. More than 3000 runners show up. A fitness run is held at the same time.

Running contacts:

Jeff Darman, National President, RRC of America, 2737 Devonshire Place NW, Washington D.C. 20008.

The DC Road Runners, C/O Ray Morrison, 120 Eastmoor Drive, Silver Spring, Maryland 20910.

The Central YMCA, 1736 G Street NW, Washington, D.C. 20006; (202-626-8250).

## WHERE TO RUN FOR FUN

If you want to see some new territory, and enter a race, you might enjoy these events. You can run backwards with sixty-four-year-old Ed Granowitz of Brooklyn, who is constantly promoting something called "The Reversible Mile." Ed also wants to start massive "cycle running"—pushing a bicycle ahead of you during races.

You can run from one country to the next. The Skylon Marathon in October starts in Buffalo, New York, and ends in Niagara Falls, Ontario, Canada. Runners must clear customs before getting a number, and if you are numberless as you pass the Customs Office on the Peace Bridge, they'll grab you. That's one way of stopping unofficial entries!

Maybe you like mountains. The Mt. Washington Road Race in New Hampshire is held every June. It's an 8-miler up the highest mountain in the Northeast—at a 12° average incline. I ran it in 1976, and it was 92° at the bottom and 52° with 40-50 mile-per-hour winds at the top, and worth the climb. Next stop will be the Pikes Peak Marathon, a 28-mile round trip, also held in June. Now that's really getting high on running!

### The Big Two: Boston, New York

The Boston Marathon, held on Patriot's Day (the third Monday in April), starts at high noon before a million people enjoying the holiday. The 1978 event was the 82nd annual race; it is sponsored by the Boston AA. The 1977 race drew more than 3000 runners despite strict entry requirements. It's a status thing to get into the Boston Marathon. It's also a great party weekend, when runners from all over the country meet and take over all the saloons. The course winds from the small town of Hopkinton through other Massachusetts towns and suburbs and ends before thousands of cheering spectators at the Prudential Center in downtown Boston. Any addicted runner knows making it to Boston is a must.

The New York City Marathon really blossomed into greatness during the 1976 Bicentennial. It expanded to touch on each of the city's five boroughs. Starting with that beautiful run across the Verrazano Bridge, the runner goes from Staten Island to Brooklyn, Queens, across the Queensborough Bridge where the view toward Manhattan's famous skyline is unequalled. After a quick trip to the Bronx, the course finishes in Central Park. New Yorkers really turn out for this race, and you'll pass more than a million of them, every one cheering you on.

The race is, best of all, a people's race—no entry qualifications are required. In 1977 more than half of the field were running their first marathon. The weekend begins with a "Meet the Marathoners" clinic where you can meet some of the world's best runners, and ends with lots of parties in "fun/run city."

It's a fast course, and lots of fun. As a member of the New York City Marathon Committee, I can attest to the fact that several hundred volunteers work thousands of hours year round to pull off this great event, which is sponsored by the Road Runner's Club of New York, Manufacturers Hanover Trust Co., the Rudin family, Etonic, Perrier and *New Times* magazine.

### Pick Your Marathon

The February issue of *Runner's World* annually includes a fifty-page marathon section with feature stories, marathon records, and a listing of all the men who broke 2:45 and all the women who broke 3:45 during the previous year. It also lists more than 200 marathons in the United States and Canada, giving the time and date of the race, a brief course description, winning times and number of finishers and whom to contact for more information. *Running Times* publishes a complete list of marathons in the East.

Also, if you'd like a list of all marathon finishers for the previous year, write: Ken Young, National Running Data Center, Institute of Atmospheric Research, University of Arizona, Tucson, Arizona 85721.

If you feel like celebrating with a race, try one (or more) of these, for fun:

- *January*  You can "Run Against Your Shadow" in the Ground Hog's Day Marathon in Little Rock, Arkansas.
- *February*  You can be patriotic and run the Washington's Birthday Marathon in Beltsville, Maryland, or go wild and run the Mardi Gras Marathon in New Orleans. If you're feeling romantic, try the Valentine's Day "Love Run" in Texarkana, Texas. It's a 6-mile dash for couples.
- *March*  You can run from one city to another in the "Bankathon," where Bill Rodgers set his world-record-breaking time for 30 kilometers. The run starts in Schenectady and finishes in Albany, New York.

- *April*  You can celebrate the Kentucky Derby in Louis-ville with a 12.8-mile run, or take the 15-kilometer Easter morning sprint up Diamond Head in Hawaii. There's the Cherry Blossom run in Washington, D.C., and, of course, the Boston Marathon on "Patriot's Day."
- *May*  You can spend a quiet Memorial Day on the 10-kilometer race in Asheville, North Carolina. Or, how about a 10-kilometer run in Somerset, Wisconsin, celebrating "Pea Soup Days." My hometown, Dansville, New York, invited me to run in their First Annual "Dogwood Fes-tival" 9-mile race a few years ago. When I showed up in running shoes and shorts, they called me a professional, but it's a good race—from the fire hall in Groveland to the first (and only) traffic light in Dansville (Groveland doesn't have a traffic light). My time was slow because the race director forgot to wind his wristwatch, and my official time was "quarter past eleven." Perhaps this is the way all races should be—informal and lots of fun. By the way, there are no dogwood trees in Dansville. You figure it out.
- *June*  Tired of seeing the same old faces? Travel to Tulsa for the "8-Mile Zoo Run."
- *July*  The annual 10-kilometer Peachtree Race in Atlanta is very popular on the Fourth. It's also very competitive, and usually has a wham-bang finish.
- *August*  There are several back-to-back 20-kilometer events this month. Try the "Sauerkraut Festival" in Phelps (up-state New York) for a good one—no hot dogs allowed. "The Fort Stanwix Day" run in Rome starts with a volley of muskets. As the leader runs around the Oriskany Battle-field Monument and heads for the fort in downtown Rome, a cannon booms, and workers back at the Y know to start icing the beer.

- *September*   Find a small town race followed by a parade and/or carnival for fun. The Fulton, New York, Fireman's 10-miler is a great outing for the entire family. Let Mom run while you buy the hot dogs and beer. The Charleston, West Virginia, 15-miler and the Lynchburg, Virginia, 10-miler attract thousands and are top races with small town hospitality. Or, try the world's largest race, the "City to Surf" run in Sydney, Australia, which had more than 10,000 finishers in 1976.
- *October*   I don't know if it's trick or treat, but there's a Hallowe'en morning fun run in Los Altos Hills, California.
- *November*   "Turkey Trots" for Thanksgiving are held all over the country. A lot of "birds" enter. The mood of giving certainly prevails in Baldwinsville, New York, where they usually have more trophies than runners for the 10-mile race. Berwick, Pennsylvania, started its 15-kilometer turkey run in 1909, but Guelph, Ontario, began their Thanksgiving Day race in 1895. Both are still held annually.
- *December*   I don't know of any races on Christmas Day, but I'm sure someone will soon organize a Bah Humbug Marathon. Two of the fastest growing marathons—for vacation and running—are the Orange Bowl Marathon in Miami and the Honolulu Marathon in Hawaii. Would you believe a midnight run on New Year's Eve? The *Runner's World* staff (Mountain View, California) hosts an annual 5-miler and in 1976 had more than 1000 entries. The starting signal is, appropriately, the pop of the champagne cork. Now that's starting the year off on the right foot!

# 18 RUNNERS MAKE BETTER LOVERS

It was a foggy, romantic morning. More than 7000 men and women crowded around the starting line for the annual Bay-to-Breakers Race in San Francisco. Most of them stayed warm by jogging in place, performing stretching exercises, or running short distances back and forth. The pre-race tension and excitement—this is more a race for fun than prizes—raised spirits and hopes; a festive feeling mingled with the fog and runners.

At the starting gun, this great mass of runners surged forward and each one began finding his or her pace. A runner, settling into his run, found himself behind an especially lovely woman whose stride matched his own. She glanced at him, he at her, and silently they paced each other for the first few miles. Finally, using an open line he had tried elsewhere, he asked, "What's a nice girl like you doing in a place like this?"

"Who says I'm nice?" she responded with a mischievous smile. He pulled closer, took her elbow, and the two of them veered off into the fog-shrouded bushes to prove that runners do indeed make better lovers.

Why do runners make better lovers? The reasons are readily apparent, the results joyful. Runners, like anyone who exercises regularly, feel and look better. They develop firm, lean bodies. With pride in your body comes a self-confidence that often carries over into your work and leisure. Sam McConnell at the age of seventy-seven runs 6 miles a day. "Running stimulates all aspects of health—physical and sexual," he says. "Most people over fifty don't have much sex, but running is a great contributor to the drive. I feel better today sexually than I did twenty years ago, and I attribute this to running."

Runners are endurance athletes, and are conditioned to pace themselves to superior performances. They participate in an activity that values endurance, versatility, overcoming obstacles (such as minor aches, pains and other discomforts), the shared experience, the ability to perform in any weather or climate, indoors or out, and of course distance over time. Runners are often more sensitive to the changes in their bodies, and from their training habits, know what it is to defer gratification. Persistence, durability, and the pleasure of each step toward a distant rewarding goal characterizes runners. Take the true story of another running friend of mine, a member of the New York Road Runner's. He had recently bedded a young woman runner, and they had quickly decided—quick for runners being a month—that runners make better lovers. To prove their point, so to speak, they made an agreeable pact: "The bet," my friend told me, "was that I could get an erection within 30 minutes after finishing a marathon. I was certain that marathon runners have extraordinary sexual prowess."

Eagerly, she accepted his bet, and the week of the marathon (held in a prestigious Eastern city) the two laid out their plans, as it were. By agreement, they abstained for two days before the race, and when he approached the starting line, it was with a more-than-usual eagerness to finish. At the gun, he jumped ahead to a fast pace, and maintained it with unusual vigor. The dreaded 20-mile marker came and went, and he was still running brilliantly. "In fact," he said, "I finished in my fastest time and didn't even think about the normal aches and pains we suffer in the closing stages of a marathon. I even carried a contented smile the last three miles. And I not only won my bet, the payoff removed every trace of my usual post-race stiffness."

Every runner we talked to for this chapter agreed that running improved his or her sexual performance. Men and women also agreed that runners are sexier, healthier, more attractive and more concerned with their bodies and their performance. In fact, running really stimulates a basic human question: How can I get my body to perform a wider range of activities? And running shows us how surprisingly versatile, strong and durable our bodies can be.

But the myth persists that running (and other sports) and sex don't mix, that if you are serious about a race you must abstain from pre-meet sex. Dr. George Sheehan, father of twelve, wrote in *Runner's World:* "Statistics on sexual activity suggest that actual energy expenditure is in the order of a 50-yard sprint. I cannot see how this would affect anyone's competitive efforts. Any problem then would be psychological. Perhaps the lowering of tension and loss of competitive drive would be a problem. However, there are some coaches and psychologists who think that such relaxation can be beneficial. My personal experience has convinced me that peak performances in middle- and long-distance runs are possible within hours of sexual activity."

Dr. Warren R. Guild of the Harvard Medical School has done extensive research on athletes, performance and sex. Discussing Muhammad Ali, the heavyweight boxer, Dr. Guild wrote, "I not only would not discourage him about sex, I would be on the positive side [and] definitely recommend and encourage him to have intercourse with his wife a night or two before the bout to ensure better sleep and have increased vigor for the competition. . . . Physical intercourse does not in any way sap one's strength or make one weak."

Dr. Craig Sharp, chief medical advisor for the British team at the 1972 Olympics, has been researching the sex-performance myth for a long time "mainly because of the bad advice that people have been getting." Dr. Sharp says that some athletes "upset their personal lives on non-physiological advice given either for puritanical reasons or through old wives' tales."

Dr. Sharp has further written, "I can find no factual evidence either in scientific literature or in discussion with many athletes and sportsmen of world class that sexual activity in moderation up to and including the night before a match has any detrimental effect on the sport in question."

He recalled the case of an Olympic middle-distance runner who set a world record an hour after making love, and that of the British miler who broke four minutes shortly after having sex. Dr. Sharp also wants to see wives accompany their husbands to the Olympic Games. Dave Wottle, the U.S. 800-meter runner, got married just before the 1972 Olympics, but once in Munich he was cloistered in Olympic Village and his wife, who spoke no German, was at a hotel almost an hour away. Dave, following the example of other athletes, began sneaking his wife into the compound. Many wives simply moved in and set up housekeeping. Although such sneaking around didn't bother Dave's performance, it might have bothered others' ideas of propriety.

Casey Stengel was right, "It isn't sex that wrecks these guys, it's staying up all night looking for it."

One woman runner told us of her excitement at the start of the 1977 New York City Marathon, when the huge crowd of noisy, thinly-clad runners bunched together on the Verrazano Bridge, tense and excited, shouting "Let's go! Let's go!" In the middle of this, our woman runner friend couldn't resist throwing her arms around a male runner who was bouncing up and down next to her. He was shocked.

"Forgive me," she told him, her arms and legs locked around his body. "I'm so turned on by all this I can't help it."

"Well," he said cautiously, "it *is* exciting." He hesitated, measuring the unexpected encounter in an unpropitious place, and then slowly put his arms around her. They kissed. They embraced. They began rocking to and fro almost as one.

The starting gun cracked the air, and, with the reflexes of trained runners, the woman and man broke apart, and began running. "About a mile or so later," she said, "it all came back to me: the urge, the embrace, the startled look. I began to laugh and laugh, and then I cried. And then I ran like hell. I never saw him again. But wherever he is, I want him to know one thing: He was dynamite on the Verazzano-Narrows Bridge in 1977."

That's almost my favorite story, but another one, heard during the 1977 Boston Marathon, offers hope for all runners. After the race, many of the men and women who completed the marathon adjoined for some post-race beer and fun at the Eliot Lounge not far from the finish line. I began interviewing some of the women and men for this chapter, and after about an hour a gray-haired man came up.

"I hear you're doing a book about running," he said, "and you've got a chapter on sex."

"Yep," I replied, and smiled.

"Well, for what it's worth, I started running when my wife died ten years ago. I was retired and had lots of time. And I was bored. I live in a retirement village, and I hate checkers and shuffleboard. So I started running. I qualified for Boston about five years ago, and I run about 60 miles a week."

At this point, I put down my beer. I was becoming most impressed with this old guy.

"Only problem is, the old ladies won't let me alone. There are damn few men my age around anyway, and one who runs 10 miles a day and keeps himself in shape is in high demand." He smiled, and chuckled. "I started wearing my old wedding ring, but that only cut down the number by a few. I find that I just can't say no. I really like young girls in their late fifties, early sixties. And when my body says 'yes' so easily, why should my head say no?"

I agreed, and we both laughed.

"Young man," he said conspiratorily, "let me tell you something. I'm getting more now than I did when I was forty or fifty years younger."

We laughed again.

"Hey," I asked him, "how old are you anyway?"

"Me? I'm seventy-two."

Now that's something to look forward to.

**APPENDICES**

RUNNING PUBLICATIONS:

*Footnotes*
Publication of the Road Runner's
  Club of America
1584 Spruce Drive
Kalamazoo, Michigan 49008

*Jogger*
National Jogging Association
1910 K Street NW
Suite 202
Washington, D.C. 20005

*New York RRC Newsletter*
P.O. Box 881
FDR Station
New York, New York 10022

*Running Times*
12808 Occoquam Road
Woodbridge, Virginia 22192

*Runner's World*
P.O. Box 366
Mountain View, California 94040

*Track & Field News*
Box 296
Los Altos, California 94022

*Yankee Runner*
P.O. Box 237
Merrimac, Massachusetts 01860

RUNNER'S AIDS
*(A partial list of hard-to-find items)*

   *Suppliers of arch supports and
   anterior crest inserts:*
**Dr. Scholl's Foot Comfort shops:**
211 North 21st Street,
  Birmingham, Alabama
160 A Del Amo Fashion Square,
  Torrance, California
21 North Wabash Avenue,
  Chicago, Illinois
21-23 Temple Place,
  Boston, Massachusetts
399 Fifth Avenue,
  New York, New York

419 Riverside,
  Spokane, Washington

   *Suppliers of heel cups:*
**M-F Athletic Company, Inc.,**
P.O. Box 8188,
  Cranston, Rhode Island 02920

   *Suppliers of glue guns for
   worn-down shoe soles:*
**Starting Line Sports,**
Box 8, Mountain View,
  California 94040
*(Also ask to see their catalogue for
a look at the full range of running
gear that they offer.)*

   *Rebuilders of worn-out shoes:*
**New Balance Company,**
38-42 Everett Street,
  Boston, Massachusetts 02135
*(They also sell their shoes by mail
and will send you a catalogue and
price list.)*

**Tred 2,** Department 125,
2510 Channing Avenue,
  San Jose, California 95131

ROAD RUNNER'S CLUBS
AND OFFICERS:
   **Executive Committee**
**Jeff Darman** (President)
2737 Devonshire Place NW
Washington, D.C. 20008
(202-462-3245)

**Don Chafee** (VP-West)
545 Kirkham Street
San Francisco, CA 94122
(415-564-1455)

**Neil Gillette** (VP-Central)
P.O. Box 1744
Greeley, CO 80631 (303-356-6671)
**Jerry Kokesh** (VP-North)
1226 Orchard Village Dr.
Manchester, MO 63011
(314-391-6712)

**Nick Costes** (VP-South)
Dept. of Health, Physical Ed.
and Rec., Troy State Univ.
Troy, AL 36081 (205-566-3159)

**Chuck Lesher** (VP-East)
Route 10, Box 38
Chambersburg, PA 17201
(717-264-5390)

**Ed Murray** (VP Programs)
3810 S. 6th Street
Arlington, VA 22204
(703-979-4362)

**Marge Rosasco** (Treasurer)
2419 Reckord Road
Fallston, MD 21047

**Les Kinion** (Secretary)
1363 Halstead Road
Baltimore, MD 21234
(301-668-3766)

**Gar Williams** (Appointed-
Past President)
6555 High Circle,
Morrison, CO 80465

**Public Relations**
Ron Adams
6913 Westlawn Drive
Falls Church, VA 22042
(703-532-1273)

CLUB ADDRESSES

*Alabama*
**Birmingham TC**
Versal Spalding
2405 Henrietta Road Court
Birmingham, AL 35223

**Huntsville TC**
Harold Tinsley, Sr.
8811 Edgehill Dr. SE
Huntsville, AL 35802
(205-881-9077)

**Troy Track Club**
Nick Costes
Dept. of Health and Rec.
Troy State University
Troy, AL 36081
(205-566-3159)

*Arizona*
**Arizona Road Racers**
John Weldy
2524 N. 69th Street
Scottsdale, AZ 85257
(602-946-3222)

**Southern Arizona RRC**
Joseph W. Cary
25 Goldfinch Circle
Sierra Vista, AZ 85635

*Arkansas*
Lloyd Walker
28 Pleasant Cove
Little Rock, AR 72211

*California*
**Ananda RRC**
George Beinhorn
900 Allegheny Star Route
Nevada City, CA 95959

**Bay Area RRC**
Bill Flodberg
12925 Foothill Ave.
San Martin, CA 95046
(408-683-2810)

**East Bay RRC**
Charles E. McMahon
154 Grover Lane
Walnut Creek, CA 94596
(415-937-0806)

**Empire Runners**
Glenn McCarthy
335 Algiers Court
Santa Rosa, CA 95405

**Lake Merritt Joggers and Striders**
John Notch
496 Mandana #4
Oakland, CA 94610

**San Luis Distance Club**
Stan Rosenfield
P.O. Box 1134
San Luis Obispo, CA 93406

**San Francisco DSE Runners**
Walt Stack
321 Collingwood St.
San Francisco, CA 94114
(415-647-9459)

*Colorado*

**Aspen TC**
Ron Nabers
Box 9609
Aspen, CO 81611

**Denver TC**
Steve Kaeuper
2263 Krameria
Denver, CO 80207
(303-388-8180)

**Colorado Masters RA**
Bill & Nancy Hamaker
1525 S. Lansing St.
Aurora, CO 80012
(303-750-9043h; 341-8032w)

**Fort Collins TC**
Ray Boyd
P.O. Box 1435
Fort Collins, CO 80521
(303-484-5076)

**Northern Colorado TC**
Neil Gillette
P.O. Box 1744
Greeley, CO 80631

**Pikes Peak TC**
Merv Bennett
Pikes Peak Y
P.O. Box 1694
Colorado Springs, CO 80901

**Rocky Mountain Road Runners**
Buzz Yancey
929 Washington #5
Denver, CO 80203
(303-831-6129)

**San Juan Mountain Runners**
Tom Haggard
Route 1, Box 221
Montrose, CO 81401

**Timber Ridge Runners**
Gary Phippen
P.O. Box 1262
Evergreen, CO 80439
(303-674-7641)

*Connecticut*
**Hartford Track Club**
Vin Fandett

11-D Fairway Drive
Wethersfield, CT 06109

*Florida*
**Fort Lauderdale RRC**
Dennis Tunks
731 Northeast 61st Street
Fort Lauderdale, FL 33334

**Gulf Winds TC**
Dr. James C. Penrod
2412 Winthrop Road
Tallahassee, FL 32303
(904-386-6294)

**Northwest Florida TC**
Ed Sears
174 Charles Dr.
Valparaiso, FL 32580
(904-678-6329)

**Pensacola Runners Assoc.**
Stuart Towns
P.O. Box 2691
Pensacola, FL 32503
(904-476-8750)

**Valparaiso-Niceville AA**
Fred Carley
177 BA, Route 1
Niceville, FL 32578
(904-897-2559)

*Georgia*
**Atlanta TC**
Billy Daniel
1760 Dyson Dr. NE
Atlanta, GA 30305

**Savannah Striders**
William Bakkeby
159 Traynor Ave.
Savannah, GA 31405
(912-354-8705)

*Guam*
**Guam Running Club**
Mike Flynn
P.O. Box 756
Agana, Guam 96910

*Hawaii*
**Mid-Pacific RRC**
Thomas Smith

203 Ihihau St.
Honolulu, HI 96734
(808-254-3944)

**Iowa**
**Cornbelt Running Club**
Karl Ungureau
203 E. Denison
Davenport, IA 52804

**Illinois**
**Club Northshore**
3272 Western
Highland Park, IL 60035
(312-432-3411)

**Galesburg RRC**
Evan Massey
1080 Tamarind
Galesburg, IL 61401
(309-342-8270)

**Glenview RRC**
Jerry Parsons
1504 Pfingsten Road
Glenview, IL 60025
(312-729-5507)

**Illinois RRC**
Alan Edgecombe
P.O. Box 2976, Station A
Champaign, IL 61820
(217-367-7711)

**Illinois Valley Striders**
Steve Shostrom
3018 No. Bigelow
Peoria, IL 61604
(309-685-3654)

**Midwest RRC**
Dick King
5600 S. Drexel
Chicago, IL 60606
(312-643-9894)

**Moraine TC**
Mike Beard
10267 Huntington Ct.
Orland Park, IL 60462

**Springfield RRC**
Tim Bonansinga
1412 South Douglas
Springfield, IL 62704
(217-782-1090)

**Indiana**
**Hoosier RRC**
Steve Kearney
205 W. Porter Ave.
Chesterton, IN 46304
(219-926-4344)

**Fort Wayne TC**
Harry Koontz
4634 Manistee Drive
Ft. Wayne, IN 46815
(219-485-9124)

**Kansas**
**Mid-America Masters T&F**
Bob Creighton
111 S. 6th St.
Atwood, KS 67730
(913-626-3679)

**Wichita Running Club**
Brent Wooten
3054 South Custer
Wichita, KS 67217

**Louisiana**
**Cajun Track Club**
Don Stuckey
627 East 11th Street
Crowley, LA 70526
(318-783-4533)

**RRC of Slidell**
Ray Durham
675 Dale Avenue
Slidell, LA 70458
(504-641-0440)

**New Orleans Track Club**
President
P.O. Box 30491
New Orleans, LA 70190

**Maryland**
**Baltimore RRC**
John Roemer
Route 1, Box 246
Evna Road
Parkton, MD 21120

**Frederick Steeplechasers**
Jim Dillon
15 Eureka Lane
Walkersville, MD 21793

**Queen City Striders**
Ray Kiddy
1916 Harrow Lane
Cumberland, MD 21502
(301-777-7391)

**RASAC**
Joseph Lacetera
1006 Whitaker Mill Road
Joppa, MD 21085
(301-877-0718)

*Massachusetts*
**Berkshire Hill Runners**
Jim Dami
17 Frederick St.
North Adams, MA 01247

**Central Mass. Striders**
Wayne Lamothe
9 Atwood Road
Cherry Valley, MA 01611

**Greater Springfield Harriers**
Brian Powell
120 Oxford Rd.
Holyoke, MA 01040

**New England RRC**
Rick Bayko
19 Grove Street
Merrimac, MA 01860
(617-346-9664)

**North Medford Club**
Julian Siegal
368 Lincoln St., Apt. 11
Waltham, MA 02154

**Poet's Seat Ridge Runners**
Edward C. Porter
26 Madison Circle
Greenfield, MA 01301
(617-774-2510)

**Sharon RRC**
Dale Van Meter
66 Summit Ave.
Sharon, MA 02067
(617-784-6348)

**Sugarloaf Mountain AC**
Ed Sandifer
P.O. Box 853
Amherst, MA 01002

*Michigan*
**Battle Creek RRC**
Robert Fischer
52½ Elm
Battle Creek, MI 49017
(616-963-9458)

**Kalamazoo TC**
Tom Coyne
1584 Spruce Drive
Kalamazoo, MI 49008

**Mid Michigan TC**
Gordon Schafer
4378 W. Holt Road
Holt, MI 48842

**Saginaw TC**
Ray Bartels
4440 Winfield
Saginaw, MI 48603
(517-793-0979)

**Upper Peninsula RRC**
Dan Lori
Box 776
Iron Mountain, MI 49801

*Minnesota*
**Minnesota Distance Running Association**
P.O. Box 14064
University Station
Minneapolis, MN 55414
(612-484-5164)

*Mississippi*
**Hattiesburg TC**
John L. Pendergrass
Box 1230
Hattiesburg, MS 39401

**Laurel Fun Runners**
Pamela J. Boyd
Route 10, Box 404
Laurel, MS 39440
(601-428-7221)

**Mississippi TC**
Walter Howell
608 Dunton Road
Clinton, MS 39056

**Ocean Springs RRC**
Terry Delcluze

1207 Londonderry Lane
Ocean Springs, MS 39564

*Montana*
**Big Sky Wind Drinkers**
Andy Blank
P.O. Box 1766
Bozeman, MT 59715

*Missouri*
**Columbia TC**
Joe Duncan
4004 Defoe Drive
Columbia, MO 65201
(314-445-2684)
**St. Louis TC**
Jerry Kokesh
1226 Orchard Village Drive
Manchester, MO 63011

*Nevada*
**Las Vegas TC**
Tony Gerardi
5020 Lancaster Drive
Las Vegas, NV 89120
(702-451-4060)

*New York*
**Hudson-Mohawk RRC**
Paul Rosenberg
124 Daytona Ave.
Albany, NY 12203
(518-489-6590)
**New York RRC**
Fred Lebow
Box 881, FDR Station
New York, NY 10022
(212-595-3389/4141)
**Greater Rochester TC**
Paul Gesell
4472 Main Street
Hemlock, NY 14466

*New Hampshire*
**North Country AC**
Paul Mailman
Box 11
Littleton, NH 03561

*North Carolina*
**Asheville TC**
Bob Wiltshire

Parish House (St. Mary's)
339 Charlotte Street
Asheville, NC 28804
(704-252-2752)

**Charlotte-Mecklenburg TC**
Bob Maydole
704 Pine Rd.
Davidson, NC 28036
(704-892-3078)

**Carolina Godiva TC**
David B. L. Royle
Box 16, Carolina Station
UNC-CH
Chapel Hill, NC 27514

**Cumberland County RR**
Roger J. Peduzzi
USAIMA-Med Trng Branch
Fort Bragg, NC 28307

*Ohio*
**Cleveland RRC**
Bill Bredenbeck
5916 Longano Drive
Independence, OH 44131

**Cleveland West RRC**
Stephen Gladis
530 Humiston Dr.
Bay Village, OH 44140

**Ohio River RRC**
Felix LeBlanc
1013 Tralee Trail
Dayton, OH 45430

**Southeast Running Club**
Roger McKain
6549 Forest Glen Ave.
Cleveland, OH 44139

**Toledo RRC**
Fred Fineske
1717 Eastfield
Maumee, OH 43537

**University of Toledo RRC**
Sy Mah
2158 Sylvania Ave.
Toledo, OH 43616

**Youngstown RRC**
Jack Cessna
269 Alameda Ave.

Youngstown, OH 44504
(216-747-3238)

*Pennsylvania*
**Allegheny Mountain RRC**
Shirley McDaniels
721 Vallevista Ave.
Pittsburgh, PA 15234
(412-343-1327)

**Chambersburg RRC**
Check Lesher
Route 10, Box 38
Chambersburg, PA 17201
(717-264-5390)

**Delco Joggers**
Byron J. Mundy
713 Beechwood Ave.
Collingdale, PA 19023

**Greater Pittsburgh RRC**
Stuart Levy
818 MacArthur Drive
Pittsburgh, PA 15228
(412-341-4141)

**Harrisburg Area RRC**
Reuben M. Smitley
3340 N. Third St.
Harrisburg, PA 17110
(717-232-8808)

**Mid-Atlantic RRC**
Chris Tatreau
Memorial Hall
West Park
Philadelphia, PA 19131

**Reading RRC**
Bruce Zeidman
211 N. 6th Street
Reading, PA 19601
(215-375-4368)

**Valley Forge RRC**
Rev. Raymond K. Reighn
Pawling Road
Phoenixville, PA 19460

*South Carolina*
**Greenville TC**
Bill Keesling
5 Rollingwood Drive
Taylors, SC 29687
(803-268-8967)

*Texas*
**Houston RRC**
J. Geller
4132 Meyerwood
Houston, TX 77025

*Utah*
**Beehive TC**
Jan Cheney
289 South at 200 East
Kaysville, UT 84037
(801-376-5072)

*Virginia*
**Rappahannock RC**
Kevin Breen
Route 1, Box 103B
Fredericksburg, VA 22401

**Tidewater Striders**
Don Grey
6429 Bridle Way
Norfolk, VA 23518

*Tennessee*
**Chattanooga TC**
Doug Hawley
Box 1167
Dalton, GA 30720
(404-226-3730)

**Eagle U. RC**
LTC Gerald L. Koch
101 Lacy Lane
Clarksville, TN 37040

*Vermont*
**Vermont Ridge Runners**
Tom Heffernan
Box 116
Killington, VT 05751

*Washington*
**Club Northwest**
Bill Roe
2557-25th Ave. East
Seattle, WA 98112
(206-325-3167)

**Walla Walla RRC**
Russ Akers
959 Olympia
Walla Walla, WA 99362

**Washington, D.C.**
**DC Road Runners**
Ray Morrison
120 Eastmoor Drive
Silver Spring, MD 20901
(301-593-3834)

**West Virginia**
**Country Roaders RRC**
Paul D. Caseman
270 Buckey Hill Road
Wellsburg, WV 26070
(304-737-3340)

**Kanawha Valley RRC**
Jim Jones
P.O. Box 2022
Charlestown, WV 25327

**Wisconsin**
**University of Wisconsin**
**at Milwaukee TC**
Clark Bowerman
36545 Colonial Hills Drive
Dousman, WI 53118

**Indianhead TC**
Dr. Doug Erbeck
707 Weshaven Rd.
Chippewa Falls, WI 54709
(715-723-7375)

**Wyoming**
**Cheyenne TC**
Greg & Mary Anne Niemiec
P.O. Box 10154
Cheyenne, WY 82001
(307-635-2033)

**Human Energy West**
Bruce J. Noble
1063 Empanada
Laramie, WY 82071

READING LIST

*Here is a carefully selected list of books that supplement this basic handbook.*

Benson, Herbert. *The Relaxation Response.* New York: William Morrow, 1975. A good, basic primer for runners interested in meditation.

Bowerman, William J., and Harris, W. E. *Jogging.* New York: Grosset & Dunlap, 1967. One of the best coaches in the world wrote this 127-page classic.

Frederick, E. C. *The Running Body.* Mountain View, California: World Publications, 1973. An interesting work on the physiology of running.

Friedman, Meyer, and Rosenman, Ray H. *Type A Behavior and Your Heart.* New York: Alfred A. Knopf, 1974. Available in paperback.

Glasser, William. *Positive Addiction.* New York: Harper & Row, 1976. How your head runs with your body.

Henderson, Joe. *Jog, Run, Race.* Mountain View, California: World Publications, 1977.

———. *The Long Run Solution.* Mountain View, California: World Publications, 1976. Running inside your head.

———. *Long Slow Distance: The Humane Way to Train.* Mountain View, California: World Publications, 1969. The basic LSD book.

———. *Run Gently, Run Long.* Mountain View, California: World Publications, 1974. More LSD.

Higdon, Hal. *Fitness After Forty.* Mountain View, California: World Publications, 1974. Hope for the middle-aged, and beyond.

Hoyt, Creig, et al. *Food for Fitness.* Mountain View, California: World Publications, 1975. Good information on nutrition.

Kostrubala, Thaddeus. *The Joy of Running.* Philadelphia and New York: J. B. Lippincott, 1976. A San

Diego psychiatrist who took up running, and found it therapeutic for himself and his patients.

Lance, Kathryn. *Running for Health and Beauty: A Complete Guide for Women*. Bobbs-Merrill, 1977. One of the best books for women who want to run, or who run short distances already.

Likoff, William; Segal, Bernard; and Galton, Lawrence. *Your Heart: Complete Information for the Family*. Philadelphia and New York: J. B. Lippincott, 1972. Another basic work.

Lydiard, Arthur, and Gilmour, Garth. *Run to the Top*. London: Herbert Jenkins, 1962. The Olympic coach describes his program for training.

Reynolds, Bill. *Complete Weight Training*. Mountain View, California: World Publications, 1977. A good, basic work for runners at the beginner competitor level and beyond.

*The Road Runner's Club Handbook: A Guide to Club Administration*. Second Edition. Edited by G. Williams. Available through the National Road Runner's Club president. An excellent guide to setting up running clubs.

Rohé, Fred. *The Zen of Running*. New York and Berkeley: Random House-Bookworks, 1974.

*Runner's World* editors. *The Complete Runner*. Mountain View, California: World Publications, 1974. From shoes to racing in your head.

Sheehan, George A. *Dr. Sheehan on Running*. Mountain View, California: World Publications, 1975. A rascally book of wisdom and hints.

————. ed. *Encyclopedia of Athletic Medicine*. Mountain View, California: World Publications, 1972. Runner's ills and cures.

Ullyot, Joan. *Women's Running*. Mountain View, California: World Publications, 1976. A woman runner-physician encourages the sisterhood to join her.

Van Aaken, Ernst. *The Van Aaken Method*. Mountain View, California: World Publications, 1976. A well-known coach's training methods.

Watts, Dennis; Wilson, Harry; and Horwill, Frank. *The Complete Middle Distance Runner*. London: Stanley Paul, 1972; revised edition, 1974. Training guides from middle distance runners.

## Bibliography

Astrand, Per-Olaf, and Rodahl, Kaare. *Textbook of Work Physiology*. New York: McGraw-Hill, 1970. The standard authority.

Cooper, Kenneth H. *The New Aerobics*. New York: Bantam Books, 1970.

————, and Cooper, Mildred. *Aerobics for Women*. New York: Bantam Books, 1972.

Costes, Nick. *Interval Training*. New York: World Publishing, 1972.

Costill, David L. *What Research Tells the Coach About Distance Running*. Washington, D.C.: American Association for Health, Physical Education and Recreation.

de Vries, Herbert A. *Physiology of Exercise for Physical Education and Athletes*. Dubuque, Iowa: William C. Brown Company, 1974. An excellent standard college text on the subject.

Doherty, J. Kenneth. *Modern Track and Field*. Englewood Cliffs, New Jersey: Prentice-Hall, 1963. A top coach's survey of training methods.

Donaldson, Rory and the National Jogging Association. *Guidelines for Successful Jogging*. Washington, D.C.: National Jogging Association, 1977.

Duffy, William. *Sugar Blues*. New York: Warner Books, 1975. Exposing sugar, the killer in your diet.

Fixx, James F. *The Complete Book of Running*. New York: Random House, 1977.

Jackson, Ian. *Yoga and the Athlete*. Mountain View, California: World Publications, 1975.

Kraus, Hans, M.D. *The Cause, Prevention and Treatment of Backache, Stress and Tension*. New York: Simon & Schuster, 1965; Pocket Books, 1969.

Myers, Clayton R. *The Official YMCA Physical Fitness Handbook*. New York: Popular Library, 1975.

Nutrition Search Inc., John D. Kirschmann, Director. *Nutrition Almanac*. New York: McGraw-Hill, 1975. A superb and detailed reference book.

*Runner's World* editors. *Age of the Runner*. Mountain View, California: World Publications, 1974.

———— *Exercise for Runners*. Mountain View, California: World Publications, 1973.

———— *New Views of Speed Training*. Mountain View, California: World Publications, 1971.

———— *Practical Running Psychology*. Mountain View, California: World Publications, 1972.

———— *Racing Techniques*. Mountain View, California: World Publications, 1971.

———— *The Runner's Diet*. Mountain View, California: World Publications, 1972.

———— *The Varied World of Cross-Country*. Mountain View, California: World Publications, 1971.

Seyle, Hans. *The Stress of Life*. New York: McGraw-Hill, 1956.

————. *Stress Without Distress*. New York: J. B. Lippincott, 1974.

Stearn, Jess. *Yoga, Youth and Reincarnation*. New York: Doubleday, 1965; Bantam Books, 1968.

Sublotnik, Steven I. *The Running Foot Doctor*. Mountain View, California: World Publications, 1977.

Wilt, Fred. *How They Train*. Los Altos, California: Track & Field News, 1959. Detailed workout schedules of 175 top runners.

| 440 | Mile | 2 Miles | 3 Miles | 4 Miles | 5 Miles | 6 Miles |
|------|------|---------|---------|---------|---------|---------|
| 57 | 3:48 | | | | | |
| 58 | 3:52 | | | | | |
| 59 | 3:56 | | | | | |
| 1:00 | 4:00 | | | | | |
| 1:01 | 4:04 | | | | | |
| 1:02 | 4:08 | 8:16 | | | | |
| 1:03 | 4:12 | 8:24 | | | | |
| 1:04 | 4:16 | 8:32 | 12:48 | 17:04 | | |
| 1:05 | 4:20 | 8:40 | 13:00 | 17:20 | | |
| 1:06 | 4:24 | 8:48 | 13:12 | 17:36 | 22:00 | 26:24 |
| 1:07 | 4:28 | 8:56 | 13:24 | 17:52 | 22:20 | 26:48 |
| 1:08 | 4:32 | 9:04 | 13:36 | 18:08 | 22:40 | 27:12 |
| 1:09 | 4:36 | 9:12 | 13:48 | 18:24 | 23:00 | 27:36 |
| 1:10 | 4:40 | 9:20 | 14:00 | 18:40 | 23:20 | 28:00 |
| 1:11 | 4:44 | 9:28 | 14:12 | 18:56 | 23:40 | 28:24 |
| 1:12 | 4:48 | 9:36 | 14:24 | 19:12 | 24:00 | 28:48 |
| 1:13 | 4:52 | 9:44 | 14:36 | 19:28 | 24:20 | 29:12 |
| 1:14 | 4:56 | 9:52 | 14:48 | 19:44 | 24:40 | 29:36 |
| 1:15 | 5:00 | 10:00 | 15:00 | 20:00 | 25:00 | 30:00 |
| 1:16 | 5:04 | 10:08 | 15:12 | 20:16 | 25:20 | 30:24 |
| 1:17 | 5:08 | 10:16 | 15:24 | 20:32 | 25:40 | 30:48 |
| 1:18 | 5:12 | 10:24 | 15:36 | 20:48 | 26:00 | 31:12 |
| 1:19 | 5:16 | 10:32 | 15:48 | 21:04 | 26:20 | 31:36 |
| 1:20 | 5:20 | 10:40 | 16:00 | 21:20 | 26:40 | 32:00 |
| 1:21 | 5:24 | 10:48 | 16:12 | 21:36 | 27:00 | 32:24 |
| 1:22 | 5:28 | 10:56 | 16:24 | 21:52 | 27:20 | 32:48 |
| 1:23 | 5:32 | 11:04 | 16:36 | 22:08 | 27:40 | 33:12 |
| 1:24 | 5:36 | 11:12 | 16:48 | 22:24 | 28:00 | 33:36 |
| 1:25 | 5:40 | 11:20 | 17:00 | 22:40 | 28:20 | 34:00 |
| 1:26 | 5:44 | 11:28 | 17:24 | 22:56 | 28:40 | 34:24 |
| 1:27 | 5:48 | 11:36 | 17:36 | 23:12 | 29:00 | 34:48 |
| 1:28 | 5:52 | 11:44 | 17:48 | 23:28 | 29:20 | 35:12 |
| 1:29 | 5:56 | 11:52 | 17:48 | 23:44 | 29:40 | 35:36 |
| 1:30 | 6:00 | 12:00 | 18:00 | 24:00 | 30:00 | 36:00 |
| 1:31 | 6:04 | 12:08 | 18:12 | 24:16 | 30:20 | 36:24 |
| 1:32 | 6:08 | 12:16 | 18:24 | 24:32 | 30:40 | 36:48 |
| 1:33 | 6:12 | 12:24 | 18:36 | 24:48 | 31:00 | 37:12 |
| 1:34 | 6:16 | 12:32 | 18:48 | 25:04 | 31:20 | 37:36 |
| 1:35 | 6:20 | 12:40 | 19:00 | 25:20 | 31:40 | 38:00 |
| 1:36 | 6:24 | 12:48 | 19:12 | 25:36 | 32:00 | 38:24 |
| 1:37 | 6:28 | 12:56 | 19:36 | 25:52 | 32:20 | 38:48 |
| 1:38 | 6:32 | 13:04 | 19:36 | 26:08 | 32:40 | 39:12 |
| 1:39 | 6:36 | 13:12 | 19:48 | 26:24 | 33:00 | 39:36 |

| Mile | 5 Miles | 10 Miles | 15 Miles | 20 Miles | Marathon | 50 Miles |
|------|---------|----------|----------|----------|----------|----------|
| 4:50 | 24:10 | 48:20 | 1:12:30 | 1:36:40 | 2:07:44 | |
| 5:00 | 25:00 | 50:00 | 1:15:00 | 1:40:00 | 2:11:06 | |
| 5:10 | 25:50 | 51:40 | 1:17:30 | 1:43:20 | 2:15:28 | |
| 5:20 | 26:40 | 53:20 | 1:20:00 | 1:46:40 | 2:19:50 | |
| 5:30 | 27:30 | 55:00 | 1:22:30 | 1:50:00 | 2:24:12 | |
| 5:40 | 28:20 | 56:40 | 1:25:00 | 1:53:20 | 2:28:34 | |
| 5:50 | 29:10 | 58:20 | 1:27:30 | 1:56:40 | 2:32:56 | |
| 6:00 | 30:00 | 1:00:00 | 1:30:00 | 2:00:00 | 2:37:19 | 5:00:00 |
| 6:10 | 30:50 | 1:01:40 | 1:32:30 | 2:03:20 | 2:41:41 | 5:08:20 |
| 6:20 | 31:40 | 1:03:20 | 1:35:00 | 2:06:40 | 2:46:03 | 5:16:40 |
| 6:30 | 32:30 | 1:05:00 | 1:37:30 | 2:10:00 | 2:50:25 | 5:25:00 |
| 6:40 | 33:20 | 1:06:40 | 1:40:00 | 2:13:20 | 2:54:47 | 5:33:20 |
| 6:50 | 34:10 | 1:08:20 | 1:42:30 | 2:16:40 | 2:59:09 | 5:41:40 |
| 7:00 | 35:00 | 1:10:00 | 1:45:00 | 2:20:00 | 3:03:33 | 5:50:00 |
| 7:10 | 35:50 | 1:11:40 | 1:47:30 | 2:23:20 | 3:07:55 | 5:58:20 |
| 7:20 | 36:40 | 1:13:20 | 1:50:00 | 2:26:40 | 3:12:17 | 6:06:40 |
| 7:30 | 37:30 | 1:15:00 | 1:52:30 | 2:30:00 | 3:16:39 | 6:15:00 |
| 7:40 | 38:20 | 1:16:40 | 1:55:00 | 2:33:20 | 3:21:01 | 6:23:20 |
| 7:50 | 39:10 | 1:18:20 | 1:57:30 | 2:36:40 | 3:25:23 | 6:31:40 |
| 8:00 | 40:00 | 1:20:00 | 2:00:00 | 2:40:00 | 3:29:45 | 6:40:00 |
| 8:10 | 40:50 | 1:21:40 | 2:02:30 | 2:43:20 | 3:34:07 | 6:48:20 |
| 8:20 | 41:40 | 1:23:20 | 2:05:00 | 2:46:40 | 3:38:29 | 6:56:40 |
| 8:30 | 42:30 | 1:25:00 | 2:07:30 | 2:50:00 | 3:42:51 | 7:05:00 |
| 8:40 | 43:20 | 1:26:40 | 2:10:00 | 2:53:20 | 3:47:13 | 7:13:20 |
| 8:50 | 44:10 | 1:28:20 | 2:12:30 | 2:56:40 | 3:51:35 | 7:21:40 |
| 9:00 | 45:00 | 1:30:00 | 2:15:00 | 3:00:00 | 3:56:00 | 7:30:00 |
| 9:10 | 45:50 | 1:31:40 | 2:17:30 | 3:03:20 | 4:00:22 | 7:38:20 |
| 9:20 | 46:40 | 1:33:20 | 2:20:00 | 3:06:40 | 4:04:44 | 7:46:40 |
| 9:30 | 47:30 | 1:35:00 | 2:22:30 | 3:10:00 | 4:09:06 | 7:55:00 |
| 9:40 | 48:20 | 1:36:40 | 2:25:00 | 3:13:20 | 4:13:28 | 8:03:20 |
| 9:50 | 49:10 | 1:38:20 | 2:27:30 | 3:16:40 | 4:17:50 | 8:11:40 |

These charts will help you determine the pace you should set over a given distance. For example, if you run the 440 in 1:30, you will run a mile in 6:00 minutes and 6 miles in 36 minutes.

# INDEX

Accessories, 177–78
  money, 177–78
  pedometers, 177
  toilet paper, 177
  watches, 177
Achilles' tendon. *See* Injuries and
    diseases: Achilles' tendonitis
Aerobic exercises. *See* Exercises
*African Running Revolution, The*
    (Sturak), 120
Age, 137–51, 156–57, 390, 393–94
Air pollution, 193–94
Alexander, Dr. Colin James, 271–72
Alexander, Dr. Ruth, 11
Ali, Muhammad, 373, 391–92
Altitude, 196
"Animal Run," 356
Arends, Dr. Joseph, 1
Arm carry, 117–19
Astrand, Dr. Per-Olof, 302, 318
Automobiles, 196–97

Bachelor, Jack, 95
*Backache, Stress and Tension*
    (Kraus), 29
Backwards running, 242, 384
Baker, Ruth, 148
Barefoot walking, 215, 231
Bassler, Dr. Thomas, 14, 285–86
Bayi, Filbert, 86, 120
Beginner runners, 21, 23, 45, 51–60,
    63–64, 70–76
  commitment, 53–55
  cool-down, 59–60
  medical examination, need for,
    51–52
  racing, 70, 71–75
  susceptibility to stitch, 266–67
  warm-up, 56–57
Bell, Jess, 11–12, 157
Bell, Julie, 157
Benson, Dr. Herbert, 340–41
Bingay, Roberta Gibb, 154
Biomechanical analysis of running,
    113
Blackistone, Zachariah, 151

Blood pressure. *See* Heart
Bonne Bell Cosmetics, 11–12, 157
Bonner, Beth, 155
Bonnet, Honore, 341
Boston Marathon, 2, 11, 68, 90, 94,
    95, 96–97, 102, 107, 149, 169,
    183, 190, 192, 278, 324, 328,
    329, 385, 387, 393–94
  women runners in, 153, 154–55
Bottinger, Dr. L. E., 146
Bowerman, Bill, 7, 17, 22, 116, 250
Breathing, 119–20
British Cardiac Society, 15
*British Medical Journal*, 253
Brunner, Daniel, 287
Buckland, Leslie, 67
Buerkle, Dick, 353
Burgess, Pamela Mendelsohn, 168
Burgess, Peter, 168

Calisthenics. *See* Exercises
Cannon, Dr. Walter B., 333
Carruthers, Dr. Malcolm, 350
Carter, Pres. Jimmy, 144
Castelli, Dr. William P., 281
Cavanagh, Dr. Peter, 192
Cerutty, Percy, 119
Childers, Tom, 68
Children. *See* Young runners
Chodes, John, 150
Cholesterol, 280–81, 305, 306–307
*Circulation*, 286
Cities, places to run:
  in Atlanta, 363–64, 387
  in Baltimore, 364–65
  in Boston, 365–66
  in Chicago, 366–67
  in Dallas, 367–68
  in Denver, 368–69
  in Detroit, 369–70
  in Eugene, 377–78
  in Honolulu, 370–71
  in Los Angeles, 371–72
  in Miami, 372
  in New Orleans, 372–73, 386
  in New York City, 373–76

in Philadelphia, 376
in Pittsburgh, 376–77
in Portland, 378–79
in St. Louis, 379
in San Diego, 380
in San Francisco, 380–82
in Seattle, 382–83
in Tulsa, 387
in Washington, D.C., 383–84
City Island Fitness and Medical
    Center (NYC), 9, 52
Cleary, Mike, 99, 270, 300
Clothing, 72, 171–77
    bras, 173–74
    chafing and, 174, 176, 178
    cold weather and, 186–88
    gloves, 187–88
    head gear, 176–77, 188
    hot weather and, 183
    night, 193
    outerwear, 175–76
    rain, 191
    rubberized, 175, 182
    shirts, 174–75, 187
    shorts, 174
    socks, 172–73, 187, 227, 256
    supporters, 173
    sweat, 175–76
    sweatbands, 176
    tight, 236–37
    underwear, 173–74, 187
    warm-up suits, 176
    windbreakers, 176, 187
    *See also* Accessories; Shoes
Colon, Tony, 68
Competition, 67–93
    attitude, 84–85
    carbohydrate loading, 304,
        318–20
    concentration, 85
    diet, 313, 317–21
    eating and drinking during,
        321–30
    first race, 71–75
    intermediate, 76–81
    passing, 88–89
    proper weight, 273, 302
    running clubs, 91–93
    stitch during, 267–68
    strategy and tactics, 86–89
    training, 70–71, 78–84
    *See also* Marathon running;
        Marathons; Races
*Conditioning of Long Distance
    Runners, The* (Osler), 97–98
Cool-down, 18, 46–48, 99, 278
    exercises, 47–48, 59–60
Cooper, Dr. Kenneth, 7, 21, 39–40,
    85, 165, 325–26
*Corbitt* (Chodes), 150
Corbitt, Ted, 150, 203, 209, 213,
    223, 241, 268
Cordellos, Harry, 102
Costill, Dr. David, 180, 324–25, 327
Coulter, Tom, 96–97
Craven, Laura, 158
Cureton, Dr. Thomas K., 5, 39–40

Dassler, Adi, 202
Dassler, Rudi, 202
Daws, Ron, 182
De Mar, Clarence, 149, 278
De Verona, Donna, 373
de Vries, Herbert, 152–53, 341–42,
    349
De Witt, Deborah, 165–66
d'Elia, Erica, 147
d'Elia, Toshiko, 147–48
De Mont, Rick, 255
Derderian, Tom, 361–62
Dickinson, Dr. L., 257
Diet, 72, 261
    absorption and, 295, 305
    alcohol, 299–300, 316
    calcium, 308, 313
    carbohydrate loading, 318–20
    carbohydrates, 294, 295, 301,
        302–304, 311–12, 316, 323
    cholesterol and, 305, 306–307
    coffee, 299
    competition and, 317–30
    digestion and, 294–95, 317

Diet (*cont.*)
    exercise and, 291–92, 301–302
    fasting, 315, 318
    fats, 294, 295, 301, 304–307,
        311–12
    heart disease and, 281–82
    iron, 307–308
    junk foods, 296–97, 298–99, 316
    magnesium, 309, 322
    meat, 304, 308, 309, 315
    metabolism and, 295–96, 303,
        304, 309, 311–12
    minerals, 307–309, 322
    nutrition and, 291, 293–94,
        301–302
    orange juice, 326, 328–29
    phosphorus, 308, 313
    potassium, 298, 309, 322, 326–27
    proteins, 294, 295, 301, 304–305,
        311–12, 315–16, 318
    salt, 298, 321, 326–27
    smoking and, 301, 313
    sodium, 298–99, 308–309, 322,
        326–27
    sugar, 297–98, 303, 316, 323–24
    vegetarianism, 315
    Vitamin A, 305, 310
    Vitamin B-complex, 297, 309,
        310–11
    Vitamin C, 257, 309, 312–13, 316
    Vitamin D, 305, 313
    Vitamin E, 305, 309, 314
    Vitamin K, 305
    water, 314–15
    weight and, 291–93, 302
    whole-wheat, 316
Dilfer, Carol, 166–67
Dixon, Don, 149–50
Dr. Scholl's products, 211, 216, 231,
    237, 242, 264
*Dr. Sheehan on Running*
    (Sheehan), 145
Doctors, 15, 222–23
    choice of, 52
Dogs, 198–200
Donahue, John, 347

Drayton, Jerome, 68, 329
Drinking, 299–300

Eating. *See* Diet
Edelen, Buddy, 182
Effects of running:
    physical, 4, 12–13, 14, 15, 16,
        275–90, 350
    psychological, 3–4, 20, 336–37,
        347–57, 389–94
Eilenberg, Carl, 7, 96–97, 212,
    296–97, 358 59, 363
Eisenhower, Dwight D., 13, 218
*Encyclopedia of Athletic Medicine*
    (Sheehan), 201
*Encyclopedia of Sports Medicine*,
    185
Epinephrine, 3
Erdelyi, Dr. Gyula, 166
ERG, 323, 326–27
Esalen Sports Center, 352, 355
Exercises, 21, 121–36, 234, 258, 264
    aerobic, 23, 38–46
    arm and torso, 127–32
    asthmatics and, 254
    back pain and, 247, 249–50
    backovers, 36
    belly breathing, 29
    calf muscle stretch, 32, 35–36,
        234
    calisthenics, 27–28
    cat back, 30, 247
    cool-down, 47–48, 59
    deep lunge, 343
    diet and, 291–92, 301–302
    flexibility, 242
    forward bend, 342
    front and back stretch, 36
    groin, 127, 262
    hamstring, 32, 35–36, 127, 234
    hanging, 247
    head roll, 29
    heart and lungs, effect on, 275–90
    hip, 264–65
    knee, 29, 30, 242–43, 343
    leg and groin, 123–27

leg limbering, 29
leg-up stretch, 36–37
multiple benefit, 132–36
pectoral stretch, 30
plough, the, 342
push-ups, 32
relaxation, 25, 221, 341–46
shin splints and, 237
shoulder shrug, 29
sitting stretch, 32–33
sit-ups, 33–34
smoking and, 283–85
soleus muscle stretch, 234
sprinter's position, 234
squats, deep knee, 28
stretching, 25–26, 221, 236,
    341–42
thigh, 243–44
types, 19, 25–26
warm-up, 29–37, 56–57
weight and, 282
yoga, 341–46
*See also* Weightlifting

Fairbank, Paul, 144–45
"Fartlek," 80–81
Feet, 201, 220, 229–31, 247, 255–56
problems with, 205–206
*See also* Injuries and diseases
Fitness, 8
Fleming, Tom, 268
Fleming, Vin, 191
"Following" tactic, 87
Food. *See* Diet
Footstrike, 113–16, 196, 210, 220,
    236, 247–48, 264
Forbes, Malcolm, 12
Foreman, Dr. Kenneth, 160
Forster, E. M., 348
Form, 112–20, 195–96
Frederick, E. C., 100–101
Friedman, Dr. Meyer, 14–15, 335–36
Front running, 86

Galloway, Jeff, 363
Gatorade, 323, 326–27, 328

Geisler, Barry, 138, 143–44
Geisler, Barry, Jr., 143
Gendel, Dr. Evelyn, 167
Gerschler, Dr. Woldemar, 82–83
"Gerschler-Reindel Law," 83
Gershman, Bennett, 140–41
Gershman, Seth, 140–41
Glasser, Dr. William, 337, 350
Robert H. Glover and Associates,
    Inc., 9
Gookin, Bill, 327
Gorman, Miki, 158, 169
Granowitz, Ed, 384
Greist, Dr. John H., 349
Guild, Dr. Warren R., 391–92
Gwinup, Dr. Grant, 282

Hall, Bob, 102
Hansen, Jacki, 108
Hartman, Hans, 102–103
Haskell, Dr. William L., 362
Haywood, Spencer, 373
HDLs, 281–82
Heart, 273–90
attacks and diseases, 10, 13–14,
    258–59, 280–90, 336
blood pressure, 276–77, 283
breathing capacity and, 277–78
exercise and, 275–90
rate, 41–44, 56, 274–75, 278, 283,
    284
smoking and, 283–85
structure and operation, 273–77
Vitamin C and, 312
Vitamin E and, 314
Heat, 178–83, 327–28
cramps, 178
exhaustion, 178, 179–80
stroke, 178–80
Heatherton, Joey, 373
Hecklers, 197–98
Heller, Joseph, 373
Hellerstein, Dr. Herman, 288–89
Henderson, Joe, 8, 17, 19, 54, 250,
    348, 352
Herskowitz, Dr. Melvin, 189–90

Hickman, James, 355
Hill training, 81–82, 194–96
Hlavac, Dr. Harry, 203, 205–206, 209
Hoffman, Dustin, 373
Holmes, Dr. Thomas H., 332
Hopi Indians, 356–57
Horowitz, Bill, 55, 105–106, 178
Humidity, 181

Indoor running, 359–61
Industry, 11–12
Injuries and diseases, 218–72
    Achilles' tendonitis, 205–206, 209–10, 214, 215, 231–34, 263
    ankle, 251–53
    arch, 210, 229–31
    arthritis, 253, 264
    asthma, 253–55
    atherosclerosis, 306
    athlete's foot, 255–56
    back, 244–50, 334–35
    ball of foot, 256–57
    blisters, 208–209, 216, 224–25, 227–29
    blood in urine, 257
    calluses, 226
    chafing, 174, 176, 178, 266
    charley horse, 240–41, 266
    chest pain, 258–59, 321
    colds, 259–60
    constipation, 262
    diabetes, 260–61
    disc, 249
    emphysema, 254, 255
    flu, 260
    groin, 262–63
    headaches, 334–35
    heart, 10, 13–14, 258–59, 280–90, 312, 336
    heel, 263–64
    high blood pressure, 336, 340
    hip, 264
    inactivity and, 218–19
    intestinal cramps, 261
    jock rash, 265–66

    knee, 241–44
    leg cramping, 239–40, 321
    leg fatigue, 238–39
    low blood sugar, 258, 261, 297–98
    neck, 335
    Osgood-Schlatter disease, 143
    sciatica, 248–49, 264
    shin splints, 206, 235–38, 269
    smoking and, 283–85
    sources of, 211–12, 219–22
    stiffness, 238
    stitch, 266–68
    stress fractures, 269–70
    tension, 248, 266–68, 331–46
    toe and toenail, 224–26
    triggerpoints, 264, 270–71
    varicose veins, 271–72
    *See also* Exercises
Insel, Dr. Paul, 349–50
Institute of Experimental Medicine and Surgery, 331
Intermediate runners, 60–66
    racing, 76–91
Interval training, 82–84
Isometrics, 15–16, 39

Jacobson, Dr. Edmund, 339
Jefferson Medical College, 15
*Jogger*, 151, 168
Jones, Mary, 152
Jumping rope, 39

Kavanaugh, Dr. Terrence, 288
Kelley, Johnny, 149
Kennedy, John F., 218
Kicking, 86
Killion, Jane, 99, 106–107, 301
Killy, Jean-Claude, 341
Kostrubala, Dr. Thaddeus, 3, 349, 350–51, 353–54, 356
Kraus, Dr. Hans, 29, 146–47, 214, 218, 223– 250, 334, 335
Kraus-Weber Minimal Muscle Tests, 218, 244, 334
Kuscsik, Nina, 67, 107, 155–57, 164, 169, 246, 272, 328

Lance, Kathryn, 161–62, 164, 169
*Lancet, The*, 271–72, 284–85
Langlacé, Chantel, 158
Lawrence, Dr. Ron, 3
LDLs, 281
Lebow, Fred, 1
Leonard, Tommy, 365
Lettis, Charlotte, 362
Lewis, Larry, 151
Liberty Athletic Club, 366
Lightning, 191–92
Liquids, 316, 322–30
  Bike Half-Time Punch, 326
  ERG, 323, 326–27
  Gatorade, 323, 326–27, 328
  Sportade, 326
Liquori, Marty, 207
*Long-Run Solution, The*
  (Henderson), 19, 352
LSD, 79–80
Lungs, 273–74, 275
  breathing capacity, 277–78
  smoking and, 283–85
Lydiard, Arthur, 7, 84, 89

McConnell, Sam, 150–51, 390
McDonough, Jim, 300
McGregor, Dr. Rob Roy, 223
McKenzie, Chris, 154
Mahrer, Jerry, 188, 323
Marathon running, 2–3, 94–109
  finishing, 101–104
  motivation, 96
  origins, 94–95
  runner types, 103–108
  training, 97–101, 103–108
  *See also* Marathons
*Marathon Man*, 373
Marathons, 386–88
  Boston. *See* Boston Marathon
  "City to Surf," 388
  Earth Day, 107
  Ground Hog's Day, 386
  Holyoke, 328
  Honolulu, 10, 370–71, 388
  Jersey Shore, 148, 190

Mardi Gras, 386
Minneapolis, 107
National AAU Masters
  Championship, 236
National Wheelchair
  Championship, 11, 102
New York. *See* New York
  Marathon
New York Mini-Marathon. *See*
  New York "Mini-Marathon"
Olympic, 7, 95
Orange Bowl, 301, 388
Pan-Am, 300
Pike's Peak, 148, 384–85
Skylon, 192, 384
White Rock, 152, 192
Yonkers, 149
*See also* Races
Marinucci, Joe, 149
Mayer, Jean, 292
Medical examination, need for,
  51–52
*Medical Times*, 326–27
Meditation, 338–41, 348–49,
  353–57
Melleby, Alexander, 9, 40, 250, 335
Merrill, Robert, 352
Metabolism. *See* Diet
Meyer, Fred, 14
M-F Athletic Company, 215
Mirkin, Dr. Gabe, 179, 314
Moore, Kenny, 95
Morris, Dr. J. N., 286
Mueller, Fritz, 236
Muhrcke, Gary, 203, 204, 207,
  209, 246
Myers, Dr. Clayton, 26–27

National Amputee Runner's Club,
  11
National Heart and Lung Institute
  Task Force, 286
National Heart, Lung and Blood
  Institute, 281
National Jogging Association, 1, 2,
  17, 151, 360

National Research Council, 298,
303, 304
National Running Data Center, 386
Nelson, Dr. Ralph, 302
Neppel, Peg, 157–58
*New England Journal of Medicine,
The*, 189–90, 278
New York Academy of Sciences,
155, 219, 336–37
New York Marathon, 2, 3, 11, 67,
85, 90, 98–99, 101–102, 107,
108–109, 149, 169, 262, 320,
385–86, 392–93
   women runners in, 155, 161
New York "Mini-Marathon," 2, 20,
71, 148, 156–58, 375
Newhouse, Stanley, 146
Niemand, Arno, 138, 156
Niemand, Kurt, 138
Night running, 193
Nutrition. *See* Diet

Obesity, 248, 282, 291–93
O'Connor, Ulick, 14, 218
Older runners. *See* Senior runners
Onassis, Jackie, 373
Osler, Tom, 97–98, 337

Pacing, 86, 87–88
   charts, 406–407
Paffenbarger, Dr. Ralph S., Jr.,
287–88
Pardo, Joe, 102
Pauling, Linus, 312
"Peaking," 90
Pedometers, 177
Pedrinan, Lauri, 99, 106–107, 229
Pheidippides, 94–95
*Physician and Sportsmedicine, The*,
351
*Physiology of Exercise* (de Vries),
152
Places to run. *See* Cities, places to
   run
*Podiatric Sports Medicine*
(Subotnik), 113

*Positive Addiction* (Glasser), 337,
350
Posture, 116–17
Prefontaine, Steve, 85, 377
President's Council on Physical
   Fitness and Sports, 15, 218
*Psychology Today*, 350
Pulsators Track Club of Anchorage,
148

Races:
   Albany Bankathon, 107, 386
   "8-Mile Zoo Run," 387
   Mt. Washington Road Race, 384
   National 50-Mile Championship,
   150
   Peachtree, 387
   San Francisco Bay-to-Breakers, 389
   Valentine's Day "Love Run," 386
   WBAI Six-Mile Race, 140
   *See also* Marathons; Competition
Rahe, Dr. Richard H., 332
Rain, 191–92, 212
Redford, Robert, 373
Reich, Leonard, 353
Reindel, Dr. Herbert, 82–83
Relaxation, 25, 221, 338–46
*Road Runner's Club Handbook: A
   Guide to Club Administration
   The* (Williams), 93
Road Runner's Club of America,
   1, 137, 359–60
   Age-Group Cross-Country
   Championship, 137–38
   *See also* Cities, places to run
Road Runner's Club of D.C., 144
Road Runner's Club of New York,
   1, 13, 70–71, 91–92, 145, 156,
   374–75
*Rocky*, 376
Rodd, Flory, 150
Rodgers, Bill, 68, 102, 107–108,
   207, 262, 329, 365, 386
Rodriguez, Mary, 70–71
Rope jumping, 39
Rosenman, Dr. Ray H., 14–15,

335–36
Ross, Browning, 1
Roth, Dr. Walton, 349–50
Royal College of Physicians, 15
Rumsey, Jim, 229, 234
Run-Easy Method, 17–49, 60
*Runner's Diet, The,* 322
*Runner's World,* 1, 8, 64, 151, 202,
    203, 205–206, 209, 219, 242,
    250, 266, 293, 386, 388, 391
"Running and Primary
    Osteoarthritis of the Hip," 253
*Running Body, The* (Frederick),
    100–101
Running Clubs, 91–93. *See also*
    Cities, places to run (clubs
    listed by city)
*Running for Health and Beauty:*
    *A Complete Guide for Women*
    (Lance), 161–62, 164
*Running Times,* 64, 314, 386

Sander, Dr. Norb, 9, 13, 52, 55, 83,
    95, 246, 254, 261, 300, 319–21
Sanders, Dr. Max, 49–50
Schuder, Pete, 114
Schuster, Dr. Richard, 8, 203, 210,
    212, 215, 219–20, 221, 223,
    225, 231, 232, 241, 242, 244,
    257, 262
*Scientific American,* 354
Segal, Erich, 326
Selye, Dr. Hans, 331, 332, 337
Semple, Jock, 154
Senior runners, 144–51, 390, 393–94
    women, 147–48, 156–57
Sex, running and, 389–94
Sex differences:
    endurance, 158
    muscles, 152–53
    style, 110–12
Sharp, Dr. Craig, 392
Sheehan, Dr. George, 8, 69, 90–91,
    141–42, 145, 193–94, 201, 220,
    223, 228, 237, 242, 250, 257,
    259–60, 261, 264, 268, 327,

347, 348, 357, 391
Shelton, Herbert, 297
Shepherd, Jack, 4–6, 44, 289–90
    *passim*
Shoes, 72, 201–17, 232
    arch supports, 216
    brands, 75, 202, 206, 208, 212
    care and repair, 212–15
    choosing, 203–205, 208–12
    Earth, 214–15, 232
    inserts, 8, 215–16, 226, 242
    insoles, 216–17
    salespeople, 217
    snow and, 191
    special problems, 205–206
Shorter, Frank, 7, 95, 207, 257, 300,
    327
Shultz, Dr. H. H., 339
Simon, Paul, 373
Slovic, Paul, 100
Smoking, 283–85, 301
Snow, 190–91, 212
Spellum, Arnold, 26
Spino, Mike, 355
*Sports Illustrated,* 218
Stallone, Sylvester, 376
Stanford Heart Disease Prevention
    Program, 282
Starting Line Sports, 213, 216
Stengel, Casey, 392
Stiller, Jerry, 373
Stillman, Dr. Irwin, 292–93
Stress. *See* Tension
*Stress of Life, The* (Selye), 331
*Stress Without Distress* (Selye), 331
Stride, 113, 116, 195–96
Stringham, Al, 8
Strudwick, Peter, 102
Sturak, Tom, 120
Style, 110–20, 248
    sex differences, 110–12
Subotnik, Dr. Steven, 113, 223
Sullivan, Tom, 102
Suncoast Nudist Camp Joggers, 170
Sweating, 15, 175–76, 181
Switzer, Kathrine, 154–55

Tarahumara Indians, 356
Tension, 331–357
  causes, 331–33
  effects, 334–36
  exercises for, 341–46
  physiology, 333–34
  relieving, 336–57
  signs, in running, 337–38
Thomashaw, Dr. David, 52
Thompson, Ian, 348
Training:
  carbohydrate loading, 318–21
  "fartlek," 80–81
  first race, 70–71
  heart and lungs, effect on, 278
  hill, 81–82, 194–96, 233
  injuries, 220–22, 235–36
  nitermediate, 78–84
  interval, 82–84
  LSD, 79–80
  marathon, 97–101, 103–108
  weight, 121–23
Traum, Richard, 11, 101–102, 347
Trent, Marcie, 148
Tuttle, Gary, 207
*Type A Behavior and Your Heart*
    (Friedman and Rosenman), 14

Ueland, Brenda, 148
Ullyot, Dr. Joan, 68, 167, 173
U.S. Masters National Track
    Championship, 147–48

Vahlensieck, Christa, 155
van Aaken, Dr. Ernst, 17, 89,
    139–40, 152–53, 158, 168,
    293, 299, 317, 332
Vegetarianism. *See* Diet
Viren, Lasse, 90
Vitamins. *See* Diet

Walking, 57–58, 113, 214–15

  barefoot, 215, 231
Warm-up, 18, 24–37, 99, 232, 266,
    275–76
  exercises, 29–37, 56–57
Weather, 178–92
  cold, 184–91, 254, 327
  hot, 178–83
Weightlifting, 15–16, 39, 121–23,
    277
Weisenfeld, Dr. Murray, 228, 231,
    244
White, Dr. Paul Dudley, 13, 289–90
Wiley, Mike, 8
Windchill factor, 184
Winds, 192
Women, 9, 152–70
  AAU and, 154–55
  anemia, 164
  contraception, 164–65
  endurance, 153
  groin pain, 262
  iron and, 308
  menopause, 169
  menstruation, 162–64
  motherhood, 168–69
  pregnancy, 152, 153, 165–68, 248
  senior runners, 147–48, 156–57
  sex differences, 152–53
  shoes, 208
*Women's Running* (Ullyot), 167,
    173
Wood, Dr. Peter, 299
Wottle, Dave, 392

*Yankee Runner*, 366
YMCA, 8, 360–61
Yoga, 338, 340–46
Young, Ken, 100, 386
Young runners, 137–44, 157

Zinn, Arden, 341